P9-AGK-590

RENEWALS 458-4574

DATE DUE

GAYLORD   PRINTED IN U.S.A.

PHILOSOPHICAL ISSUES IN PSYCHIATRY

WITHDRAWN
UTSA Libraries

PHILOSOPHICAL ISSUES
IN PSYCHIATRY
Explanation, Phenomenology, and Nosology

Edited by

KENNETH S. KENDLER, M.D.
Director, Virginia Institute for Psychiatric and Behavioral Genetics
Rachel Brown Banks Distinguished Professor of Psychiatry
Professor of Human Genetics
Virginia Commonwealth University
Richmond, Virginia

and

JOSEF PARNAS, M.D., Dr.Med.Sci.
Professor and Medical Director,
Department of Psychiatry, University of Copenhagen
Senior Researcher, Center for Subjectivity Research,
National Danish Research Foundation
Copenhagen, Denmark

The Johns Hopkins University Press
Baltimore

© 2008 The Johns Hopkins University Press
All rights reserved. Published 2008
Printed in the United States of America on acid-free paper
9 8 7 6 5 4 3 2 1

The Johns Hopkins University Press
2715 North Charles Street
Baltimore, Maryland 21218-4363
www.press.jhu.edu

Library of Congress Cataloging-in-Publication Data
Philosophical issues in psychiatry : explanation, phenomenology, and nosology /
edited by Kenneth S. Kendler and Josef Parnas.
    p. ; cm.
  Includes bibliographical references and index.
  ISBN-13: 978-0-8018-8983-7 (hardcover : alk. paper)
  ISBN-10: 0-8018-8983-9 (hardcover : alk. paper)
  1. Psychiatry—Philosophy. 2. Phenomenological psychology. 3. Psychiatry—
Classification. I. Kendler, Kenneth S., 1950– II. Parnas, Josef.
  [DNLM: 1. Psychiatry. 2. Philosophy, Medical. WM 100 P5676 2008]
  RC437.5.P4355 2008
  616.89001—dc22   2008007952

A catalog record for this book is available from the British Library.

Special discounts are available for bulk purchases of this book.
For more information, please contact Special Sales at 410-516-6936
or specialsales@press.jhu.edu.

The Johns Hopkins University Press uses environmentally friendly book materials,
including recycled text paper that is composed of at least 30 percent post-consumer
waste, whenever possible. All of our book papers are acid-free, and our jackets and
covers are printed on paper with recycled content.

Library
University of Texas
at San Antonio

CONTENTS

CONTRIBUTORS

John Campbell, Ph.D., Willis S. and Marion Slusser Professor of Philosophy, University of California at Berkeley, Berkeley, California. He received his Ph.D. from Oxford University. He is the author of *Past, Space, and Self* (MIT Press, 1994) and *Reference and Consciousness* (Oxford University Press, 2002). His interests are in the theory of meaning, metaphysics, and the philosophy of psychology. He is working on demonstrative reference and on causation in psychology.

Thomas Fuchs, M.D., Ph.D., Associate Professor, Department of Psychiatry, University of Heidelberg, Heidelberg, Germany. He received his M.D. in history of medicine and his Ph.D. in philosophy from Munich University. Professor Fuchs is head of the section for phenomenological psychopathology and psychotherapy in the Department of Psychiatry, University of Heidelberg, and chair of the philosophy section of the German Psychiatric Association. His research interests include phenomenological psychology, psychopathology, and psychotherapy. He is the author of *Leib, Raum, Person: Entwurf einer phänomenologischen Anthropologie* (Body, space, and person: Toward a phenomenological anthropology) (2000), *Psychopathologie von Leib und Raum* (Psychopathology of body and space) (2000) and *Mechanization of the Heart: Harvey and Descartes* (Rochester University Press, 2000). He is editing a book on time, memory, and the self (Oxford University Press).

Shaun Gallagher, Ph.D., Professor and Chair, Department of Philosophy, University of Central Florida, Orlando, Florida. Professor Gallagher received his Ph.D. in philosophy from Bryn Mawr College, an M.A. in economics from the State University of New York, and an M.A. in philosophy from Villanova University. He has been an invited visiting professor at the École Normale Supérieure, Lyon (2007), and the University of Copenhagen (2004–2006), and visiting scientist at the Medical Research Council's Cognition and Brain Sciences Unit at Cambridge

University (1994). His research interests include phenomenology and philosophy of mind, cognitive sciences, hermeneutics, and theories of the self and personal identity. His books include *How the Body Shapes the Mind* (Oxford University Press, 2005), *The Inordinance of Time* (Northwestern University Press, 1998), *Hermeneutics and Education* (SUNY Press, 1992), and, with Dan Zahavi, *The Phenomenological Mind: Contemporary Issues in Philosophy of Mind and the Cognitive Sciences* (Routledge, 2007). He is coeditor of the interdisciplinary journal *Phenomenology and the Cognitive Sciences* and a recent coeditor of *Does Consciousness Cause Behavior? An Investigation of the Nature of Volition* (MIT Press, 2006).

Kenneth S. Kendler, M.D., Director, Virginia Institute for Psychiatric and Behavioral Genetics, Rachel Brown Banks Distinguished Professor of Psychiatry, Professor of Human Genetics, Virginia Commonwealth University, Richmond, Virginia. He received his M.D. from Stanford University and his psychiatric training at Yale University. Dr. Kendler's major research interest is in understanding the interrelationship of genetic and environmental risk factors in the etiology of psychiatric and substance use disorders. Toward this end, he has conducted both large-scale twin studies and gene-finding molecular investigations. His work in psychiatric genetics has been widely published. He has written on issues at the interface between psychiatry and philosophy and is especially interested in problems of explanation and causation. He is the author, with Carol Prescott, of *Genes, Environment, and Psychopathology: Understanding the Causes of Psychiatric and Substance Use Disorders* (Guilford, 2006). He is also editor of the journal *Psychological Medicine.*

Sandra D. Mitchell, Ph.D., Professor and Chair, Department of History and Philosophy of Science, University of Pittsburgh, Pittsburgh, Pennsylvania. She received her B.A. from Pitzer College, M.Sc. from the London School of Economics, and Ph.D. from University of Pittsburgh. Her research focuses on the explanation of behavior of complex systems, primarily in biology. Professor Mitchell is author of *Biological Complexity and Integrative Pluralism* (Cambridge, 2003) and coeditor of *Human by Nature: Between Biology and the Social Sciences* (Erlbaum, 1997), *Ceteris Paribus Laws* (Springer, 2003), and *Komplexitäten* (Suhrkamp, 2008). She is author of numerous articles on functional explanation, laws of nature, self-organization, and pluralism.

Dominic P. Murphy, Ph.D., Assistant Professor of Philosophy, Senior Lecturer, Unit for History and Philosophy of Science, University of Sydney. Dominic Murphy studied philosophy at Dublin, London, and Rutgers universities. He is the author of *Psychiatry in the Scientific Image* (MIT Press, 2006) and several papers in philosophy of cognitive science and moral psychology. Professor Murphy is writing a book on self-knowledge.

Josef Parnas, M.D., Dr.Med.Sci., Professor and Medical Director, Department of Psychiatry, University of Copenhagen; Senior Researcher, Center for Subjectivity Research, National Danish Research Foundation, Copenhagen, Denmark. Dr. Parnas is cofounder of the Danish National Research Foundation's Center for Subjectivity Research, an interdisciplinary institute for research in philosophy of mind, phenomenology, hermeneutics, and psychopathology (www.cfs.ku.dk). His research interest centers on schizophrenia, including epidemiology, early environmental risk factors, genetics, and psychopathology. In recent years he has been working on the integration of phenomenology, philosophy of mind, and psychopathology. He has initiated a series of ongoing empirical studies of anomalies of subjective experience in the early developmental phases of schizophrenia.

Louis A. Sass, Ph.D., Professor, Department of Clinical Psychology, Graduate School of Applied and Professional Psychology and Research Affiliate, Center for Cognitive Science, Rutgers—the State University of New Jersey, Piscataway, New Jersey. He has published many articles on schizophrenia (and related conditions), phenomenological psychopathology, hermeneutics, psychoanalysis, modernism, and postmodernism. Professor Sass is the author of *Madness and Modernism: Insanity in the Light of Modern Art, Literature, and Thought* (Basic Books, 1992) and *The Paradoxes of Delusion: Wittgenstein, Schreber, and the Schizophrenia Mind* (Cornell University Press, 1994).

Kenneth F. Schaffner, M.D., Ph.D., University Professor of History and Philosophy of Science and Professor of Psychiatry, University of Pittsburgh, Pittsburgh, Pennsylvania. Dr. Schaffner received his Ph.D. from Columbia University and his M.D. from the University of Pittsburgh. His most recent book is *Discovery and Explanation in Biology and Medicine.* He is a member of the World Psychiatric Association–World Health Organization Workgroup on Classification and on International Diagnostic Systems for ICD-11. His recent work has been on philosophical issues in human behavioral and psychiatric genetics, and he is editing a book entitled *Behaving: What's Genetic and What's Not, and Why Should We Care?* (Oxford University Press).

James F. Woodward, Ph.D., Professor of Philosophy and J. O. and Juliette Koepfli Professor of the Humanities, California Institute of Technology, Pasadena, California. Professor Woodward received his Ph.D. in philosophy from the University of Texas at Austin. He works primarily in philosophy of science, and much of his recent work has focused on issues having to do with causation and explanation in various areas of science. He is the author of *Making Things Happen: A Theory of Causal Explanation* (Oxford University Press, 2003), which won the 2005 Lakatos Award, given annually for an outstanding contribution to philosophy of science.

Peter Zachar, Ph.D., Professor and Chair, Department of Psychology, Auburn University Montgomery, Montgomery, Alabama. He received his Ph.D. in psychology from Southern Illinois University at Carbondale. Professor Zachar is the author of *Psychological Concepts and Biological Psychiatry: A Philosophical Analysis* (John Benjamins, 2000). His research interests occur at the intersection of classification in psychiatry and psychology and the philosophy of science.

PREFACE

Most, but not all, of the chapters of this book are based on presentations made at a conference held in Copenhagen, Denmark, on June 25–26, 2006, and sponsored by the Danish National Research Foundation's Center for Subjectivity Research and the School of Neuroscience of the Faculty of Health Sciences, University of Copenhagen. This conference was organized and chaired by the editors of this volume, Kenneth S. Kendler and Josef Parnas.

All the material, however, has been reworked with this volume in mind.

We are grateful to the Research Foundation for providing funding for this meeting, without which this project would not have been possible. We also wish to thank Pia Kirkeman Hansen for her practical assistance.

Jill Opalesky, with skill and perpetual good spirits, assisted us in many aspects of the preparation of this book, including contact with publishers and authors, keeping all the contributions organized and up to date, and straightening out references and figures. Wendy Harris, at the Johns Hopkins University Press, was a pleasure to deal with, always helpful and encouraging.

Our deepest debt of gratitude is to the contributors to this volume. Editing this volume was very rewarding for us. Exchanging drafts of chapters, comments, and introductions back and forth among the authors was a stimulating experience. We did not have to nag authors to get their contributions to us, and they always responded with good spirits and sometimes a bit of (appropriate) guilt if they were far past their deadline. This project was, to use the philosophical term, emergent—in the end, the sum was much more than the individual parts.

Personal Thanks

From Kenneth S. Kendler: Two of the authors of this volume, Kenneth Schaffner and John Campbell, were in different ways invaluable guides for me in my rather late-life "discovery" of philosophy. Both have been generous with their time and patient in answering my questions and guiding me through the literature. I am also grateful to my coeditor, Josef Parnas, who kindly invited me to help him organize the Copenhagen conference and to work with him on this volume.

PHILOSOPHICAL ISSUES IN PSYCHIATRY

Introduction

Why Does Psychiatry Need Philosophy?

KENNETH S. KENDLER, M.D.

Assuming that you are a psychiatrist, clinical psychologist, or someone else interested in the questions considered by these closely related fields, why should you be interested in what philosophy might teach you? After all, there are still many patients to see. We have no shortage of mentally ill and troubled people. It is not as if the researchers in these fields have solved any of the major tasks before them. We have little more than a glimmer of insight into the etiology of major depression (MD), schizophrenia, or personality disorders. Although our treatments are better studied and probably more effective than those available two or three decades ago, we do not know much about how they work, and they certainly are far from curative. So, with all this work to do, do we have time for philosophy?

Let me suggest four reasons why psychiatry needs philosophy. For convenience, I will use the term "psychiatry" when I mean all the mental health fields. First, the commonsense idea that good clinicians and scientists see the world as it truly is just by attending to the facts is mistaken. Our perceptions of the world are influenced by our theoretical conceptions of it, and in no field is this more true than psychiatry. Think of the old adages "Motivation affects perception" and "You see what you look for." If you need any convincing of this, think about the experience of sitting in a crowded train station or airport waiting for an old friend. You see someone who looks likes your hoped-for friend. You jump up, with gladness in your heart, only to realize it is not your friend, just someone with a similar body type or pattern of walk. This sort of thing—our expectations influencing how we see the world—happens many times in every clinical contact we have. Human behavior and experience are so stunningly complex that if we didn't have preconceived categories—places to put things, including symptoms (such as hallucinations, anxiety), syndromes (say, bulimia, dementia), and processes (for example, transference, acting out)—we would be overwhelmed and helpless.

But it is not only in our categories that we bring strong a priori assumptions. You cannot work in the field of mental health without having some set of beliefs—examined or otherwise—about the nature of causal processes, about what constitutes a "good explanation," or about the relative value of symptom-based assessments versus deeper characterizations of psychopathological processes.

So, whether you like it or not, you have a set of tacitly operating philosophical concepts and beliefs that you use to organize your views about the nature of psychiatric illness and its treatment. You can leave these assumptions unexamined, or you can take as critical an approach to these fundamental questions as you should to the differential diagnosis or treatment planning for your patients. Thus, your choice is between following an implicit philosophical framework—which could be wrong, or overly simplistic, or at least misrepresent key aspects of our clinical and research world—and taking the time and effort to develop an explicit and coherent guiding set of theoretical concepts. As an example, I suggest that the ability to evaluate the argument made by many biological psychiatrists that neurochemical explanations for psychiatric illness are inherently better than psychological explanatory systems requires not only a grasp of important empirical information but also knowledge of philosophical principles and arguments.

The second reason psychiatry needs philosophy is that, of all the scientific disciplines currently active in most universities, psychiatry has the widest "grasp." Let us try a thought experiment. Consider reading a major psychiatry journal for a year, such as the *Archives of General Psychiatry* or the *British Journal of Psychiatry.* In that year you would be exposed to work conducted from a biological perspective at the level of molecules, cells, neural systems, and whole brains, at the psychological level involving a wide range of constructs such as mood, cognition, and memory, and at the social level involving family, relationship, cultural, ethnic, and even socioeconomic processes. For what reasons are these different approaches present in one journal, and how should they be understood to fit together? Just saying, "Well, they just do," is not a good answer because they may not fit together in the way common sense suggests. This question deserves scrutiny because getting the "fit" right could lead to progress and the wrong fit to further confusion, of which we have more than enough already.

Third, psychiatry has seen massive shifts in our central paradigms in the past 100 years. This is seen in our approach to both etiology and treatment. Popular frameworks have included psychoanalysis, phenomenology, social psychiatry, family systems theory, cross-cultural psychiatry, cognitive science, biological psychiatry, and molecular neuroscience. Driven in part by exciting advances in neuroscience and molecular genetics, a reductionist "brain-focused" paradigm is currently becoming increasingly dominant. Advocates of this paradigm argue vigorously that all "real" explanation for psychiatric illness can be found at the molecular level. Some of this persuasion might tolerate other explanatory approaches (say, at the level of systems neuroscience or even psychology) but only as a holding pattern until the necessary scientific advances render these perspectives obsolete. We have good reason to be confused!

Fourth, psychiatry treats a subject matter—human behavior—that is very close to home. We deal in both our research and our clinical work with fundamental questions about the nature of human behavior and the human experience, of love and hate, suffering and exhilaration, meaning and hopelessness, responsibility and the perception of reality. Because these issues touch so intimately on our ideas of what it means to be human, it is difficult to view them as dispassionately as we might questions about the nature of light, chemical bonds, or the origins of earthquakes. Indeed, people often come to these psychiatric issues with their own deeply held personal system of beliefs. It is a challenge to keep these personal viewpoints from being mixed up with the science and clinical practice of psychiatry.

One of the deep problems in our field is that questions that should be addressed at an evidential level—such as the role of genes versus environment in the etiology of illness or the relative efficacy of pharmacotherapy versus psychotherapy—often evoke strongly held preconceived ideas. Indeed, much of the emotion that arises in discussions about the nature and treatment of psychiatric illness comes not from disagreements about evidence but from these more deeply held—but often poorly examined— preconceptions. We need philosophy to help us critically examine the assumptions we all have about psychiatric illness and treatment. Philosophers have, after all, thought long and hard about these issues and are likely to have some ideas of value. One of the ideas underlying this book is that philosophers can be good allies and collaborators for psychiatry in the twenty-first century.

Philosophy can, however, be off-putting to the uninitiated. The vocabulary can be obscure and, *even worse,* terms can be used in a technical manner in which the working definition differs from the commonsense meaning. Two critical questions need to be considered for individuals working in mental health fields who are interested in philosophy: (1) How do I enter the field and gain access to the areas that are of interest to me? (2) How do I keep my "feet on the ground" in this endeavor and not get lost in the forest of philosophy, never to return to the practical issues of psychiatric science or practice? We think we can help with both of these dilemmas and, in the process, enrich the conceptual world of our readers and help them think more clearly about the many interesting problems with which clinical and research work in psychiatry confronts us.

1. Major Philosophical Issues in Psychiatry: A Quick Overview

In this book, we treat only a subset of the major philosophical issues confronting psychiatry. In this section of the chapter, I give an inevitably personal (or idiosyncratic) tour of the major domains, beginning with those that are the foci of this book.

Causation and Levels of Understanding

A large literature in the philosophy of science (and the specific subfield of causal models within science) has dealt with the problems of reduction and more recently the converse question of emergence. As noted above, psychiatry is exceptional in the breath of the causal claims that can be made. Certainly, the field is witnessing an increased domination of reductionist approaches being fueled partly by dramatic advances in sciences such as molecular and systems neuroscience, imaging and molecular genetics and partly by less savory forces including financial pressures to move psychiatry away from psychotherapeutic approaches and more toward strictly psychopharmacology-based practice.

Our book opens with several insightful chapters that examine how we can begin to critically interrelate arguments about the role of cultural, social, and psychological variables in the etiology of psychiatric illness with the claims that the fields of neurobiology, neurochemistry, molecular genetics, and neuroscience hold the keys to understanding the causes of mental disorders. There are many issues and questions to disentangle here. To what extent are these explanatory perspectives competing versus complementary? Even if we wanted to, is it possible to develop a conceptually rigorous pluralistic approach?

Are we at risk of degenerating into what some have argued (see Ghaemi 2003) is an uninformative "vanilla" biopsychosocial perspective—that is that "all perspectives deserve a place at the table"? Is reductionism always the strategy to be pursued or are there times when the explanatory process is inherently "higher-level," involving for example psychological or cultural factors? Should psychiatry strive for the coexistence of multiple explanatory perspectives or is true cross-level integration feasible or desirable? How can we develop a frame of reference in which we can anchor our multiple perspectives, lest our pluralism degenerate into a disorganized list of facts that could more confuse than enlighten? This is perhaps the most central task for a philosophy of psychiatry, a goal toward which we hope this book makes a contribution.

Phenomenology

The second part of this book deals with phenomenological approaches to psychiatry. One way to clearly see the interrelationship between our first and second sections is to go back to the question of "explanation" and "understanding" as articulated by Karl Jaspers in his great text *General Psychopathology* (1963). Explanation—the approach taken to the world by the "natural" science—views all phenomena from the third-person perspective and seeks to comprehend causal processes in a third-person, objective, and therefore verifiable framework. Understanding, by contrast, is a distinctly human process involving our ability, through empathy, to grasp the phenomena of meaning and connect with our fellow human beings. This is an approach typically used in literature, the arts, and other human disciplines such as history. Understanding is particular and unique rather than general, linked to the first-person perspectives, and is "story-focused." As Jaspers wrote, "The truth which understanding seeks has other criteria, such as vividness, connectedness, depth and complexity" (1963). The perennial philosophical question confronting psychiatry is how these two approaches to knowing should be related to one another.

Phenomenology is a European philosophical tradition of which Jaspers was a part that has had close links to psychiatry for several generations. (For a good introduction to this sometime difficult literature, see Sokolowski 1999.) More than any other philosophical approach, phenomenology has been intertwined with the effort by psychiatrists to develop a detailed understanding of the experiences of the psychiatrically ill. Recent years have seen an increasingly close collaboration between phenomenology and cognitive sciences and a rapprochement of phenomenology with the analytic philosophical tradition, also attentive to the issues of experience and subjectivity. The clinical approach, advocated by phenomenology, a deep and careful assessment of the inner life of the mentally ill, is now being directly challenged by the "criteria-driven" approach to clinical evaluation that is becoming predominant in much of the world. In many psychiatric services, especially in the United States, the goal of an evaluative first interview with a patient is to take a brief history and then determine the presence or absence of the criteria for the relevant *Diagnostic and Statistical Manual of Mental Disorders* (4th ed.) (*DSM-IV*) diagnosis. In what some might describe as a confusion of ends and means, the diagnostic process has become the major focus of the evaluation. Furthermore, it is seen as a sufficient basis on which to proceed to initiate treatment. Therefore the rich realm of descriptive and phenomenologically informed psychiatry is being reduced to only those symptoms and signs included in the *DSM* (or *International Statistical Classification of Diseases and Related Health Problems* [*ICD*]) manual.

Philosophers of science struggling with questions about causality and phenomenology with its focus on understanding psychopathological processes share the common concern with explanation of psychiatric illness. This rich set of issues is central to our concerns because it impacts not only the scientist struggling to understand the etiology of psychiatric disorders but equally the clinician trying to provide the best level of care to his or her patients.

Nosology

The third section of this book is about nosology—another area of this diverse field of psychiatry in particular need of philosophical attention. Focusing for a moment on the United States, the official psychiatric nosology as articulated in *DSM-II* published in 1968 (American Psychiatric Association 1968) was, in rough outline, an etiologically based system. "Organic" disorders were understood to emerge from distinct pathologically processes in the brain and "functional" conditions were seen as arising from intrapsychic conflict in accord with psychodynamic theory. *DSM-III*, published in 1980 (American Psychiatric Association 1980), broke dramatically with this tradition and tried to develop an "atheoretical" and "descriptive" nosology. Questions remain about whether such a system— which diverges from nearly all such systems in the rest of medicine—is viable, especially for the long term.

A range of other conceptual and philosophical issues arise in the field of psychiatric nosology: How do we define a psychiatric disorder? Are disorders best understood as categories or continua? To what extent should psychiatric disorders represent the constants of the human condition versus more transient cultural and historical influences? On what basis should we organize the diagnostic manual? For example, should disorders be put in the same overarching categories because of their symptomatic resemblance or because of their etiologic relationships? What should be the criteria for changing criteria? These issues are all taking on a new urgency as the international psychiatric community gears up in the coming few years for the revisions of both the *DSM* and *ICD* manuals.

Issues addressed in the third section of this book relate to those raised in the first two parts in several obvious ways, some of which have already been mentioned. Explanatory systems are typically based on diagnostic categories. The required levels of explanation will be deeply shaped by the nature of the symptoms and signs incorporated into any particular diagnosis. If we want to move from our atheoretical *DSM* approach to diagnosis toward a more etiologically based system, what level of causal explanation should we use? To what extent should we continue our focus in our nosology on "surface" symptoms and signs picked for their reliability rather than trying to develop potentially more informative or "deeper" symptoms that might emerge from careful phenomenological analysis? Can we expect the sciences to come to the rescue of nosologists showing us the joints at which we can carve our diagnoses?

The interface between psychiatry and philosophy is a broad one. Three additional areas, implicitly related to explanation, phenomenology, and nosology but also distinct and worthy of attention, are ethics, philosophically informed histories of psychiatry, and the mind-body problem.

Ethics

Psychiatry confronts a range of ethical issues that philosophy can help us frame and think through clearly. (For a good recent and concise summary of this field, see Bloch and Green 2006.) Of the many interesting issues in psychiatric ethnics, one of them—concepts of moral responsibility—is informed by both old and very difficult philosophical issues surrounding the problems of free will and determinism and recent developments in psychiatric genetics (Farahany and Coleman 2006). As we discover specific genetic variants that we show affect the risk for aggression, impulsivity, alcohol dependence, or psychosis, will they become relevant for discussions of moral and legal responsibility? If so, which seems inevitable, what will be the nature and shape of their impact on our discourse?

2. Philosophically Informed Histories of Psychiatry

Much has been written about the nature of scientific progress and the role therein of theory. (For one recent summary, see Losee 2004.) Although, as described above, psychiatry has undergone striking upheavals in its theoretical basis in the past 100 years, very few careful and well-informed historical-philosophical analyses have been attempted in the Anglophone world. In many cases, the stories are likely to be both interesting and enlightening about the range of forces that have shaped this field. Psychiatrists as individuals spend a great deal of time helping their patients understand their own personal histories, to help them gain insight into how they got where they are. It is ironic that, as a discipline, psychiatry has engaged in relatively little of such "self-examination" and much of what has been done has not been well grounded in the extensive prior work done by historians, sociologists, and philosophers of science.

3. The Mind-Body Problem

The mind-body problem cuts through the entire field of psychiatry like the intellectual equivalent of the Grand Canyon. Although it goes by many names, each of which carries a different set of nuances (for example, brain-focused versus mind-focused, scientific versus hermeneutic, organic versus functional, biological versus psychological, natural science versus human science), the broad diversity of fields and perspectives relevant to psychiatry have this key divide. More than any other professionals on earth, psychiatrists "live" the mind-body problem in their day-to-day work. Any active psychiatric clinician who uses both pharmacological and psychological treatment methods is constantly switching perspectives, seeing the dysfunction of the patients before them as a problem in brain functioning that they are seeking to treat with drugs and as a result of psychological dysfunctions in a "minded" individual, who is full of hopes, wishes, fears, and desires that they hope to help with psychotherapy. How these two perspectives interact and how these two treatment modalities can be made to synergize maximally is the bread and butter of good-quality psychiatric practice.

For those of us from a psychiatric background, it is probably helpful to distinguish two approaches toward the mind-body problem. One, which takes a metaphysical perspective asking complicated questions about issues such as "supervenience" and "the existence of qualia," continues to generate an extraordinarily large literature. My own personal sense is that, although some of this work is of great interest to psychiatry and philosophy, there is a point where the metaphysical fineries of these discussions begin to lose relevance. The second approach toward the mind-body problem is to see it more as an issue in philosophy of science (or more specifically philosophy of psychology or neuroscience). This viewpoint has generated a considerably smaller literature but one that is likely of more direct relevance to who study problems of mental health. Here the issues take on a more empirical slant and center on problems of levels of explanation and causality—the area that we examine in the first section of this book.

4. Setting the Stage: Two Clinical Examples

Another task for this introduction is to help set the stage for discussions in other parts of this book. Therefore, I here provide two examples that are grist for the mill of subsequent discussions. The first, an example of pluralistic etiologic models for psychiatric disorders, attempts to integrate diverse risk factors for MD. Several contributions to this book refer to this model in females (Kendler, Gardner, and Prescott, 2002; Kendler and Prescott 2006) or a closely related model our group developed a few years later in males (Kendler, Gardner, and Prescott 2006).

The effort begins with 1,942 females from both identical and fraternal female-female twin pairs ascertained through the birth-certificate based Virginia Twin Registry (for details, see Kendler, Gardner, and Prescott 2002). To be included in this study, the twins had to do nothing more than be born in Virginia and cooperate in our studies. These twins had been interviewed up to four times during a twelve-year period and their parents had been interviewed, so we knew a lot about them.

The goal of these analyses was to understand how genetic background, early risk factors, and proximal stressors combine to influence risk for MD in females. Our model attempted to predict the occurrence of an episode of MD (using *DSM-III-R* criteria [American Psychiatric Association 1987]) in the one-year period before the fourth wave of interviews with these twins; 9.1 percent of the twins met these criteria. From the large list of available predictors, we chose eighteen, which we organized into five developmental tiers:

Childhood—genetic risk factors, disturbed family environment, childhood sexual abuse, and childhood parental loss;
Early adolescence—neuroticism, low self-esteem, early-onset anxiety, and conduct disorder;
Late adolescence—low educational attainment, lifetime traumas, low social support, and substance misuse;
Adulthood—ever divorced and history of MD; and
Past year—past year marital problems, total difficulties, and two types of stressful life events (SLE): dependent and independent.

These risk factors included several potential levels of explanation including indices of aggregate biological factors (genes—as assessed by knowing the history of MD in co-twins, mothers, and fathers), personality (neuroticsm), self-concept (self-esteem), psychiatric disorders (anxiety and conduct disorders), interpersonal relationships, and traumatic environmental experiences (stressful life events and sexual abuse). It is important to note, however, that certain explanatory levels were not included in this model. No specific genes were measures, nor were other molecular, neurochemical, or brain imaging variables included.

In brief, we used the structural equal modeling program Mplus (Muthen and Muthen 2004) and tried to reject as many of the paths as possible with the goal of obtaining the correct balance of explanatory power and parsimony. Our final model, which fit well by several standard statistical indices, accounted for 52.1 percent of the variance in liability to develop an episode of MD. For statistical details, see the original report (Kendler, Gardner, and Prescott 2002).

The best-fit model, the parameter estimates of which are depicted in Figure I.1, is a bit daunting on first inspection but is, it is to be hoped, worth some effort to understand. The path coefficients depicted in the figure reflect the *unique relationship between variables, adjusting for all the other possible connections through other variables in the model.* One-headed arrows indicate "causal" paths (where we use this word in a statistical sense). Two-headed arrows represent correlations—the variables are associated, but it can't be assumed that one causes the other.

The figure has too many findings to here describe in any detail. Let me point out a few highlights. *High genetic risk* for MD was directly predictive of elevated levels of neuroticism (a key temperamental risk factor for later depression), substance misuse, traumatic experiences, and divorce. The level of genetic risk for MD also directly predicted both MD before the past year and the probability of a depressive episode in the past year. *Childhood sexual abuse* (CSA) uniquely predicted three of the four early adolescent and three of the four late adolescent risk factors, with its strongest effects on conduct disorder and lifetime trauma. In addition, CSA also predicted both difficulties and independent SLEs in the past year. *Neuroticism* had a particularly strong effect on low self-esteem and early-onset anxiety disorders. High levels of neuroticism also predicted low levels of social support, past year marital problems, and risk for onset of MD in the last year. *Conduct disorder symptoms* increased the risk for lifetime traumas, low social support, and, especially strongly, substance misuse.

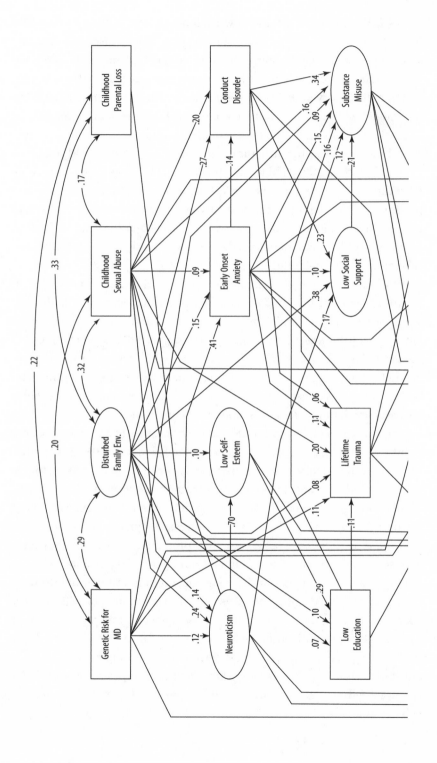

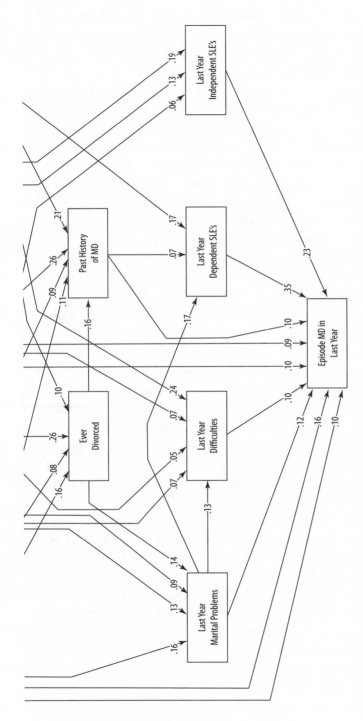

Figure I.1. Results from an integrative model for the prediction of major depression (MD) in the last year in women. Latent variables—indexed by observed variables in a measurement model—are depicted in ovals, while observed variables are depicted in rectangles. SLEs = stressful life events. All variables have estimated residual variance not depicted in the figure. See text for a description of variables.

Source: Adapted from Kendler, Gardner, and Prescott (2002).

Substance misuse was the most "connected" variable in the model. It was the second strongest predictor of a history of MD and also predicted exposure to three later environmental risk factors: divorce, past year difficulties, and dependent SLEs.

Finally, all four of the risk factors reflecting experiences in the past year were uniquely related to risk for MD, with SLEs having a stronger impact than difficulties.

Looking beyond the mass of individual path coefficients, what are the broader implications of these findings? First, they clearly demonstrate what it means to say that MD is a complex, multifactorial disorder with risk factors that reflect several different levels of abstraction. Second, they suggest three broad sets of paths connecting early risk factors to the development of an MD episode, which we termed "internalizing," "externalizing," and "adversity." Internalizing paths are anchored by two variables: neuroticism and early-onset anxiety disorders. The externalizing portion of the model is also anchored by two variables: conduct disorder and substance misuse. By contrast, the adversity paths are more extensive and diffuse, beginning with the three risk factors of disturbed family environment, childhood sexual abuse, and parental loss; flowing through low education, lifetime trauma, and low social support to being divorced; and then influencing all four of the past year's environmental risk factors. This last set of paths might be more accurately termed "adversity/interpersonal difficulties" because many of the depressogenic consequences of the earlier adversities appear to occur through troubled interpersonal relationships.

One further point about these analyses is noteworthy. These results illustrate the intricacy of the "gene-to-phenotype" pathway for complex psychiatric disorders such as MD. Two paths involve what has been termed "genetic control" of exposure to the environment in which individuals at high genetic risk for MD choose situations associated with events (such as traumas and divorce) that increase risk for depressive episodes. Another path suggests that genetic risk factors for MD act in part by influencing personality. Substance misuse is also an important intervening variable between genetic factors and MD. Finally, in addition to all these indirect pathways, genetic risk factors directly increase the probability for both prior and past years' episodes of MD.

These analyses are far from definitive. Four limitations are especially important to point out. First, the statistical model that we used included only additive relationships between risk factors. While we could have

considered interactions, the number of possible two- and three-way interactions would have been daunting indeed. Second, MD is a broad syndrome and likely to be etiologically heterogeneous. Third, all of these data
were collected using interviews and self-report questionnaires. No experimental manipulations were performed. In some cases, retrospective recall bias is possible. Thus, although the arrows in the figure imply cause
in a statistical sense, whether these relationships are truly causal is another matter entirely. In some instances we can have reasonable confidence in a direct causal relationship, but in others bidirectional relationships are at least as likely (as well as ones mediated by other factors not
included in the model). Fourth, though pluralistic, this model is far from
exhaustive and, in particular, does not include the kinds of variables studied in systems or molecular neuroscience.

Several chapters of this book also examine the association between
humiliation and depression. I could not resist adding as a second clinical
example this poignant vignette from Burton's great opus, *The Anatomy of
Melancholy* (1932):

> A grave and learned minister, and an ordinary preacher at Alkmaar in Holland
> was (one day as he walked in the field for his recreation) suddenly taken with
> a lask or looseness [of his bowels], and thereupon compelled to retire to the
> next ditch; but being surprised at unawares by some gentlewomen of his
> parish wandering that way, was so abashed that he did never show his head
> in public, or come to the pulpit but pined away with the melancholy.

5. Brief Overview of the Organization and Content of This Book

This book has three parts, each of which is focused around one of the
major themes at the interface of philosophy and psychiatry: explanation,
phenomenology, and nosology. Each chapter is preceded by a brief introduction, most commonly written by one of the editors. Each chapter is
then followed by a comment written by another one of the authors. We
structured the book in this way to simulate in print the interactive aspects
of the meeting attended by most of the authors in Copenhagen. The book
ends with a brief epilogue by one of the editors.

The chapters differ considerably in their level of philosophical difficulty. In all cases, the authors have made an effort to talk to nonspecial-

ists. For those containing more "philosophy-speak," the editor's introduction will try to break ground for the newcomer.

ACKNOWLEDGMENTS

Peter Zachar, Ph.D., and Josef Parnas, M.D., Dr.Med.Sci., provided very helpful comments on earlier versions of this chapter.

REFERENCES

American Psychiatric Association. 1968. *Diagnostic and Statistical Manual of Mental Disorders,* 2nd ed. Washington, DC: American Psychiatric Association.
———. 1980. *Diagnostic and Statistical Manual of Mental Disorders,* 3rd ed. Washington, DC: American Psychiatric Association.
———. 1987. *Diagnostic and Statistical Manual of Mental Disorders,* rev. 3rd ed. Washington, DC: American Psychiatric Association.
Bloch, S., and S. A. Green. 2006. An Ethical Framework for Psychiatry. *British Journal of Psychiatry* 188:7–12.
Burton, R. 1932. *The Anatomy of Melancholy.* Vol. 1. New York: E. P. Dutton.
Farahany, N., and J. E. Coleman Jr. 2006. Genetics and Responsibility: To Know the Criminal from the Crime. *Law and Contemporary Problems* 69:115–164.
Ghaemi, N. 2003. *The Concepts of Psychiatry: A Pluralistic Approach to the Mind and Mental Illness.* Baltimore: Johns Hopkins University Press.
Jaspers, K. 1963. *General Psychopathology.* Chicago: University of Chicago Press.
Kendler, K. S., C. O. Gardner, and C. A. Prescott. 2002. Toward a Comprehensive Developmental Model for Major Depression in Women. *American Journal of Psychiatry* 159:1133–1145.
———. 2006. Toward a Comprehensive Developmental Model for Major Depression in Men. *American Journal of Psychiatry* 163:115–124.
Kendler, K. S., and C. A. Prescott. 2006. *Genes, Environment, and Psychopathology: Understanding the Causes of Psychiatric and Substance Use Disorders.* New York: Guilford Press.
Losee, J. 2004. *Theories of Scientific Progress: An Introduction.* Routledge.
Muthen, L. K., and B. O. Muthen. 2004. *Mplus User's Guide.* Los Angeles: Muthen & Muthen.
Sokolowski, R. 1999. *Introduction to Phenomenology.* Cambridge University Press.

PART I

EXPLANATION

CHAPTER 1

Explaining Complex Behavior

SANDRA D. MITCHELL, PH.D.

In a succinct but wide-ranging essay, Sandra Mitchell grapples with an issue central to the science and clinical practice of psychiatry: how should we approach and attempt to understand a complex biological system like the human mind/brain? She begins her approach to this question, which has been tackled from several different perspectives by other authors in this volume, with a brief review of recent philosophical work on the approach to such complex systems. Then, she applies these models to the example of Major Depressive Disorder (MDD).

She begins with what she calls "a taxonomy of complexity," suggesting that we need to consider compositional complexity, dynamical complexity, and evolutionary contingency. The reader might profitably note and ponder her brief reference to an interesting literature that argues that multilevel modularity is a necessary feature of evolved complex systems—the epitome of which would be the human brain/mind.

She then turns to the main framework of her essay, which in turn is substantially influenced by the work of Bechtel and Richardson (B&R) (1993). (Theirs, by the way, is a clearly written book, nearly devoid of obscurities and full of informative historical examples that could be profitably read by clinicians interested in these issues.) Following B&R, Mitchell emphasizes the importance of two major strategies employed by scientists in their approach to complex systems: localization and decomposition. She then discusses the classification of complex systems articulated by B&R: *aggregative, component,* and *integrative.* In aggregative systems, the actions of individual components simply add together. These kinds of systems though rare, make life easy for the scientist investigating them. In component systems, the actions of modules interact, but a great deal of information can be obtained by studying them in isolation. These kinds of systems are typically called "nearly decomposable." Integrative systems are yet more complex. They have nasty properties, such as outputs from the entire system have critical top-down effects on the component parts and components interact with each other in highly nonadditive ways. Integrative systems are typically called "*minimally* decomposable." One example of this kind of nonadditivity of components of complex biological systems would be the sensitivity of the phenotypic impact of gene knockouts to the background genotype. The same gene knockout has been shown multiple times to produce quite different phenotypic effects when produced in different mouse strains.

A lovely example of top-down influences that Mitchell summarizes is Gene Robinson's work showing that state of the beehive can have a profound effect on the gene expression pattern of the constituent bees. As Mitchell summarizes, for integrative systems, "Features of the environment, both internal and external, of the entire system—a top-down perspective—will need to be invoked to determine what the system *and* its parts are doing." Mitchell then turns to an analysis of MDD, relying partly on a model my colleagues and I published (Kendler, Gardner, and Prescott 2006) and outlined in the introduction to this volume.

It will not surprise most readers that Mitchell reaches the conclusion that the etiological systems that influence MDD are of the integrative (equals *minimally* decomposable) variety. Although MDD has some classic bottom-up etiologic influences (genes, for example), there are almost certainly nasty nonadditive interactions between different causal processes. One now-classic example is the interaction between genetic risk and stressful life events. In addition, top-down influences are also likely critical. Our psychiatric patients go out into the world where, partly as a result of their personalities or the disorders themselves, they are prone to create conflictual interpersonal relationships, sometimes with their doctors. These difficulties can then feed back to stress their already fragile coping mechanisms. Drug-use disorders present an even clearer example of such effects. After all, the drug is not even introduced into the system until the individual goes out into the world, makes the needed social contacts, purchases it, and then inhales, injects, or ingests it. All that has to happen before any genes that affect drug response even get a chance to go to work.

The main conclusion of Mitchell's line of argument is that hard reductionism will not work for psychiatric disorders. We cannot treat psychiatric illness in a research or a clinical context as if they were simple *aggregative* systems. Another line of attack will be needed. One such well-articulated version would be that of integrative pluralism, an approach that Mitchell has advocated (for more details, see her useful 2003 book, *Biological Complexity and Integrative Pluralism*), which includes both top-down and bottom-up approaches.

I could not better conclude this introduction than with a short quotation from Mitchell's chapter, words that might be profitably taken to heart by any clinician or researcher who has honestly confronted the true complexity of the etiology of psychiatric illness: "Setting the standards for what is a satisfactory account to include only universal, deterministic regularities will fail to make room for the types of contingent, complex causal structures that frequent the biological world. Universality will fail when there are multiple pathways to generating the same effect in different individuals or at different times."

Kenneth S. Kendler, M.D.

REFERENCES

Bechtel, W., and R. C. Richardson. 1993. *Discovering Complexity: Decomposition and Localization as Strategies in Scientific Research*. Princeton, NJ: Princeton University Press.

Kendler, K. S., C. O. Gardner, and C. A. Prescott. 2006. Toward a Comprehensive Developmental Model for Major Depression in Men. *American Journal of Psychiatry* 163:115–124.

Mitchell, S. D. 2003. *Biological Complexity and Integrative Pluralism*. Cambridge: Cambridge University Press.

* * *

1. General Features of Complexity

There is increasing concern that reductionist programs for explaining complex behavior are inadequate. Although there have been many successes in drilling down to the more fundamental constituents of complex structures and capturing the behavior of the components, returning to the explanations of the behavior of the complex systems that they compose has not always been easy or direct. There are good reasons complete decomposition and reconstitution have failed to give us the explanations we want, but this need not entail despair. Alternative strategies exist that recognize the kinds of complexity that thwart a simple reductive strategy for generating explanations of the phenomena we aim to explain.

In this chapter I make explicit some of the reasons that complex biological systems elude the dream of simple explanations. I identify the features of complexity that are responsible. I then outline an alternative approach to sciences of complex behavior and draw some methodological inferences for the practices of investigating complex behaviors. The examples here and the target for this analysis is the explanation of clinical (or "major") depression in humans. Why will an individual, or class of individuals, have a Major Depressive Episode in a given time interval? The presumption is that a causal analysis of the precursor events and states that generate this behavior will constitute both an explanation and, if precise enough and if the precursor events are observable, the tools for predicting episodes of depression. Thus, there are both theoretical and clinical goals to be met by an account of the cause or causes of depression.

In this chapter I consider only Major Depressive Disorder (MDD), which is identified symptomatically with a characteristic set of behaviors in the fourth edition of the *Diagnostic and Statistical Manual of Mental Disorders (DSM-IV* [American Psychiatric Association 2000]). The disorder is thus inferred from an individual having one or more Major Depressive Episodes (that is, "at least two weeks during which there is either depressed mood or the loss of interest or pleasure in nearly all activities" [American Psychiatric Association 2000, p. 349]). An episode to be identified as depression must not be due directly to known physiological effects of a drug, medication, or toxin introduced into the body or better accounted for by bereavement (see *DSM-IV,* criteria D and E, p. 356).

Although *DSM-IV* states that there are no diagnostic laboratory findings for a Major Depressive Episode, it is claimed that it may involve a "dysregulation of a number of neurotransmitter systems, . . . alternations of several neuropeptides . . . [and for some] hormonal disturbances." Functional brain imaging documents changes in cerebral blood flow and metabolism for some, and sometimes changes in brain structure. Yet "none of these changes are present in all individuals in a Major Depressive Episode . . . nor is any particular disturbance specific to depression" (p. 353). In addition, there is a familial pattern with Major Depression, that is, it is 1.5–3 times more common among first-degree biological relatives of individuals with this disorder compared with the general population (*DSM-IV,* p. 373).

An individual with MDD displays a range of features characteristic of complex behavior in general. These features have important implications for how one can study the etiology of the disorder as well as the kinds of knowledge one should expect to glean from such studies.

I have proposed a taxonomy of three types of complexity that are characteristic of biological systems (Mitchell 2003). Systems, like a developing organism, an insect colony engaged in division of labor, or a slime mold transitioning from life as a collection of single-celled individuals to a single multicelled individual are, first, compositionally complex, second, dynamically complex, and, third, evolutionarily contingent. The first type, compositional complexity, points to features that, for example, Herbert Simon (1962) worried much about—namely, how complex biological structures are built from their simpler parts. This question can and has been addressed in varying degrees of abstraction. One can describe the features of many-component structures in general in terms of composition rules that range from simple additivity to hierarchal structures displaying different types of nonadditive relationship (Wimsatt 1986, 2000).

Second, the dynamical features of complex systems refer to nonlinear patterns of change in space and time. For example, chaotic dynamics incorporate extreme sensitivity to initial conditions generating unpredictability in even deterministic systems. That is, two points in a system may move in vastly different trajectories, even if the difference in their initial configurations is very small. Examples include weather phenomena. Edward N. Lorenz, a meteorologist, metaphorically termed this type of complexity "the butterfly effect," raising the possibility that the flap of a butterfly's wings in Brazil might cause a tornado in Texas (Lorenz 1996). Self-organized systems are ones in which feedback interactions among simple behaviors of individual components of a system produce what appears to be an organized group level effect. For example, individual honeybee foragers whose probability to continue to forage may be affected by the waiting time for unloading pollen in the hive, collectively generate a system that "tunes" the number of foragers to the "need for pollen" in the hive (Seeley 1988).

Third, the evolved features of complex systems record the historical contingency, variability, and path dependence of the particular array of properties and behaviors that are found in the biological systems that have occupied our planet both currently and in the past. Variability is endemic to biological populations; indeed, it is a necessary component to the evolutionary dynamics that generate adaptive change. Given certain aspects of speciation processes (for example, niche specialization) and developmental processes (for example, suppressing competition in generating higher levels of organization, such as from single-celled to multicellular organization, see Buss 1987), variations in both the distribution of traits within a population and the traits characteristic of different populations are fundamental to evolved complex biological systems.

What is evident from this discussion is that complex system behavior generally relies on multiple causes additively or interactively contributing to the production of a major effect. In addition, biologically complex systems may be organized modularly and hierarchically. Simon (1962) and Richard Lewontin (1978) have argued that modularity permits a system to remain sufficiently stable and yet at the same time evolve over time to become increasingly complex and adapted to its environment. Thus, a complex biological system will not only have a *multicomponent* causal character but also be *multilevel* in organization.

A third significant characteristic of a complex biological system that pertains to explaining its behavior is *plasticity* in the face of environmental variability. A honeybee colony, for example, is composed of workers displaying division of labor. There are four age-castes associated with four task repertoires. The youngest bees clean the cells for about 3 days and then perform brood care. From days 10 to 20, the bees engage in building activities and pollen storage and reception. At around day 20, the bees stand guard at the hive entrance, and after a few days the bees become foragers. The bees will remain foragers until they die. This pattern, however, is flexible. Young bees raised in the absence of older foragers will begin to forage precociously. In addition, experimental manipulation experiments have shown that older bees will "regress" to perform the tasks typically associated with younger bees if the younger bees are removed (Huang and Robinson 1996). Phenomenologically, a complex system can and does reorganize the properties and behavior of its component parts in the face of changing internal and external conditions. Because patterns of division of labor are variable among species and display plasticity within a species, no simple algorithmic mechanism will work to explain all the details of this complex behavior (Trainello and Rosengaus 1997).

At the same time, some components of the mechanism generating the complex social behavior of division of labor are shared across not just social insects but also other, nonsocial organisms. It is the case that some basic building blocks of organismal development, shared molecular modules found in widely divergent species can be identified. Their role in multicomponent complex causal structures thus may be regular, whereas the specific output behavior may vary in response to the variable internal and external contexts in which a given module is located. In a recent article, Gene Robinson and colleagues (2005) survey recent work on the molecular basis for social behavior. They describe the cGMP signaling pathways that are strongly conserved in the regulation of feeding behaviors in the flies *Drosophila melanogaster,* honeybee *Apis mellifera,* and worm *Caenorhabditis elegans.* However, although genes are involved in each case in contributing to variations in roaming and sitting behaviors implicated in feeding, for the nonsocial species the variation is genetic, depending on different alleles while, in the social species, the variation in behavior "is developmental, involving age-related changes in gene expression in the brain" (Robinson et al. 2005, figure 2, p. 260). This indicates that, although genes and molecular level mechanisms are operative components in the generation of a complex behavior, simply identifying a gene associated with a behavior will never be enough to causally explain the behavior. Sometimes the genotype-phenotype relation will be stable and variation will be allelic (as in fly and worm). Other times variant behaviors will be the result of interactions of the genetic- and molecular-level mechanisms as well as other factors at other levels (as in honeybee).

The failure of a causal component having a univocal contribution to a complex behavior can also be attributed to the plasticity of the organization of the complex system displaying that behavior. This has been attributed to genomic regulatory systems. Knockout experiments implement the design of a controlled experiment. In these experiments two systems are compared, one harboring a double-mutant knockout at what is thought to be an important genetic site and the other nearly identical except for the wild-type, nonmutant genetic component at that precise genetic site. But in a number of cases, as much as 30 percent according to Edelman and Gally (2001) and Ihle (2000), there is little or no evident phenotypic consequence of knocking out a gene; the two systems display nearly identical outcome phenotypic traits or behaviors. Should one infer that the knocked-out gene was not causally contributing the phenotypic trait under study? Not necessarily.

There are a number of reasons the inferences from genetic knockout techniques are difficult to interpret (see Gerlai 1996). First, the causal process involving isolated genes are extremely sensitive to genetic background. Experiments using the same strain of laboratory mice include individuals with different genetic backgrounds. Thus, part of the confounding of the effect of a gene may be by means of interaction with other genes in the background. That is, the knockout might fail to instantiate an ideal controlled experiment because of the nature of the complexity of the system.

In addition, there are different stages in the casual process from gene to protein to cell to other, more distal phenotypic expression that some of the techniques cannot distinguish. What happens late in the process may well be subject to more context-specific contributions, and so the contribution of the knocked-out gene may be difficult to identify. In addition to the complications of disentangling the contribution when there are multiple causal components, the dynamical plasticity of the structure of components can also confuse inferences about the causal upshot of any intervention or perturbation of the system. These are the cases of redundancy and degeneracy (Edelman and Gally 2001; Greenspan 2001).

Redundancy in a network, such as a genetic regulatory system, describes a situation in which there are multiple copies of a functional gene, like in an engineering failsafe or backup design. Redundancy is widespread in biological systems, though it is puzzling how it could have evolved. A copy of a functional component would induce a cost without a corresponding adaptive benefit unless it is at least occasionally called on to operate. It has been argued that there are scenarios in which redundancy is nevertheless evolutionarily stable (Nowak et al. 1997). Degeneracy, unlike strict redundancy, refers to an organization whereby alternative components and structures with distinct functions may nevertheless produce the effect of a target structure when that target is no longer operative. Degeneracy has been identified in 21 different levels of biological systems, including protein folding, biosynthetic and catalytic pathways, immune response, neural circuitry, and sensory modalities (Edelman and Gally 2001).

In the case of networks of causal components that embed causal redundancy, an experimental intervention that failed to excise *all* the copies of the redundant component would also fail to elicit a response that would indicate the typical contribution of that component. In addition, with degeneracy even when all the copies of a single genetic component are knocked out, the absence of a response in the trait product may indicate that the network itself has reorganized so that genes that typically do not issue in the target phenotype will respond to the experimental perturbation and produce some product similar, if not identical, to that of the unperturbed system. Thus, the standard inferences drawn from controlled experimental practice may not be suited to interventions on dynamically reorganizing causal networks (Greenspan 2001). Empirical research has documented the ways in which some members of gene families compensate in the absence of other members (Solloway and Robertson 1999; van Swinderen and Greenspan 2005).

These features of complex biological systems highlight what I take to be variant degrees of contingency and sensitivity of both the whole system and its component parts. That is, the behavior of a single component (a gene, say, or a worker honeybee) is not just driven from its internal capacities to act in a certain way under specific initial conditions. The behavior of the component is contingent on what other factors are also jointly acting. Activation and repression mark contingency because of genetic relativity. Degeneracy and redundancy are predicated on entire network structures to indicate internal plasticity in generating functional outcomes, and gene expression may depend on and be responsive to social influence.

2. How to Study Complex Behavior

The standard approach to making the behavior of complex systems tractable to scientific study is decomposition and localization (Bechtel and Richardson 1993). The heuristic is to dissect a complex system into its functional components, investigate and characterize the component behaviors individually, and subsequently explain the behavior of the whole in terms of the behavior of the parts and their organization. Explanations are formed "bottom up." For some systems, where the properties of the whole system are just the additive result of its components such a reductionistic strategy for generating explanations will be sufficient, but most complex biological systems violate the assumptions necessary for this strategy to be viable. They fail to be, as Bechtel and Richardson state, "aggregative." System properties of aggregative systems depend linearly on component properties (Bechtel and Richardson 1993; Wimsatt 1986). To put it differently, the organization of an aggregative system is *not* a major determinant of system functioning (Wimsatt 1986). One need know only the components and their individual behaviors in isolation to understand the behavior of the system. A pile of sand is aggregative. The mass of the whole system is linearly determined by the masses of all the grains that are its components.

Systems that are not aggregative are composite. Composite systems come in two forms, *component* and *integrative* systems (Bechtel and Richardson 1993). In component systems, the properties of the whole do depend on the organization of the parts, but the parts themselves are partially independent, or, in Simon's words, nearly decomposable. In these cases a partially reductionist strategy can work. One needs to know the properties or behavior of the components to understand the system's behavior, but one also needs to know how the components are organized together into a chain or network. For component systems the individual parts plus their organization will explain the system's behavior. The third kind of system is what Bechtel and Richardson call integrative. These are systems in which not only do the component behaviors and their organization matter to the behavior of the system but also the very behavior of the components depends on features of the whole system; "systemic organization is significantly involved in determining constituent functioning" (Bechtel and Richardson 1993). Integrative systems are minimally decomposable.

Self-organizing or self-regulating systemic behavior of integrative systems will not be derivable from a simple catalogue of the independent behavior of the functional parts. Features of the environment, both internal and external, of the entire system—a top-down perspective—will need to be invoked to determine what the system *and* its parts are doing.

There are methodological consequences for the different types of system organization. For aggregative systems, reductionism will be a successful strategy. Decompose a multicomponent system into its parts (for example, genes), investigate the parts, and their properties will determine the system's behavior. The alleles for roaming or sitting behavior in *C. elegans,* egl-4 mutant or wild, will predict the behavior of the worm. In component systems, more than the component properties are needed. A more complex reductionist strategy will be required. In addition to the properties of the parts, to explain such a system's behavior, the organization of parts is required. In such cases (for example, lactose metabolism) not just the presence of a mutant allele but also what other regulatory genes are operant is required to determine the behavior of the system. Thus, higher levels of organization above the single allele (for example, the regulatory genetic network) will set the constraints of the behavior of the single component. The well-known case of Lac operon in *Escherichia coli* studied by Jacques Monod and François Jacob is a case of regulation of gene expression. The genetic organization includes operator, repressor, and promoter regions. Lactose is metabolized when three structural genes are expressed, but their expression depends on whether or not a repressor is bound to the regulatory site on the genome. Just having the structural genes, rather than some mutant forms, is insufficient to determine the behavior of the system. In addition, one needs to know the organization of the components.

For the case of integrative organization, a bottom-up reductionist strategy will not work. Rather, a top-down approach is needed. In these systems, the behavior of the parts themselves is a function of properties of the whole system. The example of the variable behaviors for individual honeybees indicates that it is an integrative system. The genetic components and the various regulatory systems that determine their expression are themselves affected by the social context in which the individual finds herself. Whereas individual flies and worms show similar genetic structure for determining foraging behavior, for the bee, there is an additional property that regulates the behavior of the component genes (that is, the "needs" of the colony). Robinson et al. (2005) report studies indicating a change of gene expression in the brain of bees in different social contexts. Thus, to explain why an individual bee forages at a given time, one must appeal not only to the genetic components contributing to the behavior or the regulatory components of the genome that influences the expression of those genes, but also to the social situation the individual experiences.

With these general considerations at hand, I now turn to a discussion of MDD. What kind of complex system behavior is depression? What kinds of methodological consequences follow?

3. MDD

What is the causal structure of MDD? *DSM-IV* identifies various associated factors that may be involved in generating the expression of a Major Depressive Episode. As noted above, none of them was taken to be necessary factors. They included neurotransmitter systems, neuropeptides, hormonal changes, cerebral blood flow and metabolism, changes in brain structure, and familial pattern, which indicates a genetic factor.

Kendler, Gardner, and Prescott (2006) present the most comprehensive account of a top-down analysis of the etiology of MDD (see the Introduction for more details about this model). The 2006 study was targeted for the disorder in men, complementing a similar 2002 study of MDD in women. The general conclusion was that MDD is an etiologically complex disorder that involves multiple factors from multiple domains acting over developmental time.

Our best-fit model suggested three pathways to major depression in men, characterized by *internalizing symptoms* (genetic risk factors, neuroticism, low self-esteem, early-onset anxiety, and past history of major depression), *externalizing symptoms* (genetic risk factors, conduct disorder, and substance misuse), and *adversity and interpersonal difficulty* (low parental warmth, childhood sexual abuse and parental loss, low education, lifetime trauma, low social support, history of divorce, past history of major depression, marital problems, and stressful life events including genetic liability; poor parenting, traumatic experiences, predisposing personality traits, early onset anxiety disorder, poor self-esteem, low social support, substance misuse, marital difficulties, a prior history of major depression, and recent stressful life events and difficulties. . . . Major depression is a paradigmatic multifactorial disorder, where risk of illness is influenced by a range of factors.

They stratify these risk factors through an analysis of five developmental periods: childhood, early adolescence, late adolescence, adulthood, and the previous year.

In their etiological approach, Kendler et al. decompose the complex causal history of the behavioral outcome of adult MDD. Their analysis has a corresponding functional decomposition in terms of levels of organization. Marvin Zuckerman (1993) proposed a levels hierarchy for understanding personality disorders (Figure 1.1).

Joop Hettema (1995) uses this hierarchy to locate studies of depression at each level. He takes the model to imply that properties and behaviors of components at the lower levels, though necessary for depression to develop, are not sufficient. Rather, each level displays special conditions that are realized when depression occurs. The model permits there to be different routes leading to the same behavior in different individuals. This framework of levels of organization can be used to locate the risk factors identified and measured by Kender et al. in their developmental, etiological analysis (Figure 1.2).

It is clear that depression is a complex behavior of a complex system that depends on multiple causes and multiple levels. In recent years much has been learned about the components that are associated with this disorder. An important question that remains to be answered concerns the relationships between the properties and behaviors at the different levels. Even if the discovery of lower-level components is possible only by look-

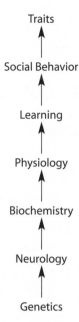

Traits

Social Behavior

Learning

Physiology

Biochemistry

Neurology

Genetics

Figure 1.1. Levels of analysis of personality.
Source: Zuckerman (1993) in Hettema 1995.

ing at higher level effects, will the explanation of the higher levels be amenable to a reductionist strategy?

That there are genetic risk factors for depression is indicated by the familial relationships and twin studies that show a higher probability of depressive disorder among related adults. The main class of drugs used to treat depression is selective serotonin reuptake inhibitors (SSRIs), which target the midbrain serotonergic neurons. The activity of these neurons is controlled at least in part by 5-HT autoreceptors (Haddjeri and de Montigny 1998), so studies have targeted the polymorphic 5-HTT (or serotonin transporter) gene in which variation in the promoter region of short and long alleles occur naturally in the human population. Hariri et al. (2005) investigated the relationship between the short-allele 5-HTT and response bias of the human amygdala, the part of the brain that is important for emotional and social behavior, to environmental threat. The results of their study, conducted on healthy subjects, indicated a relationship between the short allele and amygdala response to threat but did not lead to predictions of mood. Thus, they concluded that the 5-

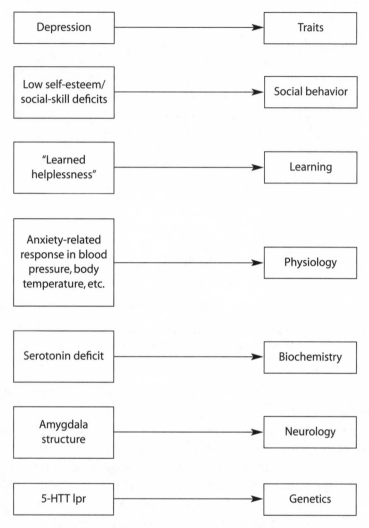

Figure 1.2. Depression and levels: mapping Zuckerman's levels for depression.

HTT gene may be best classified as a susceptibility factor in depression, not a sole determinant.

By examining the biochemical, neurological, and genetic levels of organization, one can see that MDD is not the result of an aggregative complex system. Thus, a simple reductionist strategy, in which information about the component genes, and nothing else, would lead to predictions of likelihood of depressive episode, will not be successful. This leaves open the possibility that there are other components at the lower levels whose contribution is not yet understood and thus whose organization with the identified gene might be predictive of depression. If so, it is possible that MDD is a trait of a component system and a partial reductive strategy holds out hope of working.

Recent studies, however, indicate that the plasticity and variability of MDD make it more likely to be the behavior of an integrative system. Caspi et al. (2003; see also Kendler et al. 2005) reported results of a prospective longitudinal study of 1,037 children regularly assessed from 3 years of age to 26. They were divided into three groups based on the 5-HTT genotype: those with two copies of the short allele, those with one copy of the short allele, and those with two copies of the long allele. Caspi et al. measured incidence of stressful life events for the three groups. Their results showed that stressful life events would predict depression in the groups of people who had at least one short allele but not for the homozygotic long-allele group. They concluded that "the 5-HTT gene interacts with life events to predict depression symptoms, an increase in symptoms, depression diagnoses, new-onset diagnoses, suicidality, and an informant's report of depressed behavior" (Caspi et al. 2005, p. 387). More recently, Kendler et al. (2005) replicated the Caspi study with a twin study. They also explored the mechanism by which the 5-HTT alleles would increase the probability of depression by means of increasing sensitivity to stressful life events. The results of that study indicated that individuals with two short alleles were more likely to experience depressive reactions to stressful events than were those with one or two long alleles because they were more sensitive to low-level stressful events.

What is significant about the gene-environment interaction results found for the 5-HTT gene and stressful life events is that they entail a nonreductionist approach to explaining the complex causal network leading to MDD. In rejecting a purely molecular reductionist approach, Kendler et al. state, "Our results argue against this as they suggest that understanding gene action in depression requires us to both 'go down' to individual genetic polymorphisms and 'go out' into the environment with detailed measurements of stressful experiences" (2005, p. 534).

In general, psychiatric disorders will not be amenable to purely or even partially reductionist strategies. Because evidence suggests that they are behaviors of an integrative complex system, an integrative methodology is needed to understand the etiology and causally explain such behaviors.

This is not to deny the role that genes play in the complex causal network but, rather, to understand that role as context sensitive and the system in which it operates as displaying a high degree of contingent plasticity. As Lindon Eaves said, "The classical models of inherited (or 'Mendelian') disorders which are caused by alleles at one or two loci with very little environmental influence, do not apply to most complex psychiatric disorders. The number of genes may be large, their effects may be small, and their effects on the phenotype may be many and varied as a function of other contingencies, including those of chance and the environment" (2005, p. 62).

Indeed, Kenneth Kendler (2005) detailed the ways in which "a gene for" language is likely to fail to fit psychiatric disorders because of the weak statistical association between genes and disorder, the role of environmental factors in the etiology and the complexity of the causal pathway that includes genes and concludes with a psychiatric disorder. That a simple gene-disorder causal and explanatory relation will be found is clearly precluded. This is not to deny that genes are involved, however, and associations between genes and psychiatric disorders may be found. Rather, the explanation and prediction of the presence or absence of MDD, for example, will not be projected from data about genes alone.

The weakness of the association between genes and psychiatric disorders speaks more to the variability of pathways and multiplicity of contingent factors than to the strength of genes in eliciting the disease phenotype. Under a specific range of internal and external factors, it may well be that having two short alleles at 5-HTT locus is what would make the difference between having depression and not. If that range of internal and external factors normally varies widely in a population, however, then knowing just the allele information will be insufficient to predict the occurrence of depression. In context-rich causal scenarios, both factors that have traditionally been allocated the role of cause, like the polymorphic allele, and the factors that traditionally have not been specified but rather designated only as context or background conditions will conspire to produce the outcome of interest.

The methodological upshot is to replace the purely and partially reductionist methodologies of complex psychiatric disorders with ones that are integrative. I have previously argued (Mitchell 2003) for such an integrative pluralistic approach for complex biological systems in general. It involves both top-down and bottom-up analyses. Moffitt, Caspi, and Rutter

(2005) suggested that, rather than dismissing gene-environment interactions as infrequent, new studies focused on discovering interaction may solve the puzzle of the failure of finding replicable results of the genetic contribution to complex behavior. They suggest that the failure of "gene hunting" has been attributed to the possibility of a behavior being caused by many genes with small effects so that the role of any one of the multicomponent structure is too small to be detectable. Instead of this explanation, they suggest that complex psychiatric disorders such as MDD are caused by fewer genes, but ones whose effect is contingent on the joint operation of environmental pathogens (Moffitt et al. 2005, p. 479). Certainly this type of complex interaction is possible, but it is not necessary nor is there yet sufficient evidence to determine how frequent it might be.

In light of the variability of the ways in which genes are implicated in complex behavior, that a single gene is completely deterministic of a trait may be rare but has certainly been found. The same holds for the fact that effects of individual genes may be small but still detectable. Moffit, Caspi, and Rutter's message should be taken to highlight the plausibility that in some complex behaviors the scope of study should include variability of genes and environments *and* the ways in which genes and environment interact (for a counterargument, see Eaves 2006). In short, there are many alternative scenarios that could be instantiated when there is a failure of simple Mendelian causation.

Once contingency, plasticity, and degeneracy are posited as possible characteristics of the complex causal networks leading to behaviors of complex systems, methodologies can be developed for ascertaining the causal and explanatory impact of individual or collections of individual components at different levels of organization. An integrative pluralist approach to scientific explanation presupposes the unlikelihood that there will be a simple, single causal account at the end of a reductionist investigation into the causes of behavior of complex systems. Thus, looking for only genes that act as good Mendelian players whose polymorphism directly and completely accounts for variable phenotypes will likely fail to find satisfactory accounts. Setting the standards for what is a satisfactory account to include only universal, deterministic regularities will fail to make room for the types of contingent, complex causal structure that frequent the biological world. Universality will fail when there are multiple pathways to generating the same effect in different individuals or at different times. Instead, one might expect contingent interactions among the multiple components at multiple levels of organization in a complex system in generating an effect. Deterministic pathways may be too simple to describe some types of interactions in the network of causes. When properties of the system affect the character and behavior of the component parts of that system, bottom-up explanations, the goal of reductionist strategies, will be inadequate to the task. If two short 5-HTT alleles create a condition in which an individual is more likely to experience depressive reactions to a broader range of stressful life events, the experience of those events and their effects may amplify the sensitivity so that depression is an even more likely result.

Psychiatric disorders constitute complex multicomponent, multilevel behaviors. As the type of causal structure underlying the generation of behaviors such as MDD is better understood, a methodology tuned to detecting the types of contingencies and interacting factors is more likely to yield useable knowledge. Although it would be much easier if such complex behaviors were the result of the presence of a single structural allele, which was expressed in all contexts, that is not what is found. Life, indeed, is not so simple.

REFERENCES

American Psychiatric Association. 2000. *Diagnostic and Statistical Manual of Mental Disorders,* 4th ed. Washington, DC: American Psychiatric Association.

Bechtel, W., and R. C. Richardson. 1993. *Discovering Complexity: Decomposition and Localization as Strategies in Scientific Research.* Princeton, NJ: Princeton University Press.

Buss, L. 1987. *The Evolution of Individuality.* Princeton, NJ: Princeton University Press.

Caspi, A., K. Sugden, T. E. Moffitt, J. Mill, A. Taylor, I. W. Craig, H. L. Harrington, J. McClay, J. Martin, A. Braithwaite, and R. Poulton. 2003. Influence of Life Stress on Depression: Moderation by a Polymorphism in the 5-HTT Gene. *Science* 301:386–389.

Eaves, L. J. 2005. *Psychiatric Genetics* (Review of Psychiatry). K. Kendler, and L. J. Eaves. Washington, DC: American Psychiatric Publishing.

———. 2006. Genotype × Environment Interaction in Psychopathology: Fact or Artifact? *Twin Research and Human Genetics* 9(1):1–8.

Edelman, G. M., and J. A. Gally. 2001. Degeneracy and Complexity in Biological Systems. *Proceedings of the National Academy of Sciences* 98(24):13763–13768.

Gerlai, R. 1996. Gene-Targeting Studies of Mammalian Behavior: Is It the Mutation or the Background Genotype? *Trends in Neuroscience* 19(5):177–181.

Greenspan, J. 2001. The Flexible Genome. *Nature Reviews: Genetics* 2:383–387.

Haddjeri, N. P. B., and C. de Montigny. 1998. Long-Term Antidepressant Treatments Result in a Tonic Activation of Forebrain 5-HT1A Receptors. *Journal of Neuroscience* 18(23):10150–10156.

Hariri, A. R., E. M. Drabant, K. E. Munoz, B. S. Kolachana, V. S. Mattay, M. F. Egan, and D. R. Weinberger. 2005. A Susceptibility Gene for Affective Disorders and the Response of the Human Amygdala. *Archives of General Psychiatry* 62:146–152.

Hettema, J. 1995. Personality and Depression: A Multilevel Perspective. *European Journal of Personality* 9:401–412.

Huang, Z.-Y., and G. E. Robinson. 1996. Regulation of Honey Bee Division of Labor by Colony Age Demography. *Behavioral Ecology and Sociobiology* 39(3):147–158.

Ihle, J. N. 2000. The Challenges of Translating Knockout Phenotypes into Gene Function. *Cell* 102:131–134.

Kendler, K. S. 2005. "A Gene for . . ." The Nature of Gene Action in Psychiatric Disorders. *American Journal of Psychiatry* 162:1243–1252.

Kendler, K. S., C. O Gardner, and C. A. Prescott. 2006. Toward a Comprehensive Developmental Model for Major Depression in Men. *American Journal of Psychiatry* 163:115–124.

Kendler, K. S., J. W. Kuhn, J. Vittum, C. A. Prescott, and B. Riley. 2005. The Interaction of Stressful Life Events and a Serotonin Transporter Polymorphism in the Prediction of Episodes of Major Depression: A Replication. *Archives of General Psychiatry* 62:529–535.

Lewontin, R. C. 1978. Adaptation. *Scientific American* 239(3):156–169.

Lorenz, E. N. 1996. *The Essences of Chaos.* Seattle: University of Washington Press.

Mitchell, S. D. 2000. Dimensions of Scientific Law. *Philosophy of Science* 67:242–265.

———. 2003. *Biological Complexity and Integrative Pluralism.* Cambridge: Cambridge University Press.

Moffitt, T. E., A. Caspi, and M. Rutter. 2005. A Research Strategy for Investigating Interactions between Measured Genes and Measured Environments. *Archives of General Psychiatry* 62:769–775.

Nowak, M. A., M. C. Boerlijst, and J. Cooke. 1997. Evolution of genetic redundancy. *Nature* 388:167–171.

Robinson, G. E., C. M. Grozinger, and C. W. Whitfield. 2005. Sociogenomics: Social Life in Molecular Terms. *Nature Review Genetics* April: 257–270.

Seeley, T. D. 1988. Social Foraging in Honey Bees: How Nectar Foragers Assess Their Colony's Nutritional Status. *Behavioral Ecology and Sociobiology* 24:181–199.

Simon, H. 1962. *The Architecture of Complexity: The Sciences of the Artificial.* Cambridge, MA: MIT Press.

Solloway, M. J., and E. J. Robertson. 1999. Early Embryonic Lethality in Bmp5; Bmp7 Double Mutant Mice Suggests Functional Redundancy within the 60A Subgroup. *Development* 126:1753–1768.

Traniello, J. F. A., and R. B. Rosengaus. 1997. Commentaries: Ecology, Evolution, and Division of Labour in Social Insects. *Animal Behavior* 53:209–213.

van Swinderen, B., and J. Greenspan. 2005. Flexibility in a Gene Network Affecting a Simple Behaviour in *Drosophila melanogaster. Genetics* 31(169):2151–2163.

Wimsatt, W. C. 1986. Forms of Aggregativity. In A. Donagan, A. N. Perovich, Jr., and M. V. Wedin (eds.), *Human Nature and Natural Knowledge* (pp. 259–291). Boston: Reidel.

———. 2000. Emergence as Non-aggregativity and the Biases of Reductionisms. *Foundations of Science* 5:269–297.

Zuckerman, M. 1993. Personality from Top (Traits) to Bottom (Genetics) with Stops at Each Level between. In P. J. Hettema and I. J. Deary (eds.), *Foundations of Personality* (pp. 73–100). Dordrecht: Kluwer.

Comment: Psychiatry, Scientific Laws, and Realism about Entities

Peter Zachar, Ph.D.

> It is the world around us, the messy, mottled world that we live in and that we wish to improve on, that is the object of our scientific pursuits, the subject of our scientific knowledge, and the tribunal of our scientific judgments. (Cartwright, 1999, p. 6)

Karl Popper (1974) famously argued that Darwin's theory of natural selection was not a legitimate scientific theory. As philosophers such as David Hull (1973) and Michael Ruse (1979) turned their attention to biology, it became clear that Darwin's theory was more able to withstand critical scrutiny than Popper realized. Knowing why it could withstand such scrutiny required that philosophers develop a greater level of expertise in the biological sciences. This increased expertise developed into the subfield known as the philosophy of biology. What was discovered in this endeavor has had important implications for the philosophical understanding of science in general.

Sandra Mitchell's exploration of complexity in biology and its implications for scientific explanation is a natural fit for psychiatry. After reviewing the distinction between aggregative, component, and integrative systems, she convincingly articulates why Major Depressive Disorder (MDD), because it has features of an integrative biological system, is unlikely to be explained using a conventional reductionistic framework. In this commentary I shall dig a little bit deeper into her larger body of work and some related ideas of her fellow philosophers of science, focusing on their important implications for psychiatric classification and the science of psychiatry itself.

1. Natural Scientific Laws

By convention, laws are considered to be universal and necessary statements that are required for an adequate scientific explanation. For example, the second law of thermodynamics can be formulated as the claim that *heat moves from an area of higher concentration to an area of lower concentration.* If you want to understand why your house gets cold in the winter after the heat is turned down, look to the second law. If it is zero degrees outside and you turn off the heat, because the heat will lawfully move from the inside (high concentration) to the outside (low concentration) without being replaced, your house necessarily gets colder. Scientific explanation by laws is often considered to be ideal science.

A complicating factor to science by laws (or nomological science) is accounting for exceptions. With the laws of thermodynamics, exceptions are relatively rare. When the phenomena being studied are more complex, however, as is the case in biology, psychiatry and psychology, "exceptions" are the rule.

For example, psychology's law of effect states that *a behavior that is followed by a satisfying state of affairs will be repeated.* You can reward a 9-year-old boy with chocolate for sitting still, but if there were a group of friends outside the window playing *tackle anyone who picks up the football,* even the satisfaction of chocolate may not keep him still. Sports fans continue to support losing teams, cardiac patients maintain low-salt, low-fat diets, and people repeatedly enter into the same kinds of dysfunctional, dissatisfying relationships. Higher-order mammals can also make tremendous sacrifices to enact abstract ethical principles, sometimes with no possibility of satisfaction (a soldier willing to die for her country). The law of effect is true if certain assumptions are met or "true everything else being equal" (or, *ceterus paribus*). There seem to be so many possible exceptions to the law of effect that it is hard to believe that it is a natural necessity akin to the second law of thermodynamics.

The importance of exceptions has led to the claim that there are few (if any) true laws in the "special" or inexact science such as biology, psychol-

ogy, and sociology (Beatty 1997; Smart 1968). There are natural regularities, but those regularities are limited in scope and contingent rather than
universal and necessary. The absence of universal and necessary generalizations is somehow supposed to make these disciplines lesser sciences.
The best way to make them more respectable is supposedly to show how
they can be reduced to the more exact, nomological sciences (that is, those
disciplines that explain phenomena lawfully, such as physics and chemistry). Hence, the project of reductionism.

Those entities that can be explained with respect to natural scientific
laws are traditionally called natural kinds. One commonly stated implication of widespread *ceterus paribus* conditions for classification in the special sciences is that entities such as species and psychiatric disorders are
not natural kinds. As David Hull (1989) writes, natural laws are spatiotemporally unrestricted. For example, the generalizations that are true of
gold are true everywhere and at all times.

Hull points out that species are not spatiotemporally unrestricted—
they have limited spatial distributions and beginnings and endings in
time. Furthermore, unlike gold, species change. The set of traits that
define a species in one era may not be the same set of traits that defines
that species in another era. How can there be *universal and necessary*
laws for domestic dogs, which have been around for only 10–15,000
years, presumably exist only on the planet earth, and evolve? Are there
different *laws* for German shepherds and poodles? What if a new breed of
dog was to appear—would there then be new laws to describe that breed?
Would those laws cease to exist if the dogs went extinct? Can laws of nature go extinct? The conclusion some people would draw is that, if laws
of nature cannot go extinct, there cannot be laws about German shepherds
per se and therefore neither they nor any other species should be considered natural kinds.

Although in this volume and elsewhere I have claimed that psychiatric
disorders should not be considered natural kinds, those claims have little
to do with the issue of laws (Zachar 2000, 2006b). The tradition of natural
kinds is much richer than the narrower concept of kind-specific behavior
being governed by natural laws. I have been more concerned with the
philosophical baggage of essentialism and literalist metaphors about
classification systems carving nature at the joints (Zachar 2006a).

The primary conclusion to be drawn from the role played by natural
laws with respect to the scientific understanding of species is that the

classification of biological species should not be evaluated using the classification of chemical elements as a "gold" standard. The same is true for the classification of psychiatric disorders. The principles used in the classification of chemical elements may inform other classificatory domains, but they should not serve as regulative ideals.

This argument about classification parallels Mitchell's (2003) work in the philosophy of biology, specifically her claim that the explanation of organic systems shouldn't be evaluated using the explanations of inert physical systems as the standard of adequacy. What Mitchell refers to as composite and integrative biological systems are not random occurrences; they operate according to rules. However complicated they may be, those rules are also explanatory. The complication is that these rules are conditional. Rather than examining the domains studied by the special sciences and concluding they are too complex to be subsumed under scientific laws, she argues that the conventional stipulation that scientific laws are universal and necessary is too narrow.

As an alternative, Mitchell claims that accurate generalizations exist on a continuum. On one end of the continuum are highly stable generalizations such as *mass-energy cannot be created or destroyed, but only transformed from one state to another,* whereas on the other end are less stable generalizations such as *all the coins in Nelson Goodman's pocket are copper.* Mitchell persuasively argues that philosophers have mistakenly been conceptualizing the domain of law dichotomously so that something either is or is not a law. In fact, most generalizations do not fall on either end of the bipolar continuum. Biological generalizations such as Mendel's law of segregation and its concepts of dominant and recessive genes, says Mitchell, are more like the mass-energy generalization than they are like the generalization about the coins in Goodman's pocket.

As noted, the important difference between the generalization about mass-energy and the generalization about Nelson Goodman's coins is not universality; rather, the conditions under which the mass-energy generalization applies are more stable. The mass-energy rule is contingent upon the fundamental structure of the universe that was determined shortly after the Big Bang. Generalizations about mammalian physiology are less stable. Even less stable than physiology, but more stable than Goodman's coins, are generalizations about cultural events such as observations of the rising tide of fundamentalism in both the East and West. Kendler and Zachar (this volume) explore the implications that *ontological condition-*

alities and the continuum of stability have for understanding psychiatric disorders, specifically with respect to another conventional dichotomy, that of natural kind versus social construction.

Mitchell's claim garners additional support from some careful analysis in the philosophy of science indicating that strict universality does not apply to the laws of physics either. For example, according to Rom Harré (2000), even something as important as Newton's first law does not literally describe what happens in nature—it is an abstraction (or an idealization). Newton's first law states that *an object in motion will continue moving at the same speed and direction unless acted on by an external force.* Given that there is invariably another force, objects never continue moving at a constant speed in a straight line indefinitely.

Nancy Cartwright (1983, 1999) offers similar arguments, even claiming that the laws of physics lie. Natural laws are not literally true generalizations. The useful generalizations scientists have discovered work only after specific conditions have been established. She calls these conditions *nomological machines.* Nomological machines are stable arrangements of components that have certain capacities. Examples include the solar system and chemical batteries. For example, the generalizations describing the motion of electrons in chemical batteries require components such as a nickel hydroxide plate, a cadmium hydroxide plate, and a conducting electrolyte (such as potassium hydroxide). Nickel hydroxide is the anode, meaning it has the capacity to lose electrons. The arrangement also has to be protected from extraneous influences by what Cartwright calls *shielding conditions.* Without the battery casing to shield the chemical reactions from the external influences, electricity could not be produced, stored, or discharged. Within these limits, however, the generalizations made about self-discharge rates and electrical current in batteries are more than empirical regularities, they also *explain* why the machine behaves as it does.

B. F. Skinner (1938, 1974) famously translated the law of effect into the nonpsychological and operationalist language of reinforcement and then studied the law of effect by means of a new kind of nomological machine, called a *Skinner box.* As a strict empiricist, Skinner did not favor a concept such as "scientific laws," and his research program can easily be conceptualized in Cartwright's terms. As exemplified by the earlier example of the boy and the chocolate, the problem with the law of effect is that behaviors are influenced by an ever-shifting multitude of possible reinforcers. Skinner's insight was that the basic rules of behavior couldn't be discovered unless the experimenter had complete control over all the reinforcers. The Skinner box is a shielded container in which a rat or pigeon is placed for training. It is doctrinaire among Skinnerians that behaviorist principles don't work reliably unless "stimulus control" can be achieved (that is, a nomological machine has to be constructed).

Explanatory power is an important criterion of scientific laws—the outcomes that they predict are not merely accidental, they are necessary. Mitchell (2003) cleverly suggests that philosophers have made a false analogy between the putative universal statements in science such as *all heat naturally flows from hot objects to cold objects* and universal logical statements such as *all bachelors are unmarred men.* Philosophers, claims Mitchell, have inappropriately assumed that because both universal generalizations and analytic statements have a similar logical form, both can be called "necessary." They can't. Logical necessity is not causal necessity.

Rather than necessity, Mitchell proposes using a notion of causal force to understand scientific explanation. For example, the second law of thermodynamics explains *why* it gets colder in the house after the heat is turned off. A generalization about when and why a honeybee starts to forage also has genuine explanatory force, even if the generalization does not always hold, or is a matter of probability. The age at which a honeybee begins to forage may be conditional on contextual factors and is therefore is not a *natural necessity,* but neither is it merely an accident (like the coins in Goodman's pockets). When a rule about initiating forging does apply, it works just as well any other true generalization. The job of the scientist should be to understand all the complicated reasons why the generalization is explanatory no matter how local the explanation.

Instead of defining laws essentialistically in terms of fixed properties such as universality and necessity, Mitchell contends that laws can be defined functionally in terms of the roles they play in science. She states that many of the generalizations in the inexact sciences play the roles that that laws are expected to play in the natural sciences, including explanation, prediction (supporting counterfactuals), and manipulation/intervention. Although one has to be cognizant of the conditions in which rules lower down on the continuum of stability apply, for all practical purposes, when they do apply these rules function as laws.

Mitchell's pragmatic conception of scientific law better allows philosophers and scientists to explore a wide variety of causal structures without having to categorize them using the strict dichotomy of lawful versus non-lawful. Although she highlighted the nonreductionist dimension in her chapter, another way to read it is as an exploration of what kinds of causal generalizations in specific complex biological systems can and cannot be made. For example, a generalization such as *worker honeybee ovary development and egg laying is suppressed if there is already a queen* can be made, but accurate generalizations about the function of genes using knock-out experiments are difficult to make.

2. Implications for Psychiatric Explanation and Classification

Mitchell's pragmatic account of laws has important implications for psychiatric explanation and classification. Almost everyone would agree that the reason for classifying different cases together as the same kind of thing is to draw generalizations about them. Given that psychiatric disorders are clearly complex things, the generalizations that can be drawn may always be somewhat local, based on the particular questions one is asking. The generalizations that are useful when certain conditions apply may be less useful when the conditions change. This kind of *heterogeneity* is often considered to be a flaw in psychiatric nosology, but in fact it may accurately signal inherent complexity.

This does not warrant the conclusion that we should adopt a fatalistic attitude toward heterogeneity; it can always be narrowed or widened somewhat depending on our purposes. The concept of mental disorder obviously describes a collection of conditions so heterogeneous that few, if any, useful generalizations can be drawn about mental disorders as a whole. Nosologists can narrow the scope a bit in the hope of finding better generalizations—but it is unlikely that they can titrate the scope so that generalizations about psychiatric disorders will be as stable and regimented as generalizations about copper or crystals. Considered longitudinally, the symptom profiles of conditions such as schizophrenia and bipolar disorder may be dynamic like the division of labor in honeybee colonies is dynamic, the symptom profiles of anorexia and depression even more so.

Obviously, the science of psychiatric classification is less focused on laws—rules—generalizations and more focused on entities about which those generalizations are drawn. From an entity perspective, widening the scope is often called *lumping* and narrowing the scope is often called *splitting.* Kendler and Zachar (this volume) show how in some cases widening, not narrowing, the scope can lead to more stable generalizations (that is, wide-scope categories such as internalizing and externalizing may be more stable than narrow-scope conditions such as Post-Traumatic Stress Disorder).

Although the problem of classification has to be surveyed from multiple perspectives, I suggest that the perspective advocated by Cartwright is particularly informative for psychiatric nosology's attempt to classify complex entities or conditions. Realism about entities often refers to physically concrete things such as batteries or electrons. Taking a hint from Daniel Dennett (1987), depression is also an *abstract entity*. Its level of abstraction lies somewhere between electrons and centers of gravity.

It is almost a truism among philosophers of psychiatry that a legitimate nosology has to be etiologically driven (Poland, von Eckhardt, and Spaulding 1994; Murphy 2006). One possible problem with a causal structure view of explanation is that it is easy to make causal structures into higher level abstractions, even universal processes exemplified as *the* etiology of schizophrenia or *the* etiology of MDD. In physics, Cartwright refers to that move as fundamentalism, the view that a fixed set of generalizations can always be invoked to explain what needs explaining.

An alternative to the rule-oriented causal perspective is an entity-oriented capacity perspective. Entities have capacities to behave in various ways depending on the conditions in which they are placed. The generalizations we make about them apply when the appropriate conditions occur. Cartwright focuses on the capacities such as those inherent in a planet revolving around the sun, but one could just as easily talk about the capacities of genes or personality traits.

Thinking in terms of broad capacities (which have variable outcomes) rather than well-defined dispositions (in which the outcome is predefined) results in entities being conceptualized in a developmental rather than a static framework. Psychiatric disorders are outcomes that manifest when certain conditions apply. Like cancer, much has to happen for MDD or Panic Disorder to develop. When social factors are involved, the occasioning conditions can be called *niches* (Hacking 1998).

In psychiatry the nomological machines that can produce depression are less like a machine that makes a popsicle to the same specifications every time and more like a weather system that makes snowflakes—there is always variability. The inevitability of variation does not warrant the pessimistic evaluations of "immaturity" and "soft science" commonly leveled by the hard-nosed critics of psychiatry. Mitchell teaches us that complexity is not an impassable barrier to casual understanding. Studying the variations helps, not hinders, our scientific understanding.

Popsicles vary as well, but the level at which the variation occurs is more fine grained than our interests in popsicles require. Psychiatry is about the *messy, mottled* world of individuals. As the quote offered at the beginning of this commentary suggests, making a positive intervention in the lives of patients and their various social networks is the purpose of psychiatry. With psychiatric disorders, therefore, our interests are calibrated to the levels where extensive variation exists. For practical reasons, nosologists typically select levels of abstraction that are coarse grained enough to permit useful generalizations.

Realism about entities also has implications for the problem of reification in psychiatry. The mistake of reification is not in believing that entities such as depression are real. Many psychiatric disorders, like centers of gravity, are real. The mistake is believing that the entities that are useful in a nosology are more fine grained than they are (that is, they literally represent what depression is). It is a "fundamental" misunderstanding even to believe that they should.

REFERENCES

Beatty, J. 1997. Why Do Biologists Argue Like They Do? *Philosophy of Science* 64:S432–S443.
Cartwright, N. 1983. *How the Laws of Physics Lie.* Oxford: Oxford University Press.
———. 1999. *The Dappled World.* Cambridge: Cambridge University Press.
Dennett, D.C. 1987. *The Intentional Stance.* Cambridge, MA: MIT Press.
Hacking, I. 1998. *Mad Travelers: Reflections on the Reality of Transient Mental Illnesses.* Charlottesville: University Press of Virginia.
Harré, R. 2000. Laws of Nature. In W. H. Newton-Smith (ed.), *A Companion to the Philosophy of Science* (pp. 213–223). Malden, MA: Blackwell.
Hull, D. 1973. *Darwin and His Critics: The Reception of Darwin's Theory of Evolution by the Scientific Community.* Chicago: University of Chicago Press.
———. 1989. *The Metaphysics of Evolution.* Albany: State University of New York Press.
Mitchell, S. D. 2003. *Biological Complexity and Integrative Pluralism.* Cambridge: Cambridge University Press.
Murphy, D. 2006. *Psychiatry in the Scientific Image.* Cambridge, MA: MIT Press.
Poland, J., B. von Eckhardt, and W. Spaulding. 1994. Problems with the DSM Ap-

proach to Classifying Psychopathology. In G. Graham and G. L. Stephens (eds.), *Philosophical Psychopathology* (pp. 235–260). Cambridge, MA: MIT Press.

Popper, K. 1974. Darwinism as a Metaphysical Research Program. In P. Schlipp (ed.), *The Philosophy of Karl Popper* (pp. 133–143). La Salle, IL: Open Court.

Ruse, M. 1979. *The Darwinian Revolution.* Chicago: University of Chicago Press.

Skinner, B. F. 1938. *The Behavior of Organisms.* New York: Appleton-Century.

———. 1974. *About Behaviorism.* New York: Knopf.

Smart, J. C. C. 1968. *Between Science and Philosophy.* New York: Random House.

Zachar, P. 2000. Psychiatric Disorders Are Not Natural Kinds. *Philosophy, Psychiatry, and Psychology* 7:167–182.

———. 2006a. The Classification of Emotion and Scientific Realism. *Journal of Theoretical and Philosophical Psychology* 26 (1/2):120–138.

———. 2006b. Les troubles psychiatriques et le modèle des espèces pratiques. *Philosophiques* 33:81–98.

CHAPTER 2

Etiological Models in Psychiatry

Reductive and Nonreductive Approaches

KENNETH F. SCHAFFNER, M.D., PH.D.

In this chapter Kenneth Schaffner takes on a critical issue at the center of the efforts to develop a science of psychiatry—what should be the nature of explanation in psychiatry? Are the only useful or valid explanations reductive ones—that involve molecules, synapses, and genes? Or can an important role in our understanding of the etiology of psychiatric illness be played by nonreductive explanations involving less clearly defined higher-order variables like environmental risk factors—messy things like stressful life events—and psychological constructs like personality? What is the shape of explanatory models for which we should strive in psychiatry?

Schaffner begins by contrasting two different published etiologic models for psychiatric illness, which he characterizes as, respectively, *nonreductive* and *reductive*. The first was developed empirically by Kenneth Kendler and colleagues for Major Depression (Kendler et al. 1993, 2002, 2006) and the second more speculative model proposed by Paul J. Harrison and Daniel R. Weinberger (2005) for the ways in which individual candidate genes might influence the risk for schizophrenia. The first model is a statistical one—with boxes connected by arrows. The second is a biological one focusing on neurons and synapses. The first one contains complex higher-order constructs such as "childhood parental loss" and "recent stress life events." (This model also contains a box representing "genetic risk for depression," but it reflects the effect of all genes as assessed using a twin design, not individual genes that are biologically distinct.) The second contains genes, proteins, and neurotransmitters.

He poses the question of how are we to compare these two kinds of models. Is one of them better than the other? Would we hope as our science progresses for models like the first one to develop into models like the second one?

Next Schaffner takes what might initially seem like a detour but turns out to be a relevant introduction to the "reductionist's delight"— the worm *Caenorhabditis elegans*—which has only 302 neurons in its entire nervous system. His purpose in so doing is to ask the question of how far we can push the reductionist agenda. Can we take a simple behavior—social versus solitary feeding behavior in *C. elegans*—and explain it completely in simple molecular terms? Although it might have appeared to at first, Schaffner shows that more recent work has indicated that "it ain't quite that easy." Even in this simple case, the proposed explanations are looking multilevel. This example of single-gene effects on feeding in this tiny worm can be usefully contemplated for those interested in the nature and limitations of reductive models for psychiatric illness.

Noting that "behavior is an organismic property" and suggesting that reductive models for behavior will inevitably be more "creeping" than "sweeping," more "partial" than "ruthless," Schaffner particularly emphasizes that the relationship between genes and behavior are far more likely to be of the "many-to-many" kind (that is, most genes can influence multiple behaviors and most behaviors are influenced by many genes) rather than the "one-to-one" relationship that would fit most powerfully into a hard reductionist paradigm. Schaffner gives a balanced view of the possible implications of this work for psychiatric etiologic theories. Simple explanations for psychiatric disorders are highly improbable. Rather, etiologic models will be mixed, complex, and multilevel.

He then reviews three possible ways in which causal simplification might emerge for psychiatric illness: common pathways, dominating pathways, and emergent simplifications. In each case, it remains unclear how applicable they are likely to be to psychiatric disorders.

The chapter concludes with a discussion of the relevant work of William Bechtel and Robert Richardson (1993; also discussed by Sandra Mitchell in her chapter in this volume). What are the limits of reduction? How complex can systems be and still yield to standard explanatory efforts based on the concepts of localization and decomposition? When we call systems emergent, is that a cry of despair, an invocation of the mysterious, or an admission of the limits of human intellect? Or is it instead a call for the development of more complex computational tools to begin to understand aggregate behaviors of networks, be they genes, neurons, or environments? Like Schaffner, I would, for now, advocate the latter more optimistic approach.

Kenneth S. Kendler, M.D.

REFERENCES

Bechtel, W., and R. C. Richardson. 1993. *Discovering Complexity: Decomposition and Localization as Strategies in Scientific Research.* Princeton, NJ: Princeton University Press.

Harrison, P. J., and D. R. Weinberger. 2005. Schizophrenia Genes, Gene Expression, and Neuropathology: On the Matter of Their Convergence. *Molecular Psychiatry* 10:40–68.

Kendler, K. S., C. O. Gardner, and C. A. Prescott. 2002. Toward a Comprehensive Developmental Model for Major Depression in Women. *American Journal of Psychiatry* 159:1133–1145.

———. 2006. Toward a Comprehensive Developmental Model for Major Depression in Men. *American Journal of Psychiatry* 163:115–124.

Kendler, K. S., R. C. Kessler, M. C. Neale, A. C. Heath, and L. J. Eaves. 1993. The Prediction of Major Depression in Women: Toward an Integrated Etiologic Model. *American Journal of Psychiatry* 150:1139–1148.

* * *

1. The Pros and Cons of Etiological Models

Whether there can and should be etiological models in psychiatry has been a contentious issue. In the preface to the first edition of their 1974 classic *Psychiatric Diagnosis,* Donald W. Goodwin and Samuel B. Guze (Goodwin et al. 1979) wrote, "There are few explanations in this book. This is because for most psychiatric conditions there *are* no explanations. 'Etiology unknown' is the hallmark of psychiatry as well as its bane. Historically, once etiology is known, a disease stops being 'psychiatric.' Vitamins were discovered, whereupon vitamin-deficiency psychiatric disorders no longer were treated by psychiatrists. The spirochete was found, then penicillin, and neurosyphilis, once a major psychiatric disorder, became one more infection treated by nonpsychiatrists" (1995 [1974], p. xiii). In the most recent version (1996) of their book, Goodwin and colleagues reprint that preface and do not appear to shift explicitly in favor of any etiological perspective. The 1996 edition does, however, cite a number of family studies that indicate partially genetic etiologies for psychiatric disorders such as schizophrenia and dementia.

DSM-III, -III-R, and *-IV* also embodied a prima facie antietiological position, although there it was characterized more broadly as an "approach that attempted to be neutral with respect to theories of etiology" (*DSM-IV* 1994, p. xviii). Again, like Goodwin and Guze (1996), a close reading of the specifics of some of the sections on disorders belies this neutral stance, particularly in the case of "Dementia of the Alzheimer's Type."[1]

Other psychiatrists have argued that an etiological approach in psychiatry would bring it more in line with traditional medicine. Robert Kendell, who was a proponent of this view, also maintained that an emphasis on etiology is justified on empirical grounds: "It is simply an empirical finding that the most aetiologically based classifications are more useful— because they embody a wider range of implications than purely clinical classifications" (Kendell 1989, p. 46). In a recent book, philosopher of psychiatry Dominick Murphy defends as one of his main theses that "the classification of mental illness should group symptoms into conditions based on the causal structure of the abnormal mind" (Murphy 2006, p. 11).

2. Alternative Strategies: Reductive and Nonreductive Approaches

The goal of this chapter is to explore the prospects of some candidates for etiological models in psychiatry. Elsewhere (Schaffner 2002) I have addressed the pros and cons of proceeding causally in psychiatry in a more nuanced manner than will be the case here. In this chapter, I look at a related issue of whether etiological models in psychiatry can be, should be, or must be reductive models. By a reductive model I mean an etiological account that employs standard biochemical and molecular entities and mechanisms to account for psychiatric symptoms and disorders. A nonreductive but still etiological model would use a different vocabulary but would assert causal connections between entities characterized at a higher level of aggregation.

For the purposes of this chapter, we need not dwell on the terminology of reductive versus nonreductive for two reasons. First, the main exemplars will be clear enough as representing the two types of models just described. Second, one of the concluding theses will be that "mixed" models are likely to be the most useful for the foreseeable future, thus obviating a precise definition of reductive versus nonreductive.

It will be most useful to distinguish between two broad classes of etiological models employing these reductive and nonreductive approaches. For this purpose, a typology recently published by Kenneth Kendler

(2005b) for genetics-based psychiatric studies will be a reasonable entry point. The disciplinary focus on genetics can then be easily generalized to allow this typology to function as a framework within which two detailed psychiatric etiological models can be described and evaluated. Table 2.1 is an adaptation of table in Kendler (2005b) that describes the four major paradigms of psychiatric genetics and should be clear enough in itself to serve as the basis of a general etiological framework.

Paradigms 1 and 2 are nonreductive, 3 is partially reductive, and 4 is fully reductive. The genetic focus can be relaxed to permit studies on any type of set of individuals (a population) with either qualitative or quantitative causal generalizations as the goals. Study types in psychiatry are too diverse to summarize easily in any tabular manner, but the genetic paradigms given in Table 2.1 give us a rough intuitive grasp of the two differ-

TABLE 2.1
Four Major Paradigms of Psychiatric Genetics

Number	Title	Samples Studied	Method of Inquiry	Scientific Goal
1	Basic Genetic Epidemiology	Family, Twin, and Adoption Studies Example: IQ (or SZ) heritability ≈ 0.8	Statistical (simple twin studies; no specific genes)	Quantify the degree of familial aggregation and/or heritability
2	Advanced Genetic Epidemiology	Family, Twin, and Adoption Studies Example: genetic effects double the risk that stress produces depression	Statistical (complex path analysis models; no specific genes)	Explore the nature and mode of action of genetic risk factors
3	Gene Finding	High-density Families, Trios, Case-Control Samples Example: MAOA gene affects aggression	Statistical (linkage and association studies; specific genes)	Determine genomic location and identity of susceptibility genes
4	Molecular Genetics	Individuals Example: RGS4 affects pre-synapse neuron function in schizophrenia	Biological (specific gene knockout and knockin; gene chips)	Identify critical DNA changes; trace the biological pathways from DNA to disorder

Source: Adapted from Kendler (2005b), table 1, p. 4.
Note: MAOA, monoamine oxidase.

ent approaches, 3 and 4 of which use molecular terminology. Moreover, because the two exemplars that I will use to describe nonreductive and reductive etiological models *are* in fact genetic, they can be easily situated in the table.

3. A Classical Nonreductive Etiological Account: Kendler et al. on Major Depression

Beginning in an essay published in 1993 and continuing to the present, Kendler and colleagues have been analyzing the etiology of Major Depressive Disorder (MDD), hereafter simply *depression,* using a large twin study (see the Introduction for more background on these studies). A number of different factors formulated at a variety of levels of aggregation and construct have been used in this research program. A diagram from the earliest publication will orient us in a preliminary way to the approach taken in this project (Figure 2.1).

The links, if bidirectional, represent correlation coefficients. The arrow links are path coefficients or standardized partial regression coefficients. Note that in Figure 2.1 "genetic factors" display five links to entities that represent different levels, in terms of how one assesses and describes them. "Neuroticism" is a personality trait that figures in virtually all trait theories of personality, either as an explicit factor—in Eysenck's theory used by Kendler and also in the "Big Five" theory—or implicit, as in Cloninger's theories of personality. In this study, it is assessed by using a 12-item self-administered questionnaire based on a person's views about their own emotional functioning in typical situations. The endpoint, Episode of a Major Depression in the last year, is assessed by a standard clinical interview employing *DSM* criteria for MDD based on approximately 15 symptoms of the disorder. Genetic factors represent a latent variable constructed from a composite measure of the lifetime history of major depression in the co-twin as well as in the individual's mother and father, corrected for co-twin status as monozygotic or dizygotic. It must be emphasized here that specific genes are *not* ascertained in this type of study, which uses familial history data to arrive at a measure of the risk level. It should perhaps also be emphasized that what is depicted in the diagram is probabilistic causation, not deterministic causation.

In subsequent refinements of the assessed entities, additional factors were introduced, and the model was reformulated as a developmental

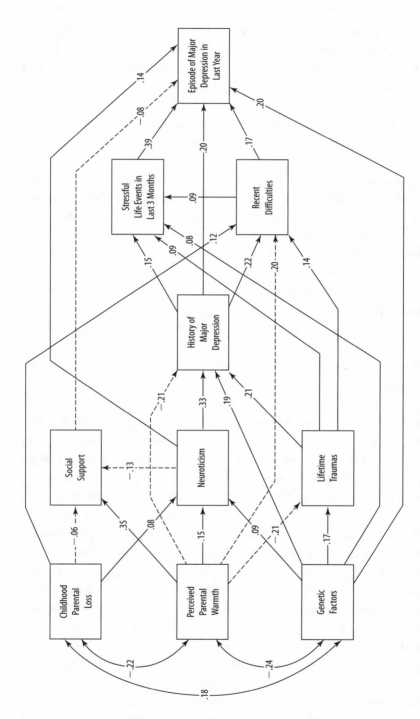

Figure 2.1. Path analysis diagram representing various factors affecting the likelihood of an episode of major depression in the last year. See text for details. *Source:* Adapted from Kendler et al. (1993).

model spanning the five life stages of childhood, early adolescence, late adolescence, adulthood, and the last year. The model has accordingly grown complicated and requires color coding to identify the life stages as well as the large number of causal links among the factors. A figure from the richest of the recent studies by Kendler et al. (2006) is given in the introduction to this volume (Figure I.1). This is a male twin study.

4. A Current Putatively Reductive Etiological Account: Harrison and Weinberger on Schizophrenia

A different type of approach is represented by current genetic models accounting for schizophrenia. The Kendler project briefly described above is the *only* such path-analytical model for a major psychiatric disorder that uses empirical data to characterize the causal influences. No such path-analytical model has ever been developed for schizophrenia, for reasons that are not fully clear. Nonetheless, flow diagrams have been published that provide a sketch of various genes that have since 2002 been identified as susceptibility genes for schizophrenia. Figure 2.2 is typical of these types of representation. These genes have various degrees of support in the psychiatric genetic literature, and here I will discuss only five, beginning with dysbindin-1.

Dysbindin-1

The dysbindin-1 (DNTBP1) gene was found by Straub et al. (2002) in the chromosome 6p22–24 region that had previously been linked with schizophrenia in the Irish high-density family study (Straub et al. 1995). The association was also confirmed in a German study (Schwab et al. 2003), a combined Irish-Welsh study (Williams et al. 2004), and additional more recent studies, providing about 11 confirmations and 3 disconfirming studies (Kendler 2004; Williams et al. 2005). The latter authors wrote in a recent article that these studies constitute "a substantial body of supportive evidence for association at a single gene [that] is unprecedented in studies of schizophrenia and is far beyond what can be attributed simply to chance" (p. 1). It is also noteworthy that Funke et al. (2004) report that, though this gene is a risk factor for white and Hispanic individuals, it may not be for African Americans. The gene is evolutionarily conserved, is 140,000 base pairs in length, and produces an approximately

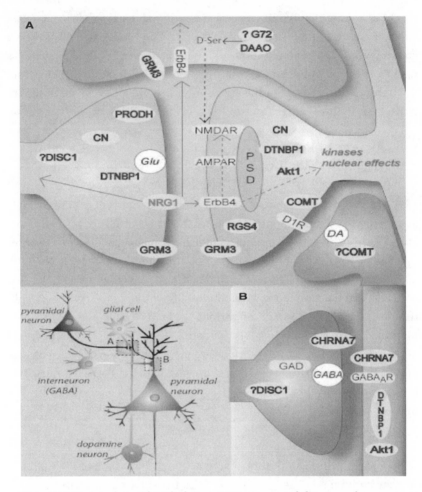

Figure 2.2. Various genes identified since 2002 as susceptibility genes for schizophrenia. This figure, from an article by two distinguished schizophrenia geneticists, is typical of these types of currently speculative representation. *Source:* Harrison and Weinberger (2005).

50,000-molecular-weight protein. The site of action is not known with full certainty, but it seems to act in both presynaptic and postsynaptic neurons and is thought to affect the release or metabolism of the neurotransmitter glutamate and perhaps also to interact with the NMDA (N-methyl D-aspartate) receptor (Owen et al. 2004; Talbot et al. 2004; Williams et al. 2005). There are, however, some differences in the haplotypes and alleles identified in the different dysbindin studies, which are thought to be due to allelic heterogeneity at the DNTBP1 locus (Owen et al. 2004). It has also been suggested that some evidence indicates that the genetic effect may lie in the regulatory region of the gene (Funke et al. 2004; see Williams et al. 2005 for an update).

Neuregulin-1

The neuregulin-1 (NRG1) gene was found on chromosome 8p21–22 by Stefansson et al. (2002) using the deCODE Icelandic population database. A whole-genome scan provided suggestive evidence for the 8p12–21 region, and a follow-up study using higher-resolution techniques focused in on two large risk haplotypes. Application of a SNP strategy then disclosed a core haplotype with a highly significant association with schizophrenia and that contained the neuregulin-1 (NRG1) gene (Stefansson et al. 2003). This gene produces a molecule affecting neuronal growth and development, as well as glutamate and other neurotransmitters, and also glial cells (see Moises et al. 2002). NRG1 may also affect myelin in the brain. Neuregulin is believed to be regulated by a postsynaptic cell receptor known as ErbB3/4. The NRG1 effect is small, accounting for approximately 10 percent of the schizophrenia risk in the Icelandic population, but the association has also been confirmed in a Welsh study and one Chinese population, though not in another Chinese population (Hong et al. 2004) or in the Irish high-density study (Thiselton et al. 2004). Specific alleles within this haplotype have yet to be identified.

G72 (and DAAO)

G72 (sometimes referred to as G30/72 because of association with another locus) was identified as a schizophrenia susceptibility linkage region on chromosome 13q, and association studies involving separate Canadian and Russian populations confirmed the gene (Chumakov et al. 2002). Another study involving Han Chinese was also confirmatory (Zou et al. 2005). The gene is primate specific and is expressed in the brain. G72's protein activates a second protein, produced by the DAAO (D-amino acid oxidase) gene, which is known to play a role in D-serine metabolism—which itself acts on the NMDA receptor known to be involved in memory and learning. This chain of events suggests that the G72/DAAO interaction is a plausible candidate gene for schizophrenia.

Catechol-O-methyl Transferase

The catechol-O-methyl transferase (COMT) gene is a plausible candidate gene because it codes for an enzyme that metabolizes dopamine, a key neurotransmitter believed on pharmacological grounds to be involved in schizophrenia. The Val(158)Met polymorphism in the COMT gene is known to affect brain frontal lobe function (Egan et al. 2001; Goldberg et al. 2003). The COMT gene is also missing in a chromosomal deletion associated with the velocardial facial syndrome, which itself increases the risk of schizophrenia. Although the mechanisms make this a plausible candidate gene for schizophrenia, the statistical genetic evidence supporting the COMT gene is thought to be weak and inconsistent and even negative in more recent investigations (Owen et al. 2004) and meta-analyses (Munafo et al. 2005), though others see it in a more favorable light (Harrison and Weinberger 2005).

RGS4

The RGS4 gene's role as a susceptibility gene for schizophrenia had its origin in a microarray study by Mirnics and colleagues (2000, 2001). Suffice it to say here that this regulator of G-protein signaling was identified in a study involving autopsy brain tissue from 10 schizophrenics and 10 normal subjects as being uniformly down regulated in those with schizophrenia. This was subsequently reconfirmed in another microarray study, and the gene had the attraction of falling within the 1q21–22 region that had in the previous year been strongly supported (LOD score > 6) as a schizophrenia susceptibility region by linkage methods (Brzustowicz et al. 2000). There were subsequently three independent replications of this gene's role in schizophrenia in one Indian and two U.S. studies. There is some difference, as there was with dysbindin, in the haplotypes and alleles identified in the RGS4 locus in the different studies. A recent meta-analysis, however, found little consistency in an RGS4 effect.

Other Genes Related to Schizophrenia

Several additional genes have been reported as linked to schizophrenia, including a gene known as PRODH2, another called 5HT2a, a PPP3CC calcineurin-related gene, a glutamate-receptor gene (GRM3), and a nicotinic-receptor gene (CHRNA7). Further attempts at replications of these, as well as the five genes discussed in detail above, are continuing in a number of laboratories. (See Harrison and Weinberger 2005 and Owen et al. 2004 for discussion and references.)

The role of NRG1 (neuregulin) has recently been further elucidated and is worth some additional discussion, to show both how this type of representation might be further developed and what the limitations of etiological inference are in this disorder using molecular methods. Even this *one* gene (and its alleles) seems to have multiple effects that may be related to the development of schizophrenia. A recent review article that looked at NRG1-erbB signaling—one of NRG1's likely main mechanisms—suggests at least four routes of influence, as depicted in Figure 2.3. (erbB is a *family* of receptor molecules that have three components, the business end of which is a tyrosine kinase that can phosphorylate and thus affect downstream molecules.) As multipathway as the diagram is, NRG1 actually is even more complex. According to Falls (2003, p. 619), "Neuregulin-mediated cell communication plays an essential role in the biology of most components of the neuromuscular system—including motor and sensory neurons, muscle fibers, Schwann cells, and major specializations (neuromuscular synapses, muscle spindles, Golgi tendon organs, and peripheral nerves)."

The specifics of how NRG1 works in schizophrenia may be significant. Thus, a bit more analysis seems in order. One possibility has been further developed recently in a communication from the Oxford and National Institute of Mental Health groups of Harrison and Weinberger, with Law as first author (Law et al. 2006). In general, these authors argue that NRG1 acts in a regulatory manner—via altered transcriptional effects that can alter both neural development as well as neural signaling in the adult. In their recent account, Law et al. write in their concluding statement,

> In summary, we provide evidence of splice variant-specific alterations of *NRG1* gene expression in schizophrenia and demonstrate that disease-associated polymorphisms in a 5′ regulatory region of *NRG1* are associated with differential *NRG1* isoform expression. We suggest that the mechanism behind the clinical association of *NRG1* with schizophrenia is altered transcriptional regulation, which modifies, probably to a small degree and in an isoform-limited fashion, the efficiency of *NRG1* signaling effects on neural development and plasticity. Such alterations may compromise cortical and hippocampal function through one or more of the roles of *NRG1* and reflect,

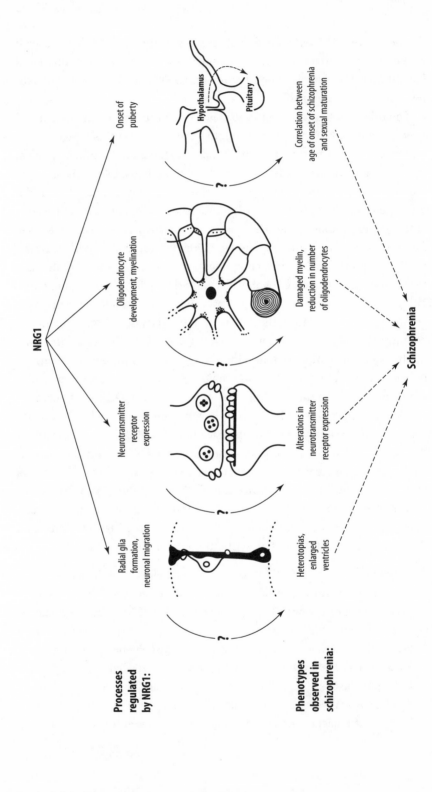

Processes regulated by NRG1:

Radial glia formation, neuronal migration

Neurotransmitter receptor expression

Oligodendrocyte development, myelination

Onset of puberty

NRG1

Hypothalamus

Pituitary

Phenotypes observed in schizophrenia:

Heterotopias, enlarged ventricles

Alterations in neurotransmitter receptor expression

Damaged myelin, reduction in number of oligodendrocytes

Correlation between age of onset of schizophrenia and sexual maturation

Schizophrenia

at least partly, the contribution of *NRG1* to the genetic risk architecture for the disease. (2006, p. 6751)

This explanation initially appears to be formulated at the Kendler level-4 of the typology developed earlier in section 2, but note that this proposal is actually a *partial molecular pathway* that bundles the effects of the allelic changes into an aggregated downstream set of effects on the dorsal lateral prefrontal cortex as well as the hippocampus, appropriately enough because both of these brain regions are implicated in schizophrenia. Thus, this chapter fills in only part of the picture of what is wanted for a complete Kendler level-4 account: in its present form it contains significant gaps as well as higher-level (organ) terminology.

In a slightly earlier article of Law's, then writing with Harrison as first author (Harrison and Law 2006), the following more critical set of comments were made that suggest that the inference to NRG1 as a susceptibility gene remains fairly weak:

> There is now substantial but not incontrovertible evidence that genetic variation in NRG1 is associated with schizophrenia. Proving this beyond all reasonable doubt will be intrinsically difficult, for two main reasons—which apply not only to NRG1 but to other putative susceptibility genes for psychiatric disorders. The first reason relates to the genetic architecture. Schizophrenia is a complex genetic disorder with multiple risk genes of small effect (e.g., for NRG1, estimated odds ratios are mostly below 1.5), none of which are necessary or sufficient, and which might influence different components of the phenotype. Moreover, even within a single gene like NRG1, allelic het-

---

Figure 2.3. (opposite) NRG1-erbB signaling—one of NRG1's likely main mechanisms—suggests at least four routes of influence, as depicted in this figure from Corfas et al. (2004), who write concerning the potential relationships between NRG1 function and schizophrenia that "NRG1 has been implicated in cortical development by regulating glia morphology and neuronal migration, in synapse formation and function by regulating oligodendrocyte proliferation and differentiation, and in the control of onset of puberty through the induction of LHRH release in the hypothalamus. All these developmental processes have been proposed to be altered or involved in schizophrenia. Thus defects in NRG1 function can potentially contribute to the disease by altering one or more of these processes. The arrows with question marks indicate the current hypothetical nature of these possible links between NRG1 function and schizophrenia." *Source:* Corfas et al. (2004).

erogeneity might well exist. In addition, the influence of NRG1 genetic variation must ultimately be considered in the context of epistasis with other susceptibility genes and potential interactions with epigenetic and environmental factors. The second reason concerns the nature of the associated genetic variants and the implications for the mechanism of their effect. If, as the present data indicate, the variants are non-coding, it is not a trivial matter to identify the specific risk-conferring alleles and haplotypes and then to demonstrate their molecular and cellular consequences and show that the latter really are the biological explanation for the association. (2006, p. 7)

Thus, showing clearly that NRG1 is a schizophrenia susceptibility gene and what its specific effects are will indeed turn out to be a daunting task.

5. A Successful "Reductive" Account: Worm Feeding

What might an etiological theory that met the requirements, such as the identification of gene interactions, that Harrison and Law just sketched look like? Because psychiatry is not currently sufficiently advanced to provide any such theory, we might consider work on the behavior of simple organisms, especially the worm, to which I now turn.[2]

The Anatomy, Genetics, and Neurology of Caenorhabditis elegans

The model organism *C. elegans,* which has attracted more than 1,000 full-time researchers worldwide, received additional recognition in 2002 when the Nobel Prize in biology and medicine went to the worm (that is, to Brenner, Horvitz, and Sulston for cell death work in *C. elegans).* The animal (researchers *do* use that term) has been called "the reductionist's delight" (Cook-Deegan, 1994), but a review of the *C. elegans* literature indicates its behavior is much more complex than originally thought: most behavior types relate to genes influencing them in a *many-many relation* (for details, see Schaffner 1998a). Nevertheless, a recent article in *Nature Neuroscience* commented on the use of the worm in the following terms: "With a circuitry of 302 invariant neurons, a quick generation time, and a plethora of genetic tools, *Caenorhabditis elegans* is an ideal model system for studying the interplay among genes, neurons, circuits, and behavior" (Potter and Luo 2003, p. 1178). Some features of the worm's anatomy are presented in Figure 2.4.

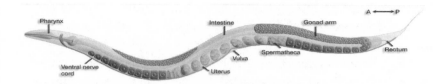

Figure 2.4. The nematode *C. elegans* has a simple cylindrical body plan that is typical of many nematode species. The hermaphrodite animal retains the same basic shape as it undergoes four molts to progress from L1 larva to adult, growing in size dramatically. At the anterior end of this simple elongated tubelike body, the two-bulbed pharynx opens with six lips while the tail ends in a tapering whiplike structure and accommodates an anal opening. Midbody is marked by a vulval opening that is used to lay fertilized eggs generated by a two-armed gonad. Along the length of the body, the animal has a uniform diameter and typically adopts a posture with only one or two shallow body bends along the dorsoventral aspect. *Source:* http://wormatlas.psc.edu/handbook/bodyshape.htm.

This 1-millimeter-long adult hermaphrodite has 959 somatic nuclei and the male (not pictured) 1,031 nuclei; there are about 2,000 germ cell nuclei (Hodgkin et al. 1995). The haploid genome contains 1×10^8 nucleotide pairs, organized into five autosomal and one sex chromosome (hermaphrodites are XX, males XO), comprising about 19,000 genes. The genes have all been sequenced. The organism can move itself forward and backward by graceful undulatory movements and responds to touch and a number of chemical stimuli, of both attractive and repulsive or aversive forms, with simple reflexes. More complex behaviors include egg laying and mating between hermaphrodites and males (Wood 1988, p. 14)—and the worm also learns—as studied by Cathy Rankin and others (Rankin 2002).

The nervous system is the worm's largest organ, consisting of, in the hermaphrodite, 302 neurons, subdividable into 118 subclasses, along with 56 glial and associated support cells; there are 95 muscle cells on which the neurons can synapse. The neurons have been fully described in terms of their location and synaptic connections. These neurons are essentially identical from one individual in a strain to another (Sulston et al. 1983; White et al. 1986), and form approximately 5,000 synapses, 700 gap junctions, and 2,000 neuromuscular junctions (White et al. 1986). The synapses are typically "highly reproducible" (approximately 85% the same) from one animal to another, but are not identical, because of "developmental noise." (For further details about this concept, see Schaffner 1998a.)[3]

An Interesting "Exception" to the Many-many Genes Behavior Relation?

A review of *C. elegans* behaviors by the author (Schaffner 1998a) suggested eight "rules" that characterized the relationship between genes and behaviors in the worm, and Table 2.2 summarizes those rules. The bottom line from the study is that the relations between genes and behaviors are not one-one but many-many. In an article in the prestigious scientific journal *Cell*, however, Mario de Bono and Cori Bargmann investigated the feeding behavior of two different strains of the worm, one of which engaged in solitary feeding, and the other in social feeding (aggregated in a crowd) (de Bono and Bargmann 1998) and appeared to discover a remarkable one-to-one relationship between a genetic mutation and two forms of feeding behavior. Figure 2.5 shows the contrasting behaviors of the two types of strain.

De Bono and Bargmann (1998, p. 679) summarized their 1998 results in an abstract in *Cell*, which I closely paraphrase here, interpolating just enough in the way of additional information that nonspecialists can follow the nearly original abstract text:

Natural subpopulations of *C. elegans* exhibit solitary or social feeding behavior. Solitary eaters move slowly across a surface rich in the bacteria (a bacterial "lawn") on which they feed and also disperse on that surface. Social eaters on the other hand move rapidly on the bacteria and bunch up to-

TABLE 2.2
Some Rules Relating Genes (through Neurons) to Behavior in C. elegans

1. Many genes → one neuron
2. Many neurons (acting as a circuit) → one type of behavior (also there may be overlapping circuits)
3. One gene → many neurons (pleiotropy)
4. One neuron → many behaviors (multifunctional neurons)
5. Stochastic [embryogenetic] development → different neural connections[a]
6. Different environments/histories → different behaviors[a] (learning/plasticity) (short-term environmental influence)
7. One gene → another gene → behavior (gene interactions, including epistasis and combinatorial effects)
8. Environment → gene expression → behavior (long-term environmental influence)

Note: The arrow (→) can be read as "affect(s), cause(s), or lead(s) to."
[a]In prima facie genetically identical (mature) organisms.

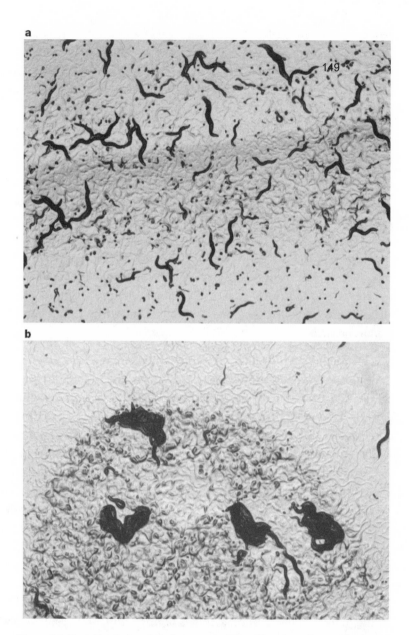

Figure 2.5. Social variants of *C. elegans.* a: solitary N2 worms; b: social AB1 strain worms, both feeding on an *E. coli* lawn. N2 worms are evenly distributed, while AB worms cluster feed in groups. *Source:* Rankin (2002), based on de Bono's work.

gether, often near the edge of a bacterial lawn. A knock-out ("loss of function") mutation in a gene known as *npr-1* causes a solitary strain to take on social behavior. This gene is known to encode a type of protein, here it is NPR-1, known as a G-protein coupled receptor, a protein that acts like a switch to open or close ion channels in nerve cells. This NPR-1 protein is similar to a family of proteins called Y receptors that are widely present in the nervous system of other organisms and relate to feeding and foraging behavior in other species. Two variants of the NPR-1 protein that differ only in a single amino acid (phenylalanine versus valine) occur naturally in the wild. One variant, termed NPR-1 215F (with phenylalanine, abbreviated as F) is found exclusively in social strains, while the other variant, NPR-1 215V (with valine) is found only in solitary strains. The difference between the F and V variants are due to a single nucleotide difference in the gene's DNA sequence (T versus G). Inserting a gene that produces the V form of the protein can transform wild social strains into solitary ones. Thus these only slightly different proteins generate the two natural variants in *C. elegans'* feeding behavior.

This remarkable report by de Bono and Bargmann made strong claims involving a genetic explanation of behavior. At the end of the introduction to this 1998 article, the authors wrote that "we show that variation in responses to food and other animals in wild strains of *C. elegans is due to* natural variation in *npr-1*" (1998, p. 679; emphasis added). The phenotype difference is actually somewhat more complex and not just related to social or solitary feeding in the presence of sufficient amount of bacterial food supply. As already indicated, the social and solitary strains also differ in their speed of locomotion. Also, the two types differ in burrowing behavior in the agar jell surface on which the worms are studied in the laboratory, but de Bono and Bargmann contended that "a single gene mutation can give rise to all of the behavioral differences characteristic of wild and solitary strains" (1998, p. 680).

De Bono and Bargmann offered several "different models that could explain the diverse behavioral phenotypes of *npr-1* mutants" (1998, p. 686) but added that "resolution of these models awaits identification of the cells in which *npr-1* acts, and the cells that are the source of the *npr-1* [*sic*] ligands [those molecules that bind to and regulate this receptor]" (1998, p. 686).

Complications and an Example of a PCMS

This wonderfully "simple" story of one gene that influences one type of behavior in the worm was told in 1998 as just described. Since then, further work by de Bono and Bargmann, who did search for the cells in which *npr-1* acts and for the source of the NPR-1 ligands, has indicated that the story is more complex, and that complexity grew even further more recently. In follow-up work in 2002 to determine how such feeding behavior is regulated, de Bono and Bargmann proposed what were, at least initially, two separate pathways (de Bono et al. 2002; Coates and de Bono 2002). One pathway suggests that there are modifying genes that restore social feeding to solitary feeders under conditions of external environmental stress. The other pathway is internal to the organism and will be briefly described at the conclusion of this section, as will a 2005 article that may synthesize the two pathways. (An accessible overview of the two initial pathways, and some possible interesting connections with fly and honeybee foraging and feeding behaviors, can be found in Sokolowski's 2002 editorial accompanying the publication of the de Bono et al.'s two 2002 papers.)

The first 2002 paper by de Bono and Bargmann, also writing with David M. Tobin, M. Wayne Davis, and Leon Avery, indicates how a partially reductive explanation works and also nicely illustrates the features of how general field and specific causal models systems work in tandem. The *explanandum* (Latin for the event to be explained) is to account for the difference in social versus solitary feeding patterns, as depicted in Figure 2.5. The explanation (at an abstract level) is contained in the title of the 2002 article "Social Feeding in *C. elegans* Is Induced by Neurons That Detect Aversive Stimuli." The specifics of the explanation appeal to the 1998 study as background and look at *npr-1* mutants, examining what *other* genes might prevent social feeding, thus restoring solitary feeding in *npr-1* mutants. A search among various *npr-1 mutants*—these would be social feeders—indicated that mutations in the *osm-9* and *ocr-2* genes resulted in significantly more *solitary* feeding in those mutant animals. (Both of these genes code for *components* of a sensory transduction ion channel known as TRPV—*transient receptor potential* channel that in vertebrates responds to the "vanilloid" (V) compound capsaicin found in hot peppers. Both the *osm-9* and *ocr-2* genes are required for chemoattraction as well as aversive stimuli avoidance. In addition, it was found that *odr-4* and *odr-8* gene mutations could disrupt social feeding in *npr-1* mutants. The *odr-4* and *odr-8* genes are required to localize a group of olfactory receptors to olfactory cilia. Of note, a mutation in the *osm-3* gene, which is required for the development of 26 ciliated sensory neurons, *restores social* feeding in the *odr-4* and *ocr-2* mutants. (Readers who have followed the account of the genetic influences on ion channels, other genes, and neurons thus far *are now entitled to a break!*)

De Bono et al. present extensive data supporting these findings in the article. Typically the reasoning with the data examines the effects of screening for single, double, and even triple mutations that affect the phenotype of interest (feeding behaviors), as well as looking at the results of gene insertion or gene deletion. This reasoning essentially follows Mill's methods of difference and concomitant variation (the latter because graded rather than all-or-none results are often obtained) and is prototypical causal reasoning. Also of interest are the results of the laser ablation of two neurons that were suggested to be involved in the feeding behaviors. These two neurons, known as ASH and ADL, are implicated in the avoidance of noxious stimuli and toxic chemicals. Identification of the genes noted above (*osm-9, ocr-2, odr-4,* and *odr-8*) allowed the investigators to look at where those genes were expressed (by using Green Florescent Protein [GFP] tags). It turned out that ASH and ADL neurons were the expression sites. The investigators could then test the effects of laser beam ablation of those neurons and showed that ablation of both of them restored a solitary feeding phenotype but that the presence of either neuron would support social feeding.

The net result of the analysis is summarized in a "model for social feeding in *C. elegans*" (Figure 2.6). The legend for the model quoted from de Bono et al. (2002) reads:

> A model for social feeding in *C. elegans*. The ASH and ADL nociceptive neurons are proposed to respond to aversive stimuli from food to promote social feeding. This function requires the putative OCR-2/OSM-9 ion channel. The ODR-4 protein may act in ADL to localize seven transmembrane domain chemoreceptors that respond to noxious stimuli. In the absence of ASH and ADL activity, an unidentified neuron (XXX) [involving *osm-3*] represses social feeding, perhaps in response to a different set of food stimuli. The photograph shows social feeding of a group of > 30 npr-1 mutant animals on a lawn of *E. coli*.

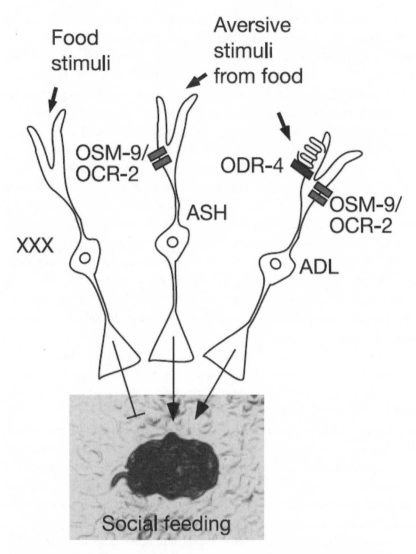

Figure 2.6. The preferred model accounting for the differences between solitary and social feeding in *C. elegans* as understood in 2002. See text for details. *Source:* de Bono et al. (2002).

This model is what I like to call a preferred causal model system (PCMS) for this *Nature* article. The model is what does the partial reduction. The model is simplified and idealized and uses causal language such as "respond to" and "represses." (The causal verbs also contain the word "act," about which much has been made in recent years in the philosophy of biology and neuroscience literature about "activities," as opposed to causation, which may be present in "mechanisms.") The *PCMS* is clearly interlevel. I think it is best to approach such models keeping in mind the scientific field(s) on which they are based and the specific "field elements" that an article proposing the model needs to refer to in order to make the model intelligible to readers. Here the fields on which the model draws are molecular genetics and neuroscience. Scattered throughout the article are occasional alternative but possible causal pathways (field elements) that are evaluated as not as good an explanation as those provided in the preferred model system presented. (One example is the *dauer* pheromone explanation, discussed on page 899 of de Bono et al. 2002; another is the "reducing stimuli production" versus "reducing stimuli detection" hypotheses on page 900 of that article.)

The preparation or *experimental system* investigated in the laboratory (this may include several data runs of the "same" experimental system) is identified in its relevant aspects with the preferred causal model system. At the abstract or "philosophical" level, the explanation proceeds by identifying the laboratory experimental system with the theoretical system— the preferred model system (PCMS)—and exhibiting the event or process to be explained (called the *explanandum*) as the causal consequence of the system's behavior. The *explanans* (or set of explaining elements) here uses molecular biology and is mainly comparative rather than involving quantitative derivational reasoning, in the sense that in this article two qualitatively different end states—the solitary and the social states of the worms—are compared and contrasted.[4] The theoretical system (the PCMS) uses generalizations of varying scope, often having to appeal to similarity analyses among like systems (for example, the use of TRPV channel *family*) to achieve the scope, as well as make the investigation of interest and relevance to other biologists (for example, via analogies of the NPR-1 receptor to Y receptors and the internal worm circuit to cyclic GMP signaling pathways found in flies and bees that control foraging and feeding behavior [see Sokolowski 2002]). For those concerned with philosophical rigor, the preferred model system and its relations to model-theoretic explanation can be made more philosophically precise (and technical), along the lines suggested in a "philosopher-speak" note.[5]

The discussion sections of scientific articles are the usual place where larger issues are raised and extrapolations are frequently found. This is also the case in this de Bono et al. (2002) article, in which the discussion section states that "food, food acquisition, and population density are important regulators of aggregation in a variety of species" (p. 902). The report concludes on an evolutionary note, tying the proximate cause model to a distal causal (that is, evolutionary) advantage, where the authors write, "The data in this paper and in the accompanying paper suggest that the regulation of social feeding behaviour in *C. elegans* is complex, involving several layers of positive and negative inputs. Such complexity may have evolved as a result of the tension between cooperation and competition that underlies social behaviour, and may be important to ensure that social behaviour is induced only when it offers a selective advantage."

Further work on the circuits that affect social and solitary feeding has been done in addition to what has just been described in detail above. Earlier I mentioned an article that appeared simultaneously with the above report in *Nature.* This second article by Coates and de Bono (2002) described a regulatory circuit that sensed the internal fluid in the worm and controlled social versus solitary forms of behavior. It involved different neurons (AQR, PQR, and URX), and was affected by *tax 2* and *tax 4* gene mutations—genes that produce components of a cyclic GMP-gated ion channel.[6]

Also, in late 2003, de Bono's group was able to identify the ligands that stimulate the NPR-1 receptor (Rogers et al. 2003). These are a class of neuropeptides known as "FMRFamide and related peptides" (FaRPs) that stimulate foraging receptors in other species. In the worm, the relevant FaRPs are encoded by 22 different *flp* genes that can potentially produce 59 FaRP peptides by alternative splicings. It was also reported in this article that comparative sequencing of the two NPR-1 variants (the F and V forms), as well as three other species of *Caenorhabditis,* suggests that the *social* form of the receptor is ancestral and that the behavior of solitary feeding arose later via a "gain-of-function" mutation. This is a preliminary conclusion, and some insect researchers find it implausible, believing that social behaviors are likely to appear later than solitary activities (de Bono, personal communication). But that may depend on the different selection pressures experienced in different environments by different species.

More recently, additional complexity affecting social versus solitary feed-

ing was discovered, which further developed the role of oxygen as a significant environmental factor identified in note 5. The internal circuit described
by de Bono in 2002 involving AQR, PQR, and URX neurons, which were
affected by *tax 2* and *tax 4* gene mutations, now seems to be a parallel pathway regulating feeding behavior. I will not detail these complications here
but will present a summary figure (from de Bono and Maricq 2005) that com-
bines several pathways of influence on aggregation behavior (Figure 2.7).

This explanation is both reductive and nonreductive. The above example (both the simpler circuit and the 2005 augmented circuit) is typical
of molecular biological explanations of behavior. Behavior is an organismic property and in the example is actually a populational property (of
aggregation), and the explanation appeals to entities that are *parts* of the
organism, including molecularly characterized genes and molecular interactions such as ligand-receptor bindings and G-protein-coupled receptor
mechanisms. Thus, this is generally characterized as a *reductive* explanation, but it represents *partial* reduction—what I termed reduction of the
creeping sort—and differs from *sweeping* or comprehensive reductive explanations in several important features:

1. The first model does not explain *all* cases of social versus solitary
   feeding; a different though somewhat related model (that of Coates
   and de Bono [2002]) is needed for the internal triggering of solitary
   behavior in *npr-1* mutants; the 2005 model does more, but is still incomplete (see below).
2. Some of the key entities, such as the signal from bacteria that is noxious to the worms and the neuron represented by XXX in Figure 2.6,
   have not yet been identified.
3. It uses what might be termed "middle-level" entities, such as neuronal cells, in addition to molecular entities.
4. It is not a quantitative model that derives behavioral descriptions
   from rigorous general equations of state, but is causally qualitative
   and only roughly comparative.
5. Interventions to set up, manipulate, and test the model are at higher
   aggregative levels than the molecular, such as selection of the worms
   by their organismic properties (feeding behaviors), distributing the
   worms on an agar plate, and ablating the neurons with a laser.

The explanation does meet the three conditions that seem reasonable for
a reductive explanation, namely:

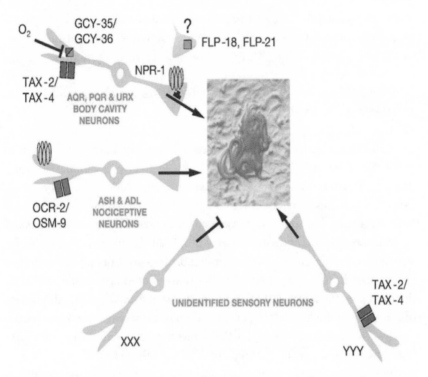

Figure 2.7. A more recent and more complex view of the neurons and signaling pathways that regulate aggregation behavior in *C. elegans* feeding.
Source: de Bono and Maricq (2005).

1. The explainers (here the preferred model systems as shown in figures 2.6 and 2.7) are a partially decomposable microstructure in the organism/process of interest.
2. The explanandum (the social or solitary feeding behavior) is a grosser (macro), typically aggregate property or end state.
3. Connectability assumptions (CAs), sometimes called bridge laws or reduction functions, are involved, which permit the relation of macrodescriptions to microdescriptions. Sometimes these CAs are causal sequences as depicted in the model figure where the output of the neurons under one set of conditions causes clumping, but in critical cases the CAs are identities (such as social feeding = clumping, and aversive stimulus = [probably] bacterial odor).

Though etiological and reductive, the preferred model system explanation is not "ruthlessly reductive," to use Bickle's phrase, even though a

classical organismic biologist would most likely term it strongly reductionistic in contrast to their favored nonreductive or even antireductionist cellular or organismic points of view. It is a *partial* reduction.

6. Model Organisms and Implications for Etiological Theories in Psychiatry

Model organisms have become vitally important tools with which to
probe the relations between genes, cells, cell circuits, and behaviors
(Schaffner 1998b; Kendler and Greenspan 2006). Their simplicity (recall
that the worm has only 302 neurons) permits interventional and manipulation strategies that can disclose causal pathways that are heavily masked
by complexity in more evolutionarily proximal organisms. Conditions for
strong causal inference—and generalizability—are thus available in the
results that have been achieved using these model organisms. As such,
they can provide a comparison case against which some of the difficulties
of achieving reductive etiological accounts in psychiatry can be sketched.

The conclusions in Table 2.1 that I reached in Schaffner (1998a) relying mainly on the worm, though partially on fly results then available,
have been deepened, grounded on additional studies in other simple organisms, and extended in an article by Kendler and Greenspan (2006).
Some of their conclusions resonate with themes developed in the present
chapter. There they wrote,

> Across the animal kingdom, individual differences in behavior are nearly al-
> ways influenced to some extent by genetic factors which in turn result from
> a substantial number of individual genes each with a small effect. Nearly all
> genes which effect behavior influence multiple phenotypes. The impact of
> individual genes can be substantially modified by other genes in the genome
> and/or by environmental experiences. Many animals alter their environ-
> ment and the nature of that alteration is influenced by genes. For some be-
> haviors, the pathway from genes to behavior differs meaningfully in males
> and females. With respect to the broad patterns of genetic influences on be-
> havior, *Homo sapiens* appears to be typical of other animal species.

The bottom line of many-many relations including environmental influence confirmed in this analysis indicates that it will be exceedingly difficult to develop any kind of simple etiological theory of brain behaviors
that can be helpful in psychiatry. However, some approaches might be

useful to consider as psychiatry attempts to harness the enormous power of molecular genetics as well as newer forms of imaging that can provide more detailed pictures of structural information and brain action.

7. Singular Etiologies and *inus* Etiologies: Searching for Etiological "Simplifications" Using Heuristics

We have seen in the account given above of *C. elegans*' behaviors that there will be only rare instances in which a single gene type is closely tied to a single type of behavior. The *npr-1* gene was introduced as representative of that kind of example and can serve as the exemplar of what kinds of "gene for" explanations molecular behavioral genetics can warrant (also compare Kendler 2005). Recall that, even though this example was taken to the molecular level regarding the type of protein and its receptor function, *no complete and fully molecularly detailed circuit for aggregation and feeding behavior* is yet available. In fact, the *npr-1* gene has now been contextualized within a set of more complicated parallel circuits in which no one gene would become a *more* sufficient type of explanation of a behavior, or first element in an etiological causal sequence. This example suggests that the kinds of explanations molecular behavioral genetics will provide for behavior in the foreseeable future are *causal-sketch explanations*. By this term, I mean that the criteria for a necessary condition explanation have been met, in the sense that appropriate controls have been identified and gene localization and expression confirmed, but no complete causal chain with identified intermediates has yet been delineated. Thus, the pathway from gene to behavior is "gappy." Furthermore, the criteria for a claim that warrants terming a single gene "a necessary condition" require the identification of a simplified isolated and localized pattern of causal influence within an otherwise complex system. In truth, the original 1998 model has become much more reticulate, and a causal factor in such a network is better characterized as an *inus* condition, to use John Mackie's terminology.

This notion of an *inus* condition was developed by Mackie on the basis of his reflections on John Stuart Mill's discussion of the plurality of causes problem (Mackie 1974). Mill recognized the complication of a plurality of causes by which several different assemblages of factors—say, ABC, as well as DGH and JKL—might each be sufficient to bring about an effect P. If (ABC *or* DGH *or* JKL) is both necessary and sufficient for P, how do we describe, for example, the A in such a generalization? Such an element, A (or any of the B . . . L factors, taken individually) is for Mackie an *in*suffi-cient but *non*redundant [alternatively *ne*cessary] part of an *un*necessary but *s*ufficient condition—a complex expression for which Mackie uses the acronym an *inus* condition on the basis of the first letters of the par-tially emphasized words. Using this terminology, then, what is usually termed a cause is an *inus* condition. In an article published in the 1970s, Paul Meehl (1977) urged more widespread consideration in the medical sciences of this notion.

Identifying a causal genetic etiology, or a key environmental factor, whether this be singular or more likely an *inus* factor, is a simplification in a bushy causal network. Such simplifications are possible, though likely rare, and when found are likely to be highly prized: they could be points of prediction and intervention, including drug therapy targets. How such valuable simplifications may be identified is the final question to which I turn in this chapter.

Three Heuristics for Obtaining Simplifications Leading to Etiological, Including Behavioral Genetic, Explanations
Common Pathways

It seems to me that, even within a complex system of the genetically influenced neural networks described for *C. elegans* and *Drosophila,* there are three ways in which causal simplification may occur that could result in something close to a single gene or only a few genes ("oligogenic") ex-planation of a type of behavior. (Although I focus on genetic etiology here, the heuristics—or guiding principles—should be generalizable to envi-ronmental factors as well.) One simplification, which can also perhaps provide points of potential intervention, occurs when a "common path-way" emerges. This is usually referred to as a *"final* common pathway" in medical and physiological etiology, in which many different parallel-acting weak causal factors (often termed "risk factors") can coalesce in a funneling toward a common set of outcomes. An example from infectious medicine is the pathogenetic mechanism by which the tuberculosis bac-terium acts in a susceptible host after parallel risk factors predispose the host to infection (Fletcher, Fletcher, and Wagner 1982, p. 190); however, investigators probably need to be attentive to the possibility of common pathways emerging at *any* stage (early, intermediate, or final) in the temporal evolution of a reticulate network involving multiple causes and complex "crosstalk."[7] Determining the effects of factors in complex networks is methodologically difficult and typically requires complicated research designs with special attention to controls.[8] The existence of a common pathway, perhaps a specific neural circuit with a specific set of metabolites, might permit intervention by manipulation of the metabolites in such a common pathway.[9]

This notion of a coalescing common pathway was further elaborated and reconceptualized by Mirnics, Levitt, and Lewis (2006) as part of an analysis of microarray/transcriptome results in psychiatry. In their article, Mirnics and colleagues introduce the notion of a *convergent molecular hub model* of gene effects in psychiatry. They write,

> Many of the putative disease susceptibility genes also are major transcript network convergence points, or "molecular hubs." For example, RGS4 expression levels may depend on the expression and function of a wide range of upstream proteins, including various G-protein coupled receptors, heterotrimeric G-protein subunits and RAS-RAB system components. Alteration in the DNA sequence in any of these upstream genes that has functional consequences may result in downstream RGS4 expression changes, and reduced RGS4 levels could compensate for reduced presynaptic drive (Mirnics et al. 2001). By a similar mechanism, the expression of other hub genes could be affected by multiple, pathway-dependent genetic insults. (2006, p. 29)

They add,

> The convergent hub hypothesis can influence our thinking about genetic susceptibility and the pathophysiology of psychiatric disorders. First, this model raises the possibility that some neuronspecific molecular hubs also are susceptibility genes for specific diseases. Combining data from genome-wide scans for chromosomal location with functional relevance, hub-status and gene expression data from postmortem studies could more readily prioritize candidate genes that deserve targeted testing in association studies. Second, the disease-affected molecular hubs, and their cellular contexts, may serve as correlates of the behavioral features that are associated with a disease. While altered expression of molecular hubs could explain the similarities in the behavioral features shared across individuals with schizophrenia, the patient-specific clinical symptoms would depend on alterations

in a set of non-hub genes that could be specific to affected individuals [though environmental and individual psychology will very likely also be important here—KFS]. Third, as large-scale transcriptome profiling data accumulate, we will be in a better position to attempt a hub-based molecular classification of brain disorders. These data may prove much more reproducible than comparing single gene expression changes across datasets. (2006, pp. 29–30)

Figure 2.8 summarizes the convergent hub approach of Mirnics et al. (2006).

Dominating Pathways

Another type of simplification that may be differentiated from the common pathway or molecular hub model of simplification and that can emerge in a complex network of interactions is the appearance at any given stage of a *dominating* factor. Such a dominating factor exerts major effects downstream from it, even though the effects still may be weakly conditioned by other interacting factors. I suspect that different neurotransmitters at different points in a complex causal chain may be dominating factors. This type of simplification is distinguished from the coalescing pathway simplification in that multiple pathways may continue to persist, but one of these several parallel pathways grows significantly in influence in comparison to the other parallel lines of influence.

Manipulation of such a dominating factor may thus have major effects on the future course of the complex system, though such effects can be specific and affect only a small number of event types. Such factors are major leverage points that can permit interventions, as well as simpler explanations, which focus on such factors. The distinction between common pathways and dominant pathways is not always sharp: in a parallel system, the limiting case of a single dominant pathway will be a common pathway.

Whether such dominating factors exist, as well as whether any common pathways exist, is an empirical question to be solved by laboratory investigation of specific systems. This is, in fact, where the power of model organisms is likely to become most evident. Carrying out an investigation in an organism several orders more complex than *C. elegans* becomes considerably more difficult. One might hazard a guess that the difficulty may increase exponentially with the numbers of genes and neurons. The prospects of recognizing highly specific single-gene and single-neuron effects

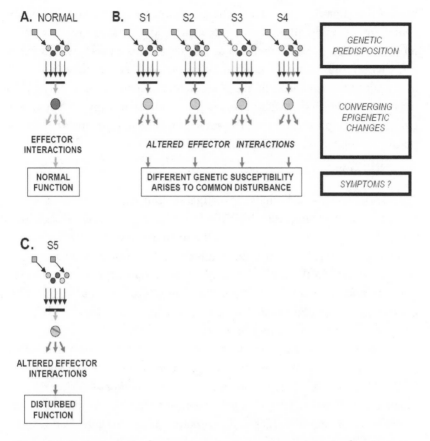

Figure 2.8. Distinct genetic changes may arise to common, epigenetic alterations that may be related to the common symptoms of the disease. A: In a normal tissue, five genes directly (five clustered small symbols) and two upstream genes indirectly (small squares and circles) regulate the expression of a common cellular hub (big circle). B: Four subjects with schizophrenia (S1–4) have altered DNA sequence in distinct genes (asterisk), but their effect converges on a cellular hub gene. This convergence gives rise to similar downstream effects and may ultimately give rise to the common symptoms of the disease. C: In contrast, subject S5 has a specific DNA sequence in the hub gene itself, which directly alters its expression, giving rise to similar downstream effects as seen in subjects S1–4. *RGS4* and *GAD67* are good candidates for such molecular hubs, where the expression changes may arise by both genetic and epigenetic mechanisms. *Source:* Adapted from Mirnics et al. (2006).

in complex organisms is likely to be accomplished only if highly homologous and strongly conserved genes can be identified in much simpler model organisms. Such identifications can give us powerfully directive hints where to look for such genes in more complex organisms and may help begin to characterize dominating factors or common pathways.[10] As in connection with the behaviors of even simple organisms such as *C. elegans* and *Drosophila,* however, the answer thus far appears to be that dominating factors and common pathways will be rare.[11]

Emergent Simplifications

In certain areas of biology, investigators can capture what might be termed "emergent simplifications" that transcend the specific workings of the molecular details. This is akin to the ideal gas law, $PV = nRT$, which is an emergent simplification of the underlying stochastic molecular collisions described in the lower level theory of statistical mechanics. Molecules do not per se have a "temperature"—only average translational kinetic energy. A gas, however, has a temperature that is ascertainable in the usual ways with various thermometers.

In a sense, a more abstract mechanism, usually formulated at a higher level of aggregation, can even be a "basic mechanism," even if it is clearly realized that there are as yet unknown molecular details of the mechanism. Possibly such a basic mechanism is more like a "prototypical" mechanism, which identifies and characterizes salient core features of a biological entity and its actions.

In some circumstances, the core features of those simplifications can be generated by quantitative investigations and represented by mathematical equations as in those equations that were used to develop the Hodgkin-Huxley (H&H) model of action potential propagation. But such equations do lack that broad universality and instead serve their functions by being prototypes for analogical modeling to similar prototypes, albeit in this case, analogical modeling to other quantitative prototypes. In addition, they are not usually unilevel but instead mix levels of aggregation, as in the PCMS systems described for worm aggregation. In the H&H work, the discussion is focused on current flows and potential difference changes due to ions and inferred ion channels but as situated in an axon of a particular species. Elsewhere I have proposed that further reflection of the H&H systems–level methodology may provide important generalizable heuristics that can inform biology pursued at the level of general systems (Schaffner 2006).

These levels of emergent simplification are not, I think, equivalent to the interesting tripartite set of levels that David Marr suggested in *Vision* (1982) may be helpful in the computational neurosciences. Although the lowest level (3) of molecular processing or physical realization may be the same in Marr's analysis and the one that I favor, Marr's next two higher levels of (2) computational, algorithmic representation and (1) computational theory—the goal and logic of a computation—seem more appropriate to computer science theorizing. In biology, and medicine, and a fortiori, psychiatry, we must take our levels as we find them—as heuristic aggregations where generalizations are findable and causal processing traceable. This heuristic approach to levels, complementing the heuristic search for causal simplifications, is more akin to William Wimsatt's (1976) characterization of levels than to Marr's account.

In terms of our psychiatric examples, Kendler and colleagues' model for MDD summarized in section 3 may be an emergent simplification and one that might provide downward pointers toward molecular interactions and more specific etiologies that could be searched for at Kendler levels 3 and 4. Some of Caspi and Moffitt's work on GXE in depression (Caspi et al. 2003) might be seen in this light.

Bechtel and Richardson on Decomposition and Localization

In addition to the three heuristics just described, it is worth considering two heuristics that have been discussed as aids to isolating and localizing causal pathways in complex systems. These might include what I have termed above common and dominating pathways, and they can be found in Bechtel and Richardson's *Discovering Complexity* (1993). In their monograph, Bechtel and Richardson state that one of their aims is to understand how to arrive at mechanistic explanations in the context of "complex systems in biology" (1993, p. 17). Their main strategy is to examine how far what they refer to as two heuristics can take them in formulating "mechanistic" explanations. These two heuristics are what they call "decomposition" and "localization." Roughly, decomposition means that an investigator can divide up the system of interest into separate subprocesses. In their words, decomposition "assumes that one activity of a system is the product of a set of subordinate functions performed in the system . . . , that there is a small number of such functions, . . . and that they are minimally interactive" (1993, p. 23). Localization means that the investigator can point to the component parts (in the cell or in the brain, for example) where these subprocesses occur. That is, localization "is the identification of the different activities proposed in the task decomposition with the behavior or capacities of specific components" (1993, p. 24). These guiding principles of decomposition and localization work well in some contexts, and Bechtel and Richardson provide examples of Wieland's localization of cell respiration in dehydrogenase enzymes and Warburg's competing localization of respiration in membrane iron (1993, pp. 72–92). But as Bechtel and Richardson proceed through a number of rich examples of increasing complexity, they eventually come to systems where decomposition and localization "fail" (pp. 172, 199–201, 228). Of special interest to us is Bechtel and Richardson's claim that decomposition and localization fail when they are applied to "'emergent' phenomena in interconnected networks," represented, for example, by connectionistic neural nets (and also by genetic regulatory networks of the type investigated by Kauffman [1993]).

Neural Networks

A claim of the failure of the decomposition heuristic would *seem* to represent a counsel of despair; Bechtel and Richardson are more nuanced on this issue. They argue that, although decomposability (and near decomposability) would be "hopeless, or even misguided" as applied to interconnected networks (p. 202), nonetheless "there is a clear sense in which . . . [network models] are mechanistic . . . [:] the behavior of the system is a product of the activities occurring within it" (p. 228). Such networks validate the concept of "emergent" properties, but "without waxing mysterious" (p. 229). They add, underscoring the innocuous character of *this* notion of emergence, that "in calling the systemic properties of network systems emergent, we mark a departure from the behavior of simpler systems and indicate that traditional mechanistic strategies for understanding neural network systems may simply fail. But the behavior of the systems is not unintelligible or magical: it follows from the nature of the connections between the components within the system" (p. 229).

Using a neural network approach, then, according to Bechtel and Richardson, is not obviously a *simplification* strategy, which is how I tend to view their heuristics of decomposition and localization. And perhaps it needs to be emphasized that the networks discussed by Bechtel and Richardson are actually far simpler than the neural networks found in *C. elegans*—not in terms of numbers of network connections, but in terms of the inner complexities of the neurons, the effects of gene products on the neurons, the types of synapses, and the effects of short- and long-term environmental influences. In spite of this complexity of the biological system, for *C. elegans* researchers a kind of near decomposability also seems to hold, in that various neural circuits are isolable (though they overlap) *within C. elegans,* and can be analyzed with standard neuroscience tools. Thus, behavior is explicable in terms of the interacting parts, and these neural networks offer one of the most promising keys to explaining behavior.

There is a sense, however, in which Bechtel and Richardson do acknowledge that even a network approach, as powerful as it may be in explaining complex behaviors, may fail to yield any type of mechanistic explanation and become "mysterious." They write, "We may not be able to follow the processes through the multitude of connections in a more complex system, or to see how they give rise to the behavior of the system. We may fail in the attempt to understand such systems in an intuitive way" (p. 229). At this point Bechtel and Richardson's position appears to merge with Rosenberg's (1985, 1994) then antireductionist view: as a *pragmatic* failure of human intellect. Whether *C. elegans* researchers will encounter this problem—or, if they do not, whether it will be met in *Drosophila,* or in mice, or in humans—is only food for important speculation at present. It is possible, however, as even Rosenberg (1985) seems to admit, that increasingly powerful computers and software will enable scientists to manage and deal with this complexity, should behavioral neuroscience and psychiatry begin to enter this "mysterious" realm. Complexity need not necessarily lead us to what some philosophers of mind characterize as the "new mysterianism" position.[12]

8. Summary and Conclusions

I began this chapter by noting that a quest for etiological models in psychiatry was controversial. Some have thought that premature, or inappropriate (Goodwin and Guze), while other authors have viewed an etiological analysis of mental disorders as the only legitimate scientific approach (Kendell and Murphy). I then considered two contrasting approaches within etiological perspective: reductive and nonreductive forms of analysis, where reductive approaches roughly aimed at a molecular causal description, and nonreductive accounts were formulated at much higher levels of aggregation. A framework from psychiatric genetics from Kendler was used to situate these two types of approaches. One extended example of a nonreductive etiological theory (the Kendler et al. 1993–2006 program examining MDD) was summarized. This was a genetically informed path-analytical model. A contrasting etiological theory of schizophrenia was juxtaposed to the MDD example, this drawing on work by Harrison and Weinberger, but also many others. We considered several putative susceptibility genes for schizophrenia as etiological factors for that disorder, the nature of the evidence for those generic factors was summarized, and the roles of one gene, neuregulin1 (NRG1), were elaborated to indicate the complex nature of just one etiological actor in this model. The schizophrenia model was found to be weak and incomplete, and, for a contrast case, I reviewed some recent studies of genetic factors affecting two forms of worm feeding behavior—social versus solitary. Although these two forms of feeding were initially thought to be governed by one gene, *npr-1,* subsequent research has shown that this is at least an oligogenic system, with several distinct genes playing roles in affecting the nature of the neuronal circuits that result in downstream types of feeding behaviors. An important lesson from that extended example is that even in highly inbred simple model organisms, the etiological theories (more accurately models) are actually mixed, not purely molecular, models. Such models intertwine cellular and organ causal pathways and are only partially molecular.

I closed the chapter speculating on how the confounding complexity that is found in bushy networks in higher organisms might be better studied and understood and sketched three types of heuristics that may clarify results in such partially molecular etiological studies. These included common pathway models (including the Mirnics et al. 2006 molecular hub proposal), dominating factors, and searching for emergent simplifications. Two additional heuristics—decomposition and localization, which have been explored by Bechtel and Richardson—were also discussed. The take-home lesson from the analysis in the present chapter is that etiological accounts in psychiatry are possible, will be difficult to develop and test, will be mixed (interlevel) models, and will likely focus on narrow areas of application in their initial stages.

NOTES

1. This sense of "antietiological" is probably designed to achieve the broadest possible consensus among psychiatrists and other users of the *DSMs* by bracketing possible competing theoretical etiologies. The text preceding this quotation cites

the change from *DSM-I* to *DSM-II* that eliminated the widespread use in *DSM-I* of the term "reaction," based on Adolf Meyer's psychobiological theory (p. xvii). Also see Faust and Miner (1986) for a critique of the antitheoretical approach of *DSM-III*.

2. This section borrows from my recent account of reduction and emergence (Schaffner 2006).

3. De Bono (personal communication) indicates that "there may also be more plasticity in synapse number/size than indicated in the mind of the worm—difficult to say as only 2–3 worms were sectioned in the John White's em [electron micrograph] studies."

4. A quantitative derivation of a path of *C. elegans* motion that agrees with the experimentally observed path can be computed based on neural theory, though the explanation quickly becomes extraordinarily complicated—see my summary of Lockery's results using this type of approach (Schaffner 2000).

5. The following philosophically general account parallels the discussion in my 1993 book. It assumes an analysis of biological explainers as involving models representable as a collection of generalizations of variable scope instantiated in a series of overlapping mechanisms as developed in chapter 3 of the 1993 book. As described in that chapter, we can employ a generalization of Suppes's set-theoretic approach and also follow Giere (1984) in introducing the notion of a "theoretical model" as "a kind of system whose characteristics are specified by an explicit definition" (1984, p. 80). Here entities $\eta_1 \ldots \eta_n$ will designate neurobiological objects such as neuropeptide receptors, the Φ's such *causal* properties as "ligand binding" and "neurotransmitter secretion," and the scientific generalizations $\Sigma_1 \ldots \Sigma_n$ will be of the type "This odorant activates a G-protein cascade opening an ion channel." Then $\Sigma_i(\Phi(\eta_1 \ldots \eta_n))$ will represent the ith generalization, and

$$\prod_{i=1}^{n}[\Sigma_i(\Phi(\eta_1 \ldots \eta_n))]$$

will be the conjunction of the assumptions (which we will call Π) constituting the preferred model system or PMS. Any given system that is being investigated or appealed to as explanatory of some explanandum is such a PMS if and only if it satisfies Π. We understand Π, then, as implicitly defining a kind of natural system, though there may not be any actual system that is a realization of the complex expression Π. To claim that some particular system satisfies Π is a theoretical hypothesis, which may or may not be true. If it is true, the PMS can serve as an explanandum of phenomena such as "social feeding." (If the PMS is potentially true and well confirmed, it is a "potential and well-confirmed explanation" of the phenomena it entails or supports.)

6. Subsequently, de Bono's lab showed that the internal circuit involves soluble guanylate cyclases in that pathway (see Cheung et al. 2004). These appear to be activated by oxygen (see Gray et al. 2004).

7. The term *crosstalk* for complex regulatory interactions is used by Egan and Weinberg in their description of the *ras* signaling network (1993, p. 783).

8. See my 1993, esp. pp. 142–52, for a discussion of this type of problem.

9. It might be that focus *only* on common pathways could lead to an overly simplistic, reactive, and reductionistic approach to health care and to a downgrading of more complex "risk factor" types of influences. For cautionary comments along these lines, see Rose (1995).

10. A good example of the utility of model organisms is the discovery of the DNA repair gene in humans, termed hMSH2, that is strikingly similar to the MutS gene in *Escherichia coli* and to the MSH2 gene in the eukaryotic yeast *Saccharomyces cerevisiae*.

11. Bargmann takes a more optimistic view and believes not only that dominating factors will become evident as research proceeds, but also that "dominant genes will be quite common in behavior once we succeed in breaking behavior down into small precisely defined components" (personal communication, August 1995).

12. From Wikipedia: "New Mysterianism is a philosophy proposing that certain problems will never be explained or at the least cannot be explained by the human mind at its current evolutionary stage. The problem most often referred to is the hard problem of consciousness; i.e. how to explain sentience and qualia and their interaction with consciousness." See Colin McGinn's *The Mysterious Flame: Conscious Minds in a Material World* (2000).

REFERENCES

Bechtel, W., and R. C. Richardson. 1993. *Discovering Complexity: Decomposition and Localization as Strategies in Scientific Research*. Princeton, NJ: Princeton University Press.

Brzustowicz, L. M., K. A. Hodgkinson, E. W. Chow, W. G. Honer, A. S. Bassett. 2000. Location of a Major Susceptibility Locus for Familial Schizophrenia on Chromosome 1q21–q22. *Science* 288(5466):678–682.

Caspi, A., K. Sugden, T. E. Moffitt, A. Taylor, et al. 2003. Influence of Life Stress on Depression: Moderation by a Polymorphism in the 5-HTT Gene. *Science* 301(5631):386–389.

Cheung, B. H., F. Arellano-Carbajal, I. Rybicki, M. de Bono. 2004. Soluble Guanylate Cyclases Act in Neurons Exposed to the Body Fluid to Promote *C. elegans* Aggregation Behavior. *Current Biology* 14(12):1105–1111.

Chumakov, I., M. Blumenfeld, O. Guerassimenko, L. Cavarec, et al. 2002. Genetic and Physiological Data Implicating the New Human Gene G7, 2 and the Gene for D-Amino Acid Oxidase in Schizophrenia. *Proceedings of the National Academy of Sciences USA* 99(21):13675–13680.

Coates, J. C., and M. de Bono. 2002. Antagonistic Pathways in Neurons Exposed to Body Fluid Regulate Social Feeding in *Caenorhabditis elegans*. *Nature* 419 (6910):925–929.

Cook-Deegan, R. 1994. *Gene Wars*. New York: W. W. Norton.

Corfas, G., K. Roy, J. D. Buxbaum. 2004. Neuregulin 1-erbB Signaling and the Molecular/Cellular Basis of Schizophrenia. *Nature Neuroscience* 7(6):575–580.

de Bono, M., and C. I. Bargmann. 1998. Natural Variation in a Neuropeptide Y Receptor Homolog Modifies Social Behavior and Food Response in *C. elegans*. *Cell* 94(5):679–689.

de Bono, M., and A. V. Maricq. 2005. Neuronal Substrates of Complex Behaviors in *C. elegans*. *Annual Review of Neuroscience* 28:451–501.

de Bono, M., D. M. Tobin, M. V. Davis, L. Avery, and C. I. Bargmann. 2002. Social Feeding in *Caenorhabditis elegans* Is Induced by Neurons That Detect Aversive Stimuli. *Nature* 419(6910):899–903.

DSM-IV (2000) *Diagnostic and Statistical Manual of Mental Disorders DSM-IV-TR*, 4th ed. Washington, DC: American Psychiatric Publishing.

Egan, M. F., T. E. Goldberg, B. S. Kolachana, J. H. Callicott, et al. 2001. Effect of COMT Val108/158 Met Genotype on Frontal Lobe Function and Risk for Schizophrenia. *Proceedings of the National Academy of Sciences USA* 98(12):6917–6922.

Egan, S. E., and R. A. Weinberg. 1993. The Pathway to Signal Achievement. *Nature* 28;365(6449):781–783.

Falls, D. L. 2003. Neuregulins and the Neuromuscular System: 10 Years of Answers and Questions. *Journal of Neurocytolology* 32(5–8):619–647.

Faust, D., and R. A. Miner. 1986. The Empiricist and His New Clothes: DSM-III in Perspective. *American Journal of Psychiatry* 143(8):962–967.

Fletcher, R. and E. Wagner. 1982. *Clinical Epidemiology: The Essentials*. Baltimore: Williams and Wilkins.

Funke, B., C. T. Finn, A. M. Plocik, S. Lake, et al. 2004. Association of the DTNBP1 Locus with Schizophrenia in a U.S. Population. *American Journal of Human Genetics* 75(5):891–898.

Giere, Ronald N. 1984. *Understanding Scientific Reasoning*. 2nd ed. New York: Holt, Rinehart and Winston.

Goldberg, T. E., M. F. Egan, T. Gscheidle, R. Coppola, et al. 2003. Executive Subprocesses in Working Memory: Relationship to Catechol-O-Methyltransferase Val158Met Genotype and Schizophrenia. *Archives of General Psychiatry* 60(9):889–896.

Goodwin, D. W., and S. B. Guze. 1979. *Psychiatric Diagnosis*. New York: Oxford University Press.

Gray, J. M., D. S. Karow, H. Lu, A. J. Chang, et al. 2004. Oxygen Sensation and Social Feeding Mediated by a *C. elegans* Guanylate Cyclase Homologue. *Nature* 430(6997):317–322.

Harrison, P. J., and A. J. Law. 2006. Neuregulin 1 and Schizophrenia: Genetics, Gene Expression, and Neurobiology. *Biological Psychiatry* 60(2):132–140.

Harrison, P. J., and D. R. Weinberger. 2005. Schizophrenia Genes, Gene Expression, and Neuropathology: On the Matter of Their Convergence. *Molecular Psychiatry* 10(1):40–68.

Hong, C. J., S. J. Huo, D. L. Liao, K. Lee, et al. 2004. Case-Control and Family-Based Association Studies between the Neuregulin 1 (Arg38Gln) Polymorphism and Schizophrenia. *Neuroscience Letters* 366(2):158–161.

Kauffman, S. A. 1993. *The Origins of Order: Self-Organization and Selection in Evolution.* New York: Oxford University Press.

Kendell, R. E. 1989. Clinical Validity. *Psychological Medicine* 19(1):45–55.

———. 2004. Schizophrenia Genetics and Dysbindin: A Corner Turned? *American Journal of Psychiatry* 161(9):1533–1536.

Kendler, K. S. 2005a. "A Gene For . . . ": The Nature of Gene Action in Psychiatric Disorders. *American Journal of Psychiatry* 162(7):1243–1252.

———. 2005b. Psychiatric Genetics: A Methodologic Critique. *American Journal of Psychiatry* 162(1):3–11.

Kendler, K. S., C. O. Gardner, and C. A. Prescott. 2006. Toward a Comprehensive Developmental Model for Major Depression in Men. *American Journal of Psychiatry* 163(1):115–124.

Kendler, K. S., and R. J. Greenspan. 2006. The Nature of Genetic Influences on Behavior: Lessons from Simpler Organisms. *American Journal of Psychiatry* 163: 1683–1694.

Kendler, K. S., R. C. Kessler, M. C. Neale, A. C. Heath, and L. J. Eaves. 1993. The Prediction of Major Depression in Women: Toward an Integrated Etiologic Model. *American Journal of Psychiatry* 150(8):1139–1148.

Law, A. J., B. K. Lipska, C. S. Weickert, T. M. Hyde, and R. E. Straub. 2006. Neuregulin 1 Transcripts Are Differentially Expressed in Schizophrenia and Regulated by 5' SNPs Associated with the Disease. *Proceedings of the National Academy of Sciences USA* 103(17):6747–6452.

Mackie, J. L. 1974. *The Cement of the Universe: A Study of Causation.* Oxford: Clarendon Press.

Marr, D. 1982. *Vision: A Computational Investigation into the Human Representation and Processing of Visual Information.* San Francisco: W. H. Freeman.

McGinn, C. 2000. *The Mysterious Flame: Conscious Minds in a Material World.* Jackson, TN: Basic Books.

Meehl, P. 1977. Specific Etiology and Other Forms of Strong Inference: Some Quantitative Meanings. *Journal of Medicine and Philosophy* 2:33–55.

Mirnics, K., P. Levitt, and D. A. Lewis. 2006. Critical Appraisal of DNA Microarrays in Psychiatric Genomics. *Biological Psychiatry* 60(2):163–176.

Mirnics, K., F. A. Middleton, A. Marquez, D. A. Lewis, and P. Levitt. 2000. Molecular Characterization of Schizophrenia Viewed by Microarray Analysis of Gene Expression in Prefrontal Cortex. *Neuron* 28(1):53–67.

Mirnics, K., F. A. Middleton, G. D. Stanwood, D. A. Lewis, and P. Levitt. 2001. Disease-Specific Changes in Regulator of G-Protein Signaling 4 (RGS4) Expression in Schizophrenia. *Molecular Psychiatry* 6(3):293–301.

Moises, H. W., T. Zoega, and I. I. Gottesman. 2002. The Glial Growth Factors Deficiency and Synaptic Destabilization Hypothesis of Schizophrenia. *BMC Psychiatry* 2(1):8.

Munafo, M. R. L. Bowes, T. G. Clark, and J. Flint. 2005. Lack of Association of the COMT (Val158/108 Met) Gene and Schizophrenia: A Meta-Analysis of Case-Control Studies. *Molecular Psychiatry* 10(8):765–770.

Murphy, D. 2006. *Psychiatry in the Scientific Image.* Cambridge, MA: MIT Press.

Owen, M. J., N. M. Williams, and M. C. O'Donovan. 2004. The Molecular Genetics of Schizophrenia: New Findings Promise New Insights. *Molecular Psychiatry* 9(1):14–27.

Potter C. J., and L. Luo. 2003. Food for Thought: A Receptor Finds Its Ligand. *Nature Neuroscience* 6(11):1178–1185.

Rankin, C. H. 2002. From Gene to Identified Neuron to Behaviour in *Caenorhabditis elegans. Nature Review Genetics* 3(8):622–630.

Rogers, C., V. Reale, K. Kim, H. Chatwin, et al. 2003. Inhibition of *Caenorhabditis elegans* Social Feeding by FMRFamide-Related Peptide Activation of NPR-1. *Nature Neuroscience* 6(11):1178–1185.

Rose, S. P. 1995. Aggression in Mice and Men? *Science* 270(5235):362–364.

Rosenberg, A. 1985. *The Structure of Biological Science.* New York: Cambridge University Press.

———. 1994. *Instrumental Biology; or, The Disunity of Science.* Chicago: University of Chicago Press.

Schaffner, K. F. 1998a. Genes, Behavior, and Developmental Emergentism: One Process, Indivisible? *Philosophy of Science* 65:209–252.

———. 1998b. Model Organisms and Behavioral Genetics: A Rejoinder. *Philosophy of Science* 65:276–288.

———. 2000. Behavior at the Organismal and Molecular Levels: The Case of *C. elegans. Philosophy of Science* 67:S273–S288.

———. 2002. Clinical and Etiological Psychiatric Diagnoses: Do Causes Count? In J. Sadler (ed.), *Descriptions and Prescriptions: Values, Mental Disorders, and the DSMS* (pp. 271–290). Baltimore: Johns Hopkins University Press.

———. 2006. Reduction: The Cheshire Cat Problem and a Return to Roots. *Synthese* 151(3):377–402.

Schwab, S. G., M. Knapp, S. Mondabon, J. Hallmayer, et al. 2003. Support for Association of Schizophrenia with Genetic Variation in the 6p22.3 Gene, Dysbindin, in Sib-Pair Families with Linkage and in an Additional Sample of Triad Families. *American Journal of Human Genetics* 72(1):185–190.

Sokolowski, M. B. 2002. Neurobiology: Social Eating for Stress. *Nature* 419(6910): 893–894.

Sulston, J. E., E. Schierenberg, J. G. White, and J. N. Thomson. 1983. The Embryonic Cell Lineage of the Nematode *Caenorhabditis elegans. Developmental Biology* 100(1):64–119.

Stefansson, H., J. Sarginson, A. Kong, P. Yates, et al. 2003. Association of Neuregulin 1 with Schizophrenia Confirmed in a Scottish Population. *American Journal of Human Genetics* 72(1):83–87.

Stefansson, H., E. Sigurdsson, V. Steinthorsdottir, S. Bjornsdottir, et al. 2002. Neuregulin 1 and Susceptibility to Schizophrenia. *American Journal of Human Genetics* 71(4):877–892.

Straub, R. E., Y. Jiang, C. J. MacLean, Y. Ma, et al. 2002. Genetic Variation in the 6p22.3 Gene DTNBP1, the Human Ortholog of the Mouse Dysbindin Gene, Is

Associated with Schizophrenia. *American Journal of Human Genetics* 71(2): 337–348.

Straub, R. E., C. J. MacLean, F. A. O'Neill, J. Burke, et al. 1995. A Potential Vulnerability Locus for Schizophrenia on Chromosome 6p24–22: Evidence for Genetic Heterogeneity. *Nature Genetics* 11(3):287–293.

Talbot, K., W. L. Eidem, C. L. Tinsley, M. A. Benson, et al. 2004. Dysbindin-1 Is Reduced in Intrinsic, Glutamatergic Terminals of the Hippocampal Formation in Schizophrenia. *Journal of Clinical Investigation* 113(9):1353–1363.

Thiselton, D. L., B. T. Webb, B. M. Neale, R. C. Ribble, et al. 2004. No Evidence for Linkage or Association of Neuregulin-1 (NRG1) with Disease in the Irish Study of High-Density Schizophrenia Families (ISHDSF). *Molecular Psychiatry* 9(8): 777–783.

White, J. G., E. Southgate, J. N. Thomson, and S. Brenner. 1986. The Structure of the Nervous System of the Nematode *C. elegans*. *Philosophical Transactions of the Royal Society of London Series B, Biological Science* 314(1165):1–340.

Williams, N. M., C. O'Donovan, and M. J. Owen. 2005. Is the Dysbindin Gene (DTNBP1) a Susceptibility Gene for Schizophrenia? *Schizophrenia Bulletin* 31(4):800–805.

Williams, N. M., A. Preece, D. W. Morris, G. Spurlock, et al. 2004. Identification in 2 Independent Samples of a Novel Schizophrenia Risk Haplotype of the Dystrobrevin Binding Protein Gene (DTNBP1). *Archives of General Psychiatry* 61(4): 336–344.

Wimsatt, W. 1976. Reductionism, Levels of Organization, and the Mind-Body Problem. In G. Globus, X. Maxwell, and I. Savodnik (eds.), *Consciousness and the Brain* (pp. 199–267). New York: Plenum.

Wood W. B. (Editor). 1988. The Nematode *Caenorhabditis Elegans*. Cold Spring Harbor, N.Y: Cold Spring Harbor Laboratory Press.

Zou, F., C. Li, S. Duan, Y. Zheng, N. Gu, G. Feng, Y. Xing, J. Shi, L. He. 2005. A Family-Based Study of the Association between the G72/G30 Genes and Schizophrenia in the Chinese Population. *Schizophrenia Research* 73 (2–3): 257–261.

Comment: Understanding Causes and Reversing Outcomes

Dominic P. Murphy, Ph.D.

In his chapter, Kenneth Schaffner, as he usually does, exhibits a familiarity with the gory details of his chosen science that is, frankly, unfair. And, being Schaffner, he has added philosophical value to it. In particular, he has highlighted the significance of model organisms, which have not been treated by philosophers of biology to the extent they deserve, given their importance in the life sciences. So I shall ask some questions about model organisms and their special status. I also want to pick up on a question Schaffner begins with but to which he does not fully return, which is why we want causal explanations at all. Schaffner has named me as someone who thinks that psychiatry should strive for causal explanations—indeed, I think that the search for causal structure is what science is all about, but I agree with him that causal explanations in psychiatry, though possible, are hard to formulate, difficult to test, and interlevel rather than fully reductive. So I won't quarrel much with the chapter. Indeed, I think Schaffner's earlier work has taught us that this is how it usually goes in the life sciences, and my concluding remarks will echo the main themes in Schaffner's discussion of the lessons of the reductive explanations he peruses. I am not interested in criticizing Schaffner, but in amplifying some themes in his chapter. I will start by asking why we want a science that represents causal relations, and then I will consider model organisms in the light of the answers I give to that question.

To begin with, then, why do we want causal explanations at all? Why look for causal relations rather than just correlations? In some cases, certainly, a correlation can provide us with valuable predictive information, and if your idea of the goals of science is that they are limited to prediction and control, you might feel happy enough with correlations. A VRAG (Violent Risk Appraisal Guide) score, for example, gives a probability that a violent offender will reoffend within a specified period back in the community. It is strikingly reliable as a predictive instrument, especially when compared to the predictions of a parole board or some other group of human judges, no matter how expert. The VRAG is an actuarial tool. Its predictions are based on the observed correlations between violent recidivism and twelve measured variables, including age, early separation from a parent, marital status, criminal record, and past episodes of a small number of relevant mental disorders (for a full discussion, see Quinsey et al. 2006).

The VRAG is a powerful instrument, but it is far from perfect and it is, as Bishop and Trout say (2005, pp. 47–49), ungrounded. That is, we don't know why it succeeds to the extent that it does, because we don't why the correlations obtain or why they should influence recidivism. It is natural to think that there are causal stories to be told here. The VRAG probably does not work because it reflects the operation of one neat underlying causal mechanism, but it seems that, to the extent it works, it must do so in virtue of causal relations between what it measures and what it predicts. In the absence of causal understanding about why the VRAG works as it does, we may be unclear about its success and reluctant to apply it to populations other than the North American (Canadian, in fact) population that served as the source of the data. The reason why that set of correlations has the predictive power it does is because there is a stable set of causes tying whatever realizes the variables in actual cases to the properties of violent reoffenders. If the predictions aren't made true by the underlying causal framework, what does make them true? And if we find the underlying framework, our predictive power may well be enhanced.

This is why I agree with Michael Strevens (2006), who suggests that the point of thinking causally is to search for mechanisms. The reason why predictive success often turns on causal understanding is that, if one member of a kind has a property, it does so in virtue of the mechanisms that distinguish that kind and typically (though not invariably) cause it to have the observable properties of the kind. Prediction in that sense, as Strevens points out, is the inverse of categorization, which assumes that entities belong to the same kind if they have the same properties, because the presence of those shared properties is taken to be evidence that the entities share the mechanisms that make members of that kind into the things they are. It is these relations between causal relations, mechanisms, categorization, and prediction that make theorists such as Kendell argue that nosology should be based on causes, and I have defended that idea at length (Murphy 2006). (Interventionist models such as Woodward's are another route into this problem; we want to know about causes so we can intervene in the world—not just predict. See Woodward [2003; this volume].)

The details, of course, are likely to be messy, especially in light of the fact that causal understanding does not have to be reductive. Indeed, it probably can't be, for reasons that Schaffner outlines. His paradigm of a reductive explanation is the search for genetic pathways underlying feeding behavior in *Caenorhabditis elegans,* and he points out that the explanation, even of one behavior in so simple an organism, is not completely reductive. When it comes to more complex organisms, including paradigmatically humans, we find that many, many relationships between genes and traits are the norm. Biological and environmental influences are mixed up together in causal networks that are, as Schaffner says, bushy.

So the problem of building causal models looks intractable, but Schaffner has some suggestions for how we might tract it. Schaffner's strategy is to look for heuristics that reveal "a simplified isolated and localized pattern of causal influence within an otherwise complex system."

One cautionary point I want to emphasize is that Schaffner ties the search for causal pathways to the search for opportunities to intervene, and I think here things are more complicated. Now it's only common sense to assume that the more causal influences we uncover, the more opportunities we will have for intervention and manipulation, both experimentally and in therapy. However, I don't think that the search for dominant causal pathways—the main explanatory relation among all the many relations in the bush—should be seen as directed to therapeutic payoffs in the first case. Even if we can identify a causal pathway that seems to bear most of the explanatory burden, what causes the problem and what is best targeted to rectify it may not be the same. Although a condition may be best modeled via molecular representations of its causes, nothing follows about how best to treat it. The factor that best explains a condition may not be the factor that is most easily manipulated in therapy. However, it is also true that the search for a reductive causal explanation might lead to an inappropriate stress on some causes and the neglect of others when we think about remedies.

For example, Schaffner cites the tuberculosis bacterium as a final common pathway, but eradicating tuberculosis might be more easily accomplished through attacking environmental factors, like cleaning up the air or improving working-class nutrition. Richard Lewontin (1993, pp. 44–45) concludes that because, historically, Western societies got rid of tuberculosis through such environmental improvements, it is wrong to cite the bacillus as the cause. He thinks it is more accurate to say that tuberculosis was caused by the conditions of nineteenth-century capitalism. Similarly, Alexander et al. (1981) devised rich, stimulating environments for the rats in their lab, and their happy rats did not exhibit the usual addiction to morphine that laboratory rats come to exhibit. Alexander (2000) took this to show that prior animal models of addiction were wrong to see addiction as a neurological condition. Rather, in rats it was due to the physically and socially impoverished circumstances of their housing, and in humans to the same process on a broader scale, which he attributed to the dislocating effects of industrialization.

Arguments such as Lewontin's and Alexander's are supposed to demonstrate the poverty of reductionism for finding the causes of the conditions. A better lesson to draw is that the search for the one true cause is not always sensible, because most interesting human phenomena are caused by a huge natural conspiracy between factors inside and outside the organism. In particular, note that these arguments don't at all discredit the strategy for figuring out how the world works by searching for mechanisms. Rather, it shows that causal mechanisms can exist at many levels of explanation. Our theories of mechanism and causation must be general enough to capture this, perhaps by introducing a manipulationist element into our concept of mechanism, because the manipulationist (Woodward 2003) speaks of relations among variables, which in principle might be identified at any number of levels. And sometimes we find the right causal path but cannot intervene on it (for example, the gene we have found gets turned on and off in development in utero, so by the time we get to the patient the damage is already done).

Examples like these also drive home Schaffner's point about the bushiness of causal networks. So, if genetic pathways don't have a monopoly on either causal influence or therapeutic convenience, why do they seem so special, and what explains our devotion to model organisms?

Simply compare the relative ease and precision with which one element of a descriptive model of the mouse nervous system can be manipulated to the extreme difficulty involved in changing some of a person's beliefs without any psychological ramifications, and you can see why reductionist molecular strategies offer a manipulative power that higher level theorizing lacks. We simply do not understand cognitive capacities at computational or other high levels in ways that are analogous to descriptive molecular models in terms of power and precision.

One way in which gene expression is special is that it gives us a precise understanding of some biological processes that can be experimentally manipulated. But part of the drive for reductionism in this area is surely a belief that reductive explanations are somehow more fundamental, in that they show what everything is made of, or what is really going on.

The question, then, is whether the greater precision and manipulation of descriptive genetic models also picks out a specially privileged level of root causes in nature that makes explanations at this level somehow fundamental. One might think that the durability of multilevel bushy networks in our theories, and their environmental embedding, merely reflect our ignorance of how, ultimately, the physical composition of the component causes works. I think a number of people are tempted by the idea that the further down you go, the more fundamental are the forces you encounter, and hence the more fundamental are the explanations you can build.

If there is a fundamental physical level, it is subatomic. Yet perhaps within biology we should think of the molecular level as relatively fundamental—fundamental for organisms—and molecular explanations as privileged on that account. I think that there is a sense in which the explanations derived from genetic models are privileged, but it is unclear that they are privileged because they are about something metaphysically fundamental. Fundamental explanation is a slippery concept, but I do think there is a sense in which reductive, gene-driven explanations are fundamental, and one way of putting Schaffner's conclusions is that there aren't many such explanations in psychiatry.

Let's start with the case of Huntington disease, where what we know about the clinical genetics does look like it singles out a fundamental cause, even though the causal story is still just a gappy sketch, to use Schaffner's terms. Huntington disease is associated with a gene, IT15 or "Huntingtin," on the short arm of chromosome 4, characterized by an abnormally long CAG trinucleotide repeat. There is a strong correlation between repeat length and age at onset of the disease—people with 39 and 40 repeats have an average age of onset of 66 and 59 years, respectively, whereas for people with 49 repeats the average age at onset is 28 years and, for 50 repeats, 27 years. One can have the gene and not show the symptoms, but this occurs only in rare cases for low values of the repeat.

That does not mean that there is a fully deterministic relation between Huntingtin and the symptoms of Huntington disease, such that anyone born with the repeat will get the disease. Huntingtin is not fully penetrant, and even if it were you could die of something else before the disease develops. In the case of such "single major locus" (or SML) conditions, it makes sense to think of the genetics as the fundamental explanation. But suppose we contrast the Huntingtin story with a different cause of mental illness, stress. Stress is frequently involved in episodes of many different conditions, and the presence or intensity of stress makes a difference to the form that symptoms take. But stress levels alone do not predict who will come down with, for example, depression, because your reaction to stress depends on a lot of other facts about you. In that sense, stress is not a robust explainer—a model that assigns great causal significance to stress will need to make a large number of additional assumptions. And stress may explain, say, why insomnia features as a symptom in Fred's latest depressive episode, but it may not explain many other symptoms, so it lacks what we might call causal reach; it affects only a few of the properties of the condition that we want to explain. Stress as a cause of mental illness, however, is general in a way that Huntingtin isn't. Huntingtin is implicated in only one disorder, and stress is implicated in many (including many physical disorders). So Huntingtin is a robust cause that explains a lot, but it is highly specific. Stress is a general cause, but it is not robust because it is sensitive to small perturbations in context, and it lacks reach because in each case it may explain only a small number of symptoms.

There look to be many conditions for which we should not expect fundamental explanations but will build up explanations piecemeal from causes like stress rather than discover one big dominant pathway like that which leads Huntingtin to have its terrible effects. The complexity involved in the multiple-path models of depression that Schaffner discusses makes it difficult to make sense of the notion of fundamental explanations. The complexity implies that the idea of a fundamental explanation in psychiatry is generally misguided. The exceptions will occur, as Schaffner suggests, in those cases where we can find a dominant pathway.

With a dominant pathway, if the system is left alone, we can predict the outcome with great confidence because we have identified the key mechanism. All the variety in the culture, psychology, and physical attributes of people with the Huntingtin gene seems to make almost no difference to the gene pathway. Even though the brain of a person with Huntington disease, like any other brain, is the outcome of a huge number of causal interactions, it seems that, to a strong approximation, none of those interactions can change the brain in a way that stops the repeat from wreaking havoc. Only if the system collapses altogether (as in premature death from some other cause) will the h-H relation (the relation between the Huntingtin gene and Huntington's syndrome) be prevented for most values of the repeat.

This imperviousness to real-world variation is what makes the Huntington disease long repeat a fundamental explanation. Obviously the explanation picks out a process that goes on in a context, but there are hardly any ways of specifying the context that make a difference to the explanation that cites the h-H relation. There are exceptions that we can invent:

you can't put a string of CAGs in a Petrie dish and give the dish Hunting-ton disease. But the exceptions are usually beside the point, because we are interested in the h-H relations in humans. From human to human the physical context is usually the same, because it is a matter of facts about human biology, which, thanks to evolutionary and developmental proces-ses, will come out more or less the same every time. The differences don't rob the explanation of its power. So in my sense, fundamental explana-tions in psychiatry are those that (1) cite maximally robust causal rela-tions (including relations that cross levels of explanation) and (2) have what we might call causal reach—they explain all (or at least many) of the symptoms of a condition. Such an explanation identifies what Schaffner calls a maximally dominant pathway, and I think his account captures much of what seems fundamental about a genetic explanation and shows why the depth of understanding that model organism gives us is so allur-ing. The property of being a fundamental explanation, though, does not attach to an explanation at a given level but to an explanation with the properties of robustness and causal reach. It is an open question whether a maximally dominant pathway could be found at higher levels, but, al-though we may have more chance of finding them at the molecular level, we should still not expect to find many.

We should expect to see few fundamental explanations in psychiatry and lots of models that explain disorders in terms of interacting, nonfun-damental explanations. In some cases, we might ask a question about some property of the disorder, such as an epidemiological difference, that is best explained by only one causal factor. So in that sense there could be lots of explanations that are fundamental relative to one explanatory in-terest. Contrastive explanations, which say why something rather than something else occurred, might cite a causal pathway that is specifically dominant or fundamental in a given context, if the other sufficient condi-tions in the INUS analysis are held constant. In general, though, the other conditions will exhibit great variety, and the same pathway might have much less explanatory power when the context shifts. So explanations that are fundamental without qualification—dominant causal pathways—are likely to be rare in psychiatry, and this is because of the complexity of the system as it behaves in nature, not just our ignorance. Model organisms give us knowledge about control, intervention, and prediction, but not metaphysical insights into a fundamental level of organization in nature.

REFERENCES

Alexander, B. K. 2000. The Globalization of Addiction. *Addiction Research* 8: 501–508.

Alexander, B. K., B. L. Beyerstein, P. F. Hadaway, and R. B. Coambs. 1981. Effects of Early and Later Colony Housing on Oral Ingestion of Morphine in Rats. *Pharmacology, Biochemistry, and Behavior* 15:571–576.

Bishop, M., and J. D. Trout. 2005. *Epistemology and the Psychology of Human Reasoning.* New York: Oxford University Press.

Lewontin, R. 1993. *Biology as Ideology.* New York. HarperPerennial.

Murphy, D. 2006. *Psychiatry in the Scientific Image.* Cambridge, MA: MIT Press.

Quinsey, V. L., G. T. Harris, M. E. Rice, and C. A. Cormier. 2006. *Violent Offenders: Appraising and Managing Risk,* 2nd ed. Washington, DC: American Psychological Association.

Strevens, M. 2006. Why Represent Causal Relations? In A. Gopnik and L. Schulz (eds.), *Causal Learning: Psychology, Philosophy, Computation* (pp. 245–260). New York: Oxford University Press.

Woodward, J. 2003. *Making Things Happen.* New York: Oxford University Press.

Levels of Explanation in Psychiatry

DOMINIC P. MURPHY, PH.D.

In chapter 3, Dominic Murphy takes a systematic look at the key issue of levels of explanation in psychiatry. His viewpoint is that of cognitive neuroscience, and his entry point into this question is the seminal work by the neuroscientist David Marr. Marr's book—now nearly 25 years old—still well deserves reading, especially the earlier, more philosophical parts, which are a model of clarity of thinking and presentation (Marr 1982). (Marr's work is also explored from a somewhat different perspective in the chapter by Campbell in this volume.) Although Marr's approach is simple and appealing and commonly invoked in cognitive neuroscience, Murphy queries its applicability to the problems of psychiatry. He points out that the more common view of the "Marrian levels" is epistemic. That is, his three levels (roughly, functional, algorithmic, and implementational) represent different ways of knowing about the same process. But Murphy points out that there is another view of levels—one that he suggests may be more applicable in psychiatry—in which the levels represent qualitatively different causal processes. For example, one can understand the causes of major depression at the "levels" of genes and environmental adversity. These "levels" do not represent different epistemic perspective on the same process; rather, they are substantively different processes. A Marrian approach would run into trouble in figuring out how to reduce, to the implementation stage, environmental risk factors. The problem of levels in psychiatry doesn't seem to fit Marr's model.

Murphy suggests that Marr's three-level picture is too neat and tidy for psychiatry. We cannot, he argues, be too strongly guided by a priori assumptions about what the explanatory levels in psychiatry would be. We have to understand the lower-level processes and see how they will constrain what could be going on at higher levels. Our top-down preconceptions might be wrong.

Murphy's approach reflects the deep tension between bottom-up and top-down perspectives in psychiatry. That is, how do we relate the functional descriptions of what the mind does with biological explanations of how the brain works? Which way and with what force these two processes will work themselves out over time is uncertain. It is interesting that philosophers, neuroscientists, and psychiatrists alike often have strong intuitive judgments about how things will develop that are sometimes held with emotional fervor.

Murphy is an advocate of reductive approaches—as seen in his account of mouse models of intrauterine viral infections and their impact on risk for schizophrenia. He nevertheless also appreciates their limits. In particular, he suggests, such approaches will never yield in psychiatry the beauty, power, and simplicity of those seen in the harder sciences such as physics. In particular, the environment will be hard to "reduce." This sounds right.

Murphy differs from Marr and agrees with Schaffner in suggesting that most explanations in psychiatry will end up being cross levels rather than solely within levels, as initially visualized by Marr. But, in accord with a Marrian view, he suggests that the lower-level explanations (that is, implementation) will leave the higher levels of generalization intact. We won't, he thinks, hear a great sucking sound as the molecular clarification of the etiology of psychiatric disorders subsumes and replaces psychosocial explanatory systems. That is, he is asserting that we obtain explanatory power at a variety of levels of explanation.

He points out another limitation of the Marrian perspective. It does not well allow for interactions across levels. Murphy singles out "organism-environment interactions" as being particularly likely in psychiatry and not well captured in Marr's account of levels.

The example he uses are the well-known genetic and cultural effects on risk for eating disorders. This reflects a paradigmatic case, he argues, where hard reductionism will not work because no one level is the "fundamental" one. Rather, each modifies the other.

Is Murphy asking too much of Marrian models? He developed them, after all, to explain the mammalian visual system. A positive aspect of his model, less emphasized in Murphy's chapter, is that it provides a framework in which to see how psychological or functional level descriptions of mind can provide a structure for biological explanations of brain. In this sense, Marr's model provides an integrative and possibly realistic picture of how neuroscience and psychology can work together in explaining psychiatric disorders. This approach has the virtue of avoiding the extremes of both hard reductionism (mind will be completely reduced to brain, and all psychology will become neuroscience) and dualistic or behaviorist viewpoints on the other (psychology can and should operate entirely independently of that gelatinous gray mass inside our skulls).

Having concluded that explanation in psychiatry will inevitably be "multilevel," Murphy then turns to a subsequent logical question—what sort of things are we trying to explain in psychiatry? In answering this question, he raises the issue of the use of exemplars in psychiatry. (This discussion bears some relationship to the diagnostic issues raised by Peter Zachar in his chapter in this book.) The issue of exemplars arises, Murphy suggests, when we confront on the one hand the diversity of clinical reality and on the other the goal of simplification of scientific research. That is, science will have to look at modal processes. We have to study exemplars (pathogenic features in the phraseology of Birnbaum [1974]) because the diversity of individual psychiatric phenomenon is just too great. Our science has to search for the broad commonalities and not get lost in the individual flurry of details that are unique to each individual.

So, as Murphy points out, our models are twice divorced from raw clinical reality. We make artificially simple models in our research (only, for example, ever examining a small fraction of the relevant risk factors). However, the subjects of our research (or the dependent variable in statistical terms) are exemplars that are themselves abstractions taken from a much messier clinical reality.

Will the model of simple neurological exemplars—where we can understand all the resulting neurological deficits as arising from a single simple pathologic process—work for psychiatry? Probably not, he concludes. If you look at the history of schizophrenia research, there are many efforts to describe such a pathological process. They are, however, typically described at such a vague level—such as "synaptic slippage"—that they are nearly useless as scientific hypotheses. Perhaps some day we will understand one simple pathologic process—a defect in neuronal cell migration during development—that can be articulated at a useful degree of specificity. But at least as likely is that the clinical state of schizophrenia reflects the concatenation of multiple pathologic processes. This "multiple hit" model for schizophrenia might resemble some etiologic theories for cancer formation. One hope, often expressed in the past and now most recently by genetics researchers, is that we will "carve nature at its joints" and find subforms of schizophrenia that are etiologically homogeneous, where the disorder is the result of a single well-defined process. Many have been trying to do this since the days of Kraepelin with limited success to date.

Also of note, Murphy contrasts schizophrenia—the psychiatric equivalent of a "multisystem disorder" that affects cognition, perception, mood, and volition—with panic disorder, which is considerably more circumspect in its impact. Is it a different kind of illness with a potentially much simpler etiologic story more analogous to simple neurological exemplars?

Thus, Murphy's chapter can be seen as coming in two integrated parts. First, he asks in general how will explanatory systems work in a "mature" psychiatry? Second, he asks what are the sorts of things that these explanatory systems will try to explain?

Readers who want to study more of Murphy's thoughts about psychiatry and psychiatric illness could profitably consult his recent book, *Psychiatry in the Scientific Image* (Murphy 2006).

Kenneth S. Kendler, M.D.

REFERENCES

Birnbaum, K. 1974. The Making of a Psychosis: The Principles of Structural Analysis in Psychiatry. In S. R. Hirsch and M. Shepherd (eds.), *Themes and Variations in European Psychiatry: An Anthology* (pp. 199–238). Charlottesville: University Press of Virginia.

Marr, D. 1982. The Philosophy and the Approach. In *Vision: A Computational Investigation into the Human Representation and Processing of Visual Information* (pp. 3–38). San Francisco: W. H. Freeman.

Murphy, D. 2006. *Psychiatry in the Scientific Image (Philosophical Psychopathology)*. Cambridge, MA: MIT Press.

* * *

Suppose we think of psychiatry as "the discipline within cognitive neuroscience that integrates information from all these related disciplines in order to develop models that explain the cognitive dysfunctions of psychiatric patients based on knowledge of normal mind/brain function" (Andreasen 1997, p. 1586).

In this chapter I explore this idea. In particular, I want to think about explanation in psychiatry based on how explanation works in cognitive neuroscience, although my conception of cognitive neuroscience will be broad. It includes the systems underlying visceral states, emotional appraisals, and other affective processes. The basic assumption I make is that the brain is a cognitive organ, in the sense that information processing is involved in all states, not just "cold" cognition. Normal psychology depends on cognitive parts (Glymour 1992)—physical structures in the brain that process different kinds of information—functioning as they are supposed to. To explain breakdowns within and between cognitive parts, we need to understand and be able to model the operation of cognitive parts at different levels of explanation. I contrast the picture in psychiatry with the traditional picture in the philosophy of the cognitive sciences. My way in is the picture of explanation that all of us philosophers of mind learned from David Marr, a cognitive scientist. I start with the basic Marrian picture of levels of explanation in the cognitive sciences and noting the ways in which neuroscientific practice has departed from Marr. The result, as applied to psychiatry, is a mechanistic but still broadly reductive account that fits the idea that psychiatry should look for explanations in terms of systems neuroscience. In the course of studying these questions, I examine the problems involved in trying to generalize this picture to all the different causal histories, both proximal and distal, that are involved in psychiatry.

I have little to say about what levels of explanation actually are, beyond a sketchy, preliminary typology. Marr thought of levels as primarily epistemic—he actually calls them "levels of understanding." They are abstract descriptions of what a system does, with a theoretical apparatus that is appropriate to each type of description and that lets us understand a system in different ways. So you can think of a level of explanation as a way of understanding how a system works in terms of the functions characterized at each level of description, without making many commitments about what components actually exist in the system and discharge its functions. Another way of thinking of levels is that they specify actual forms of *organization in nature:* higher levels are made up of lower-level things, and at each level things interact with each other (Wimsatt 1976) rather than with things at lower levels. Both these ways of thinking about levels fail to do justice to the complexity of things in psychiatry, because in psychiatry we have different systems interacting. Therefore, the levels are not rival descriptions of the same process, but descriptions of different processes. Also, the levels interact with each other—explanations cross levels, as Kenneth Schaffner emphasized. I think, however, there is something to the idea that levels are a matter of different sorts of entity. Rather than thinking about patterns of interaction or organization, I want to think of each kind of entity as behaving in ways that are explained by the sorts of causal mechanism that characterize them. Rather than trying to make this more precise here, I will turn to Marr.

1. Levels of Explanation

David Marr famously advocated (Marr 1982, pp. 24–25) viewing the mind at three levels of explanation. The highest level specifies, in functional terms, the computational task accomplished by the psychological system that a theory is concerned with. The topmost level, said Marr, would show you the computational problem that is solved by the particular information-processing algorithms the system uses: these are described at the second (middle) level. The information constituting the system's input and output is represented at this middle level, and here too we specify the algorithm that transforms the input into the output. The lowest level is that of implementation, which asks how computational processes are realized in the brain. Marr called this the level of detailed computer architecture. The lowest level describes the physical implementation of the algorithms in the brain. Marrian levels of explanation specify different vocabularies and methods in which generalizations are formed about the same entity, the central nervous system. Levels-talk, however, is often used in another way in psychiatry, to specify processes that operate across different phenomena. Many mental illnesses, for example, are caused by a complex interaction of proximal causes within the organism, such as neurochemical disturbances or genetic vulnerabilities, and distal, environmental causes, such as dysfunctional families or stressful life events.

Marr's biological and computational levels are ways of representing the same process that are useful for different purposes: for example, we can generalize across the same psychological processes even if the underlying biology differs somewhat. Suppose that an interaction of genetic endowment and long-term unemployment conspires to make someone depressed. In this case, we are dealing with radically different processes, not the same process realized in different ways, even though being unemployed affects the brain.

On a Marrian picture we might ultimately expect to replace higher-level cognitive generalizations with lower-level ones in terms of genes or other biological entities, in the same way that we learned to understand chemical bonds in terms of their underlying physics. Such a vision makes sense when we are talking about generalizations that apply at different levels to the same structures, but a replacement project aimed at a complete molecular explanation of most forms of mental illness would require a molecular specification of not just cognitive processes within the brain but also environmental causes. The Marrian picture might still apply to the processes going on within the skin, although even here I think there is some room to doubt. It nevertheless doesn't fit the general picture of the development of mental illness, which typically involves a mixture of internal and environmental factors.

Marr imagined that we could understand psychological processes in the abstract without worrying about the biology used to perform them, just as we can understand flight without knowing anything about the anatomy of a bird's feathers. That point remains uppermost in the minds of philosophers who try to understand cognition in the abstract. However, if one is interested in the details of human biological cognitive organization, one obviously needs to see how our mental processes are realized in the body, just as one needs to investigate feathers if one wanted to understand not just flight in general but also the specific workings of birds that enable them to fly. When we try to understand the engineering of the human organism—as opposed, perhaps, to the nature of intelligence in the abstract—we look for the physical structures in the brain that carry out information-processing jobs, our cognitive parts. First, theories are presented, preferably in the form of "box-and-arrow" diagrams, and detailed hypotheses are then derived and tested experimentally. Historically, intentional or behavioral theories have marked the starting point, and neurological investigation has attempted to understand the realization of a mental taxonomy taken off the psychological shelf, not one built up from brain investigation (Hatfield 2000).

The methods of cognitive neuroscience do not make the intentional level as autonomous as the Marrian approach expected. The functional decomposition of the human mind into its components cannot be the autonomous analysis of the abstract tasks that minds carry out, but the decomposition assumption is vindicated as part of the twin processes of decomposition and localization (Bechtel and Richardson 1992; Zawidski and Bechtel 2004). Although mental capacities can be distinguished functionally, the final decomposition of our mental life into components should be guided by the interrelation of cognitive hypotheses and physical facts. Compared to the Marrian picture, this is a reductionist view that puts much tighter constraints on the relations between levels—our understanding of realization feeds back into and constrains our understanding of the abstract demands of cognition. As Schaffner (this volume, ch. 2) says, we have to take our levels where we find them. We should not, as in the Marrian approach, be guided by a set of assumptions about what generalizations must exist at different levels for the system to meet the abstract demands of a task. Rather, we assume that there are causal mechanisms at lower levels that realize the functions described at higher levels, but our description of those higher-level functions must be constrained by what we discover about the properties of the lower-level systems and the sorts of functional roles that they can support. The actual engineering of the system may realize functions in ways that would not occur to us if we remained content with abstract specifications of the functions from the point of view of the most elegant engineering solution.

Because the description of and relation between levels depend on actual engineering facts rather than theoretical assumptions, it might be possible to link up molecular accounts with the emerging cognitive ones in ways that fit the "partially reductive" picture of explanation that Schaffner wrote about. For example, researchers working with records of the 1957 Helsinki flu outbreak have found an elevated incidence of schizophrenia among children of mothers who were infected during the second trimester (Green 2001, pp. 27–28). No such increase has been found among children exposed during their first and third trimesters *in utero*. Some, but not all, other studies support the conclusion about the second trimester, and similar results have been obtained for measles and rubella and other mental illnesses, including autism (Green 2001, pp. 31–32; Patterson 2002). Paul Patterson and colleagues at Caltech (Patterson 2002; Shi et al. 2002) explored the possible pathways between infection and behavioral change by infecting mice with the flu and measuring their offspring on a variety of tests. The results showed that mice born to infected mothers were less likely than controls to interact socially and explore novel environments. They also had a further property of great interest to schizophrenia researchers: they had a lowered prepulse inhibition (PPI) that could be corrected by antipsychotic medication. Let me explain.

The startle reflex includes several measurable responses, such as eyeblinks. The strength of eyeblinks can be measured by electrodes placed around the eyelids. A prior exposure to a quieter, unstartling noise (the PPI) lessens the subsequent startle response. This is not the case in schizophrenics, who typically are deficient in PPI; that is, their startle response is not lowered to a normal degree by the prior stimulus (Green 2001, p. 77). Patterson and colleagues found the same effect in the offspring of infected mice and also found that it could be corrected by clozapine, to which the mice were abnormally sensitive. PPI deficits were also found in the offspring of mothers that had been injected with synthetic RNA to induce an antiviral immune response. This immediately suggests a line of research on the interaction of maternal infection (as an environmental risk factor) and genetic predisposition to schizophrenia, as well as the possibility of tracing the mechanisms in the immune system that mediate the relationship, and developing technologies aimed at targeting that relationship in therapy. So here we have a case in which a mouse model might be something that we can hook up with some aspects of a cognitive model, but aiming for not just genetic analogs of human traits in mice but also cognitive analogs.

Patterson's lab, for example, is currently studying the brain activity of mice that receive different sensory stimuli, to see if definite patterns of activity can be correlated with different inputs. The hope is then to monitor neuronal activity in the brain by using "immediate early" genes—genes that turn on when the state of the cell is altered. This is a familiar technology. The object will be to see whether giving the mice a drug that induces hallucinations in humans induces activity in the visual or auditory cortex of the mice in the absence of sensory input. If this is the case, we ask whether a mouse model of mental illness also displays activity in these areas in the absence of sensory input. Perceptual activity without specific input is used as the operationalization of hallucination. There are obviously all sorts of interesting questions about human cognition that are left unanswered when we move from endogenous perceptual activity in mice to hallucinations in humans. The experiment is not intended as a complete explanation of hallucination, merely a way of asking precise questions about its biological basis and manipulating the perceptual system so as to make its causal pathways more perspicuous.

Comparison of the relative ease and precision with which one element of a descriptive model of the mouse nervous system can be manipulated to the extreme difficulty involved in changing some of a person's beliefs without any psychological ramifications demonstrates why reductionist molecular strategies offer a manipulative power that higher-level theorizing lacks. We simply do not understand cognitive capacities at computational or other high levels in ways that are analogous to descriptive molecular models in terms of power and precision.

We might still be able to link molecular, neurological, and cognitive generalizations to provide a systems-level account of mental illness. We might expect to see more or less efficient reductions of different higher-level traits to their molecular bases. For some aspects of human cognitive biology, we might see something like the picture that Marr expected, as amended by recent theories. The visual system, for instance, may well admit of a precise characterization in terms of information processing and its cellular and molecular basis. In that case, a systems-level account of schizophrenia could avail itself of reductive accounts of our perceptual systems that might explain the form, if not the content, of some hallucinations. It is unlikely, however, that we will be able to replace all cognitive generalizations with molecular ones, and even more unlikely that we will be able to replace *all* generalizations—including environmental ones—with molecular ones.

We should continue to see, then, the multilevel causal models that Schaffner (1994) identified as the rule in biomedical science; causes described in genetic vocabulary will be related to effects described in terms of behavioral tests, for example, and generalizations will cross levels, relating elements of a model at one level to elements of a model at another. What we achieve by molecular means is not the elimination of higher-level generalizations but rather the articulation of extra low levels in a way that interacts with the existing structure but leaves it basically in place. Reduction in cognitive neuroscience will probably complicate matters rather than simplify them: it furnishes molecular models that illustrate the underlying workings of information-processing systems without replacing them and, in effect, adds extra structure instead of reinterpreting the existing structure. Such a reductive account, however, is not going to be generally forthcoming.

Some conditions may indeed be almost exclusively explained in molecular terms, notably conditions such as Huntington disease, which are tied to specific genes that bear most of the explanatory load. But as Schaffner (1994) in particular has stressed, biomedical theories in general typically cross levels, with effects from one level being related to causes from a different level, and this shows up the limitations of Marr's picture in psychiatry.

David Lykken (1995), for example, argues that the biological basis of psychopathy is a genome that makes some individuals difficult to socialize and that this genome typically leads to the development of psychopathy in early adulthood. But the claim that the "hard-to-socialize" genome causes psychopathy holds only for the most part, "because really talented parents or, more likely, a truly fortuitous combination of parents, neighborhood, peer group, and subsequent mentors, can socialize even these hard cases" (Lykken 1995, p. 12). The extent and severity of psychopathy varies according to both the genetic load and the socialization process. Molecular biology cannot aim at replacing generalizations about environmental factors like a socialization process with generalizations about the molecular basis of those environmental factors. Most of the causal relations that psychiatry will need to understand will be these organism-environment interactions that cross levels. These are not processes that Marr's account of levels fits very well. Marr was thinking about processes, such as the construction of a visual representation, that can be described in different ways. His levels are different perspectives on the same process. In psychiatry we often want to relate different processes, not the same process described in different ways. The genome and the environment are different causes of the same outcome, whereas Marr's levels are different ways of understanding one cause.

The reductionist urge might seem to stand a better chance of satisfaction if it is limited to the processes that Marr had in mind, where a higher-level story can be reformulated in lower-level terms. Yet in fact there is little reason to bet on it even here, because autonomous higher-level explanations show little sign of being reductively explained out of existence within the cognitive sciences. From the fact that all psychological phenomena involve gene expression, it does not follow that higher-level phenomena don't really exist or don't really matter or that generalizations across those phenomena are not autonomous, because they prescind from fine-grained differences in the molecular processes within individuals. There is enough plasticity and difference in brain structure development across individuals to make higher-level generalizations, which smooth out those differences, indispensable. Similarly, there is variation across individuals at the level of functional organization, so we also need to employ top-level generalizations that cite cognitive capacities but abstract away from the details of the realizations of those capacities in different people.

Above all, we need a variety of generalizations to answer different questions. In studying eating disorders, for example, we find that the explanations we need in a given case depend on the relevant question: social factors may explain particular epidemiological patterns, such as variance in eating disorder levels across populations. Social factors alone, however, don't tell us why, out of all the girls in a family within an at-risk group, only one daughter develops an eating disorder. To explain her case, her membership in a class of people who share a particular brain chemistry or childhood trauma may be more relevant than her membership of a specific culture.

Not everyone responds to trauma by becoming bulimic, and those who do may share a biological property, but that does not establish that neurobiology is fundamental. Rather, nothing is fundamental. The trauma may require biological mediation to have its pathological effect, and viceversa. A full explanation needs to mention both biology and psychic trauma, even though particular questions can be answered by citing one or the other. Neither one should be considered fundamental, except relative to a question.

I conclude that there are several reasons for thinking that psychiatric explanations will continue to employ different types, or levels, of explanation. I now ask what the multilevel explanations in a mature psychiatry will look like.

2. Exemplars

Psychiatric explanation, I suggest, is best seen as the attempt to explain exemplars. Exemplars are idealizations. We can think of an exemplar as an imaginary patient who has, in canonical form, the disorder we wish to explain. (Or we can think of an actual patient as an exemplar of a disorder enriched with a set of real-world facts.) In an exemplar we are interested in only a restricted range of properties of our imaginary patients: what's distinctive about them as individuals is ignored, because we are interested in their condition. For the sake of parsimony, we assume that an exemplary patient has only one disorder at a time. This is a note that is sounded recurrently in the history of psychiatry, as scholars acknowledge the utility of thinking about a disorder as an ideal type, or essence, that can be realized in individuals in different ways. Charcot ([1887–88] 1987) distinguished between *archetypes,* or the basic forms of a disorder, which could be decomposed into component parts, and *formes frustes,* in which the disorder appeared in individual subjects with some of its components missing or altered. Birnbaum (1923) argued along similar lines that a disorder typically manifested pathogenic features, which defined its essential structure, and a mix of pathoplastic features, which are caused by the personal circumstances of a given patient. Neuroscientists who talk about the effect of a tumor, lesion, or other pathological process must do something similar, because different patients will exhibit slightly different forms of the same abnormality. The task for the neuroscientist is to extract the core deficit that is shared across similar cases and then go on to explain the result of an insult to a cognitive part that can be manifested in different ways depending on its precise location in the brain and the prior history of the patient.

The idea of an exemplar shares a lot with these approaches. What we need to explain in theory is a picture of the core aspects of a disorder built up from studying a population that shares that core aspect but also exhibits idiosyncratic features that we must prescind from when we build the model, although they are of the first importance to a clinician dealing with members of the population. In reality, the picture is more complex, because an exemplar itself can be modeled in several different ways. In that sense, we construct idealizations to explain idealizations, because what we are trying to explain is highly variable. Disorders look different according to the different biographies, circumstances, and other psychological properties of the people who have them, so when we impose a certain order on the phenomena, we trade off epistemic tractability and fidelity to the facts. The aim is to identify robust processes (Sterelny 2003) that are repeatable or systematic in various ways across individuals rather than the actual processes that occur as a disorder unfolds in one person rather than another. Once an exemplar for a disorder is constructed, we can construct further models designed to explain it. In that sense, psychiatric theory building is doubly indirect. It aims to represent what's going on in idealizations that are themselves representations of a messier reality.

The first form of idealization occurs because mental illnesses take different forms in different patients, and this natural variation means that modeling the biology directly is too awkward. Instead, we can use as the explanatory target an idealization that abstracts away from the variation and try to model that idealization. It is then up to clinicians to translate our knowledge of exemplars into hypotheses about a particular patient who has the condition in a nonideal form. When we move from the biological perspective to the clinical one (to adopt Guze's 1992 formulation), we move from a more abstract to a more precise model, because we are shifting from a general description of a disease process to a specific description of the biology and psychology of an individual. That is, in Sterelny's (2003) terms, we move from robust processes to actual sequences, in an attempt to trace the particular causal history that realizes a given exemplar in a given patient. We do this by ignoring some aspects of the original model, making others salient and defining the salient aspects more precisely.

Exemplars specify a number of features or symptoms for the various disorders. They have slots left open at various levels of explanation for the causal explanation of symptoms at that level by a causal model of the abnormal processes. That explanation, in turn, is derived from a model of how the system normally works. In the normal case we explain the process by showing how relations in the model resemble real-life processes. In the abnormal case, we explain by showing those normal relations are frustrated. Thus, the exemplar for major depression might include lowered affect, negative (but complicated) self-assessment, and lethargy and lack of motivation, allowing for corresponding explanations in terms of interactions among the biology of mood, cognitive distortions that skew perceptions of reality in ways that maintain depressed mood, and failures of the behavioral activation system (which produces exploratory and reward-seeking behavior). The same process can be applied recursively to symptoms themselves within the wider structure. Thus, for instance, "hopelessness," a symptom of depression and other mood disorders, might have as stereotypical features "automatic cognitions" that lead one to make persistent, wide-ranging negative evaluations that attribute life-impairing problems to oneself ("I got a bad grade because I'm stupid, I've always been stupid and that's why I can't find a girlfriend"). Hopelessness might itself be explained by an interaction of an inherited temperament and stressful, aversive early experiences, together with a general cognitive style that leads one to overestimate one's ability to control the course of one's own life and, hence, one's responsibility. The result is an ecumenical picture, with numerous explanations of different types, at different levels, jostling together in the same structure. The overall idea, though, is that the medical model is vindicated by the general endeavor of tracing abnormalities in behavior and cognition to specific causal factors that are realized in, or mediated by, brain tissue.

A mental disorder is a destructive process that takes place in a human being, and an exemplar represents one such process and its typical outcome. I am not claiming this is a general picture of explanation in science, or even in the life sciences more broadly. I do claim that it preserves most of what's attractive in contemporary psychiatry, makes sense of many of the semiarticulated theoretical claims of psychiatrists, and gives the whole business a realist slant instead of the official operationalist one.

An explanation might not include information at every level of explanation, because, although in general we should identify causal mechanisms at different levels, there may be disorders for which a given level doesn't apply: it may be just a brute fact, for example, that some forms of brain damage produce a given pattern of cognitive deficits in more or less random ways without there being a decomposition of the deficit in terms of underlying cognitive parts that normally carry out components of the overall process.

To explain a mental disorder, then, is to explain an idealized picture of that disorder, to show what causes and sustains it, abstracted away from many of the details of its realization in individual patients. The detailed forms that pathologies take in individuals are the focus of a clinical project, not the scientific one. The scientific project generalizes, whereas the clinical one uses the resources of the science to help individuals.

When we explain a mental disorder, we show that some biological processes cause the symptoms and course. The exemplar represents the syndrome and course, and the model explains the relations between features of the exemplar in terms of a representation of causal processes that occur in a patient. This is what introduces the second indirect relation into the picture. Depending on our knowledge and needs, the model that aims at explaining the exemplar will be more or less idealized. The model-exemplar relation can be manipulated to fit clinical demands as well as scientific constraints, and it can be more or less metaphysically committed. Let me take these points in turn.

If the model is a good one, its structure resembles the processes taking place in subjects who exhibit the symptoms that go into the exemplar. This resemblance relation is adjustable in two respects. First, the model presents opportunities for therapeutic actions. The model defines a set of relations that differ from those present in a patient in two ways. One is precision: qua idealization, the model contains a certain looseness, in that the causal relations it represents need to be made more precise when we look at a patient. The degree to which a symptom is present, for example, might need to be specified precisely in a clinical setting, whereas in the exemplar the symptom can be defined as inhabiting some range of values, any one of which might apply in nature and can be used diagnostically to compute the probability that a given symptom arises in a given category. Also, not every patient instantiates every feature of an exemplar, so not every part of a model will apply to a given patient. Once we understand the relations that exist between parts of the model and the exemplar, we can try to manipulate the model to change or forestall selected outcomes in the real world.

Second, the model can be more or less realistically construed, depending on the information available to the model-builders as well as their general intellectual commitments. The lesion method, for example, correlates biological insults with symptoms, but it does not show that the site of the lesion is responsible for the normal form of the behavior, in the sense of being the piece of tissue where the disturbed computations occur. A model that relates lesions to features of the exemplar thus is not a thoroughgoing realist's model of causal structure, but it does provide predictive utility. In some cases, this might be all we get or all we want. In other cases, the model may depict the actual causal relations responsible for the symptoms. This is what biomedical model building aspires to in general, and I assume it is the goal of psychiatry, but the utility of the lesion method shows that less realistic models can still be of great use. The picture, then, is one in which a clinical description and an account of the natural history of a disorder give us an exemplar: they tell us what has to be explained. The explanation should proceed by displaying causal relations. The causes are diverse biological and nonbiological factors, often interacting in complicated ways, and typically they raise the probability that something will happen, but they do not make it certain. Modeling exemplars is not a search for laws governing mental phenomena, but a search for the causal relations that explain the presence of exemplary features. The assumption is that those relations in the exemplar mirror relations that obtain in actual humans who meet a diagnosis, but an exemplar is a representation of an imaginary, prototypical patient.

The slant is realist even though the relation between explanation and reality is indirect, mediated as it is by the exemplar, which idealizes away the natural variation in clinical phenomena. The relations that hold between bits of the exemplar track relations that obtain between entities in the patient, and these entities include not just observable symptoms but also unobserved causal processes. Not every relation in the exemplar exists in the patient, because some processes do not occur in a given case.

An exemplar is a faithful depiction of causal relations in nature, but not all cases exhibit all causal relata: that is, people usually instantiate only some aspects of the exemplar. People may also instantiate more than one exemplar at a time.

Some exemplars may be simple, with few symptoms and an uncomplicated course. Symptoms include any measurable or observable characteristic, so a lesion is a symptom, as is a behavioral test score, a brain scan, or a biopsy result. Simple exemplars need few additional assumptions to apply to individuals. Disorders that we currently see as neuropsychological rather than psychiatric often have simple exemplars. Associative agnosia, for example, is defined as the inability to recognize an object by sight even though one can recognize it in other ways (by touch, say). That definition, plus associated information about lesions, is a simple exemplar.

Even here there are individual differences in symptoms, because some patients are more disabled than others and there are differences in the form of the disorder, with some patients being especially poor at face recognition and others doing worse at printed-word recognition. Furthermore, the exemplar for associative agnosia, as with many neurospychological conditions, abstracts away from other cognitive deficits and therefore offers us a partial picture of the total symptomatology, even if it offers a complete depiction of part of it.

As well as information about the presentation of a patient at a time, exemplars include information about the course of diseases. Biological psychiatry is often called "neo-Krapelinian" in honor (or not, depending on who's using the term) of Emil Kraepelin. Kraepelin ([1896] 1987, [1899] 1990, 1919) argued that different mental disorders had characteristic histories and kept detailed records on the progress of his patients until he felt able to generalize across them, classifying individuals together on the basis of their shared histories. This emphasis on following the course of a disorder led him to distinguish what we now call schizophrenia from similar conditions. It started, he argued, with a slow decline of general psychological function, accompanied by headaches and physical lassitude. Over time, a progressive dementia set in, at different speeds in different individuals. In some, it did not progress very far. In others, it was swift and calamitous. A stage of excitement and euphoria occurred, followed by a period of calm that appeared to indicate improvement, but soon disease progression showed itself with the onset of severe and profound mental collapse. Kraepelin pointed out that this progressive deterioration characterized a number of patients who had, on the basis of their clinical presentation, been previously thought to exhibit different conditions, including Kraepelin's own diagnosis of dementia paranoides, as well as catatonia and hebephrenia.

Discrimination among conditions via information about their histories is characteristic of theory building in immature medicine: Sydenham used information about course to distinguish similar syndromes in the seventeenth century. Contemporary psychiatry still uses this method to disentangle related diagnoses or support a unitary interpretation of a category. Disagreement over whether a diagnosis is unitary or a collection of several subtypes often turns on the extent to which we can distinguish distinct populations of patients based on separate outcomes. Jellinek (1960), for example, argued that there were several classes of alcoholics, each with a characteristic natural history. Yet Vaillant (1995, pp. 38–39), on the basis of a decades-long study, argued that, "when a longitudinal view of alcoholism is substituted for the cross-sectional view, there do not appear to be many different alcoholisms."

So the course of a disease should be represented in the exemplar along with its symptoms. Exemplar explanation works by displaying the causal relations among pathogenic processes that produce the symptoms and cause them to occur when they do and unfold as they do. The issue I turn to now is whether this ideal can be realized once we move beyond simple neurological cases. In cognitive neuropsychology, we may hope to associate a pattern of physical trauma with a circumscribed, measurable symptom that can be treated in isolation by the theory even if it seldom shows up in isolation in the data. For example, in apperceptive agnosia a description of a neurological deficit and information about accompanying lesions set the explanatory job, which is to make clear how the lesion causes normal relations among cognitive parts to be interrupted or otherwise deformed. This is the basic picture of exemplar explanation in neuropsychology: describe a deficit, find a physical correlate, and explain their real-world relation. How plausible is the hope that the much more complicated exemplars we will generally need in psychiatry could work well enough to make this method a useful general approach? Let me turn now to sketch out some of the complications.

Most psychiatric diagnoses incorporate diverse symptoms and great variation across subjects. In Major Depression, for example, there are nine possible symptoms: depressed mood most of the day; diminished pleasure in all activities most of the time; unexplained changes in weight or appetite; abnormal sleep patterns; psychomotor agitation or retardation; fatigue; feelings of worthlessness; inability to concentrate; thoughts of death or suicide. To merit the diagnosis of major depression, at least five of the nine symptoms must present together during a two-week period, and at least one of the presenting symptoms must be depressed mood or loss of pleasure (American Psychiatric Association 2000, pp. 349–56).

Our current categories often group together very different symptom profiles as manifestations of the same disorder. Thus, one can qualify as having a Major Depressive Episode even though one does not experience a depressed mood, provided that one does exhibit a markedly diminished interest in daily activities, and by one reckoning there were 56 different ways to satisfy the *DSM-III* criteria for Borderline Personality Disorder (Clarkin et al. 1983). As one might expect, these heterogeneous categories are often poor predictors of the patients' future trajectory or of their response to treatment and thus the vast majority of *DSM* categories remain unvalidated. As knowledge progresses, we may hope to see more order imposed on some of these messes, and the proliferation of subtypes that will be more tractable. It is likely that exemplars will always, in general, need to recognize considerable variation, because underlying systems, once disrupted, can manifest in a variety of ways. We should expect patients who share an exemplar to share a disruption to a mechanism that can produce one of a range of results on a test, depending on the context.

Consider the fact that depressives tend to sleep either a lot more or a lot less than average. Imagine this is due to individual differences that cause the circadian mechanism to reacts to stress by either overexpressing or underexpressing the relevant genes (mammalian *per* and *tim*). In that case, we can figuratively imagine a mechanism (the suprachiasmatic nuclei, in fact) with a switch that reacts to stress by moving up or down the dial. We might, for instance, explain the tendency of depressives to sleep a lot more or a lot less than others by citing a circadian mechanism that moves either up or down depending on the other processes at work in the mind or brain of the depressed person. That lets us associate a large range of outcomes with damage to only one underlying mechanism; for example, those who tend to sleep more also tend to eat more and respond better to monoamine oxidase inhibitors.

The goal, then, is to understand the relation between properties of the circadian system and states of the rest of the mind and brain, such that, when the overall cognitive system is working normally the circadian system has an output within normal bounds. However, if the cognitive system gets into some abnormal state, its relation to the circadian system ensures that the latter system is pushed out of its normal state, too, with the result that sleep is either excessive or insufficient. We can readily imagine a feedback effect in which disruptions to normal rhythms have an adverse effect on psychological capacities, like reaction times, that degrade in step with sleep deprivation. Such a behavioral outcome could feed back into the cognitive systems, making one more anxious and thus pushing the circadian mechanism even further askew.

The story about people with depression I envisioned just now would, if we could get it, reflect a robust relation that holds as other conditions change. Indeed, I assumed that changes in the values of cognitive variables, like reaction times, and circadian variables, like hours of sleep, vary in step because they reflect a systematic causal relationship. The relationship continues to hold even when one or the other end is pushed out of normal function by some pathogenic process.

The story is probably false. But it illustrates an important idea that we can exploit when we try to generalize the strategy lying behind the modeling of a simple exemplar that I referred to earlier. In the simple story, a behavioral deficit is associated with a lesion and our job is to explain why a lesion *there* should have a robust relationship with *that* behavioral outcome. On the more complicated story about depression I just made up, we explain the causal process linking some neurocomputational abnormality in one cognitive part to a second cognitive part (the circadian regulator) that mediates between the first part and the behavioral effects and can generate a range of outcomes.

The identification of cognitive parts, which is the job of cognitive neuroscience, is thus central to generalizing the strategies that explain simple neurological exemplars across all psychiatry, bearing in mind, again, that emotional or other affective dysfunction underlies psychiatric illness at least strongly as cognitive pathologies. Cognitive parts produce the symptoms of the exemplar when their normal cognitive or affective functioning is disrupted. That is, a systemic breakdown produces a change in the observable properties of the subject's behavior. If variation in behavioral outcomes reflects the variety of possible outputs of a cognitive part, we can generalize across patients at the level of cognitive parts, even if we cannot do so at the level of outcomes.

The recent enthusiasm for endophenotypes reflects an explanatory bet on a small number of mediating variables rather than a large array of causes and outcomes. As such, it is a way of looking for a crucial level at which maximal tractability can be found. The endophenotype (Gottesman and Gould 2003) is an unobserved intermediate between phenotype and genes. Given the typically large number of genes involved in complex traits and the variation in phenotype across individuals within a diagnosis, Gottesman and Gould advocate a search for endophenotypes as a simplifying heuristic. They suggest that a complicated set of symptoms probably depends on a smaller set of abnormalities at various levels, and each of those underlying abnormalities are built out of what are, relative to the symptoms, a smallish set of genes. Rather than look for a great variety of genes and a great variety of phenotypes, we should look for endophenotypes, which depend on a set of genes and give rise to sets of symptoms.

Gottesman and Gould see endophenotypes as uncovering the genetic causes of disorders. We can liberalize their idea to accord with the presumption that the explanatory task in psychiatry is to look for cognitive parts that mediate between two sets of complicated biological processes. There are so many different levels between the total genotype and the ultimate phenotype that there is little reason to assume that we must restrict our search to only a genetic endophenotype, conceived of as a small set of genes. The hope is that by identifying systems that mediate between causes and symptoms we can impose some tractability amid all the variation, and the correct level at which to mediate depends on theoretical concerns. If exemplar explanation is to work in the face of empirical variation, it will do so by tracing systemic relationships among underlying factors that cause the variation, not trying to deal with each variation. To get a sense of how things might go, let's take schizophrenia, a disorder with many different cognitive, motor, and affective symptoms, and see what the prospects and problems are.

There are two broad explanatory approaches to uncovering the defective mediating systems in schizophrenia. Modular models of the schizophrenia exemplar assign a discrete part of the exemplar to a breakdown in a particular cognitive part. The crucial supposition is that all the diverse genetic, developmental, and environmental factors involved in schizophrenia conspire, in the final state, to produce a set of computational failures in cognitive parts, with failures in different parts explaining different aspects of the disorder. Modular approaches tend to go symptom-by-symptom, tying parts of the syndrome to distinct systems. Modular approaches provide a clear sense of the various tasks that the mind or brain performs and how they can be disrupted.

Global models of schizophrenia, on the other hand, look for a generic biological or cognitive deficit and work bottom-up, identifying a widespread flaw that explains a lot and affects many cognitive parts. More narrowly cognitive models drawn fairly directly from existing practices in cognitive neuroscience currently dominate the field. These do work especially well for schizophrenia, but they must also, in the end, explain flattened affect, the absence of motivation, and the other noncognitive phenomena that characterize schizophrenics. Global models often cite abnormal computational properties of neurons but have not so far connected mathematical models of neurocomputation with psychological processes or symptoms. In light of the great diversity and heterogeneity of problems in schizophrenia, this may be the best we can do. That is, it could just be that, although we can come up with descriptions at the intentional and behavioral level of the various deficits that schizophrenics display, we may not be able to explain them other than as the different manifestations of an underlying failure of communication between neurons, or some other large-scale biological problem. Perhaps the relation between cellular processes and cognitive manifestations is chaotic, with an interaction of genetic susceptibility and environmental factors leading to a failure of normal communication among brain cells, with the consequence that, cognitively, everything falls apart and that looking for distinct explanations for discrete cognitive and affective failures is a fool's errand.

Something like this is obviously part of the truth about schizophrenia. As Meehl (1990, p. 14) puts it, the big fact about schizophrenia is that something is haywire pretty much everywhere, in all systems, at all levels. Perhaps when the system slips out the space of functional states, random biological and environmental factors play the largest role in determining where in the space of nonfunctional states it ends up, and there are no useful causal generalizations to be made, just descriptive ones. On this view, there is one big problem—crudely, poor communication between neurons—that can produce many different results. This is a limited explanation, which essentially points to a robust process at the neurobiological level and says that, as a result of this, all hell breaks loose in the mind.

The history of schizophrenia research is studded with terms like "synaptic slippage," "loosening of associations," or "cognitive dysmetria"

(Andreasen et al. 1999) that are really just fancy names for the process of all hell breaking loose in the mind. A model of the schizophrenia exemplar that connects deficits in particular cognitive parts to discretely assessable aspects of the underlying neurobiological insult (and its many environmental precipitators) may not be attainable, and detailed psychological modeling could be beyond us.

There could, nevertheless, still be models of intermediate scope, somewhere in between the big picture and the individual history. There might be reasons to differentiate subtypes of schizophrenia in terms of the deficits they share, even if they don't share a causal history that is less complicated than the generic schizophrenic causal history. Subtyping schizophrenia in terms of systemic deficits might sort patients into classes that are useful for predictive or therapeutic classes. Similarly, there might be histories that some patients just happen to share, and tracing types of pathways that realize the generic history of schizophrenia might also be useful, even if it doesn't explain much. There could be many different ways to get to the same set of symptoms, so tracing particular pathways would not answer the question of how those symptoms arise, but useful knowledge might be gained by grouping actual sequences together into families. A model like this takes the symptoms of the schizophrenia exemplar and divides them up into families that reflect failures of normal relations to hold among parts of cognition. It then looks to connect those failures with the developmental story by specifying the end state of abnormal brain development even if there is no shared history to that particular deficit. The big model involves a lot of small ones. At the intentional level the smaller models that fit into the overall model each represent a part of the exemplar in terms of functional failure among parts of the human cognitive decomposition. These models track, but may not explain, specific forms that the global neurocomputational breakdown takes. Most of the explanatory burden is likely to be borne by the specification of the neurocomputational problem, so in that sense this picture model is a version of a global approach to explaining schizophrenia. Even so, modular models at an upper level are necessary. The modular approach at the cognitive level can sort disjunctions of fine-grained specifications of neurological breakdown.

Although the neurocomputational story in terms of cellular disconnection probably tells us what makes schizophrenia happen, cognitive characterizations of failures can have a vital role to play in tracking types of

pathology. Rather than looking for generalizations across cellular relationships, we can sort people into classes at the level of systems neuroscience.
Just as talking about beliefs allows you to group physically different set-
ups together in terms of the difference they make to behavior, so talking
about failures of normal intentional relations allows us to group patterns
of neural connections together in terms of the difference they make to
which aspects of the schizophrenia exemplar are displayed.

The upshot, then, is that some exemplars may work for psychiatry as
they do for cognitive neuropsychology at the moment. The aphasias, for
example, are all forms of damage to language systems, and their variety is
explicable in terms of particular lesions within the system. Some psychiatric disorders may yield similarly satisfying systemic explanations. Panic
disorder, if Clark's influential theory is vindicated, might be an example
(Clark 1986, 1988, 1997). Clark argues that panic attacks are triggered and
sustained by catastrophic misinterpretations of bodily signals, such as the
dizziness one may feel when standing up too quickly. Overinterpreting
this as evidence that something is seriously wrong causes your system to
become even more intensely activated, with corresponding physiological
effects that are in turn detected, thus increasing the sense that something
is badly wrong and causing further panicking. Although as many as a quar-
ter of us may experience the occasional episode, persistent panic attacks
are rare, leading Clark to hypothesize that only some people have a tendency to perceive autonomic nervous system events as indications of im-
pending disaster. Clark does not offer a view about why some people are so
sensitive but does cite some evidence that the tendency can be seen as abnormal sensitivity in an evolved monitor of autonomic activity. If it is true
that the susceptibility to panic is a matter of an overtuned cognitive system, we may be able to model the condition effectively as a deficit in a system designed to monitor the body's internal milieu. There are plausible
candidates for the neurological realization of such a system, including
core brainstem regions. (See Damasio 1999 for a general treatment of the
importance to cognition of regulation of the body's internal workings.)

Identifying a bodily monitoring system and tying abnormalities therein
to the symptoms and experimentally derived results on panic that we already have would be, in my terms, to find a systems-level model of the
panic exemplar. If there is a distinct bodily monitoring system comprising
a small number of well-understood cognitive parts, we would have a clear
case of a psychiatric condition receiving an explanation in terms of a mal-

function at the level of systems neuroscience. Many other disorders, such as, probably, schizophrenia, will most likely not be smoothly explicable in this way in terms of a damaged underlying system. Schizophrenia is much more behaviorally diverse than the fairly restricted manifestations of panic, and the diversity is not a product of poor diagnosis but of a wide-ranging, large-scale biological breakdown that has diverse environmental and genetic antecedents. Computational stories might then serve to make the intentional profile more precise and let us track physical causes more perspicuously, but they might not explain much. In other cases, computational, or even cultural and normative factors, may bear most of the explanatory burden. In light of the interaction of so many different factors in a full explanation of most mental illnesses and the many possible ways to go about treating it that these interacting facets offer us, we should not expect any kind of explanation to be fundamental.

ACKNOWLEDGMENTS

For my thinking about models, I owe much to Peter Godfrey-Smith (2005, 2006) and conversations with Michael Weisberg.

REFERENCES

American Psychiatric Association. 2000. *Diagnostic and Statistical Manual of Mental Disorders,* 4th ed. Washington, DC: American Psychiatric Association.

Andreasen, N. C. 1997. Linking Mind and Brain in the Study of Mental Illnesses: A Project for a Scientific Psychopathology. *Science* 275:1586–1593.

Andreasen, N. C., P. Nopoulos, D. S. O'Leary, D. D. Miller, T. Wassink, and M. Flaum. 1999. Defining the Phenotype of Schizophrenia: Cognitive Dysmetria and Its Neural Mechanisms. *Biological Psychiatry* 46:908–920.

Bechtel, W., and R. Richardson. 1992. *Discovering Complexity.* Chicago: University of Chicago Press.

Birnbaum, K. 1923. The Making of a Psychosis. Trans. H. Marshall. In S. R. Hirsch and M. Shepherd (eds.), *Themes and Variations in European Psychiatry* (pp. 197–238). Bristol: John Wright 1974.

Charcot, J.-M. (1887–88) 1987. *Charcot, the Clinician: The Tuesday Lessons.* Trans. C. G. Goetz. Philadelphia: Lippincott, Williams & Wilkins.

Clark, D. M. 1986. A Cognitive Approach to Panic. *Behavior Research and Therapy* 24:461–470.

———. 1988. A Cognitive Model of Panic Attacks. In S. Rachman and J. Maser (eds.), *Panic: Psychological Perspectives* (pp. 71–90). Hillsdale, NJ: Erlbaum.

———. 1997. Panic Disorder and Social Phobia. In D. M. Clark and C. G. Fairburn (eds.), *The Science and Practice of Cognitive Behavior Therapy* (pp. 121–153). Oxford: Oxford University Press.

Clarkin, J., A. Widiger, S. Francis, S. W. Hurt, and M. Gilmore. 1983. Prototypic Typology and the Borderline Personality Disorder. *Journal of Abnormal Psychology* 92:263–275.

Damasio, A. 1999. *The Feeling of What Happens*. New York: Harcourt.

Glymour, C. 1992. Freud's Androids. In J. Neu (ed.), *The Cambridge Companion to Freud* (pp. 44–85). Cambridge: Cambridge University Press.

Godfrey-Smith, P. 2005. Folk Psychology as a Model. Philosophers Imprint, vol. 5, no. 6 (www.philosophersimprint.org/005006/). Accessed May 25, 2007.

———. 2006. The Strategy of Model-Based Science. *Biology and Philosophy* 21: 725–740.

Gottesman, I. I., and T. D. Gould. 2003. The Endophenotype Concept in Psychiatry: Etymology and Strategic Intentions. *American Journal of Psychiatry* 160: 636–645.

Green, M. F 2001. *Schizophrenia Revealed*. New York: W. W. Norton.

Guze, S. B. 1992. *Why Psychiatry Is a Branch of Medicine*. New York: Oxford University Press.

Hatfield, G. 2000. Mental Functions as Constraints on Neurophysiology: Biology and Psychology of Vision. In V. Hardcastle (ed.), *Where Biology Meets Psychology* (pp. 252–271). Cambridge, MA: MIT Press.

Jellinek, E. 1960. *The Disease Concept of Alcoholism*. New Haven, CT: Hillhouse Press.

Kraepelin, E. (1896) 1987. Dementia Praecox. In J. Cutting and M. Shepherd (eds.), *The Clinical Roots of the Schizophrenia Concept* (pp. 13–24). Cambridge: Cambridge University Press.

———. (1899). *Psychiatry: A Textbook for Students and Physicians,* 6th ed. J. Quen (ed.). Trans. H. Metoui and S. Ayed. Canton, Mass: Science History Publications 1990.

———. 1919. *Dementia Praecox and Paraphrenia*. Trans. R. M. Barclay. Edinburgh: E & S. Livingstone.

Lykken, D. 1995. *The Antisocial Personalities*. Hillsdale, NJ: Erlbaum.

Marr, D. 1982. *Vision*. San Francisco: W. H. Freeman.

Meehl, P. E. 1990. Toward an Integrated Theory of Schizotaxy, Schizotypy, and Schizophrenia. *Journal of Personality Disorders* 4:1–99.

Patterson, P. 2002. Maternal Infection: A Window on Neuroimmune Interactions in Fetal Brain Development and Mental Illness. *Current Opinion in Neurobiology* 12:115–118.

Schaffner, K. F. 1994. Reductionistic Approaches to Schizophrenia. In J. Sadler, O. Wiggins, and M. Schwartz (eds.), *Philosophical Perspectives on Psychiatric Diagnostic Classification* (pp. 279–294). Baltimore: Johns Hopkins University Press.

Shi, L., S. H. Fatemi, R. W. Sidwell, and P. H. Patterson. 2003. Maternal Influenza

Infection Causes Marked Behavioral and Pharmacological Changes in the Offspring. *Journal of Neuroscience* 23:297–302.

Sterelny, K. 2003. *Thought in a Hostile World: The Evolution of Human Cognition.*
Oxford: Blackwell.

Vaillant, G. 1995. *The Natural History of Alcoholism Revisited.* Cambridge, MA.:
Harvard University Press.

Wimsatt, W. 1976. Reductionism, Levels of Organization, and the Mind-Body Problem. In G. G. Globus, G. Maxwell, and I. Sadovnik (eds.), *Consciousness and the
Brain: A Scientific and Philosophical Inquiry* (pp. 205–267). London: Plenum.

Zawidski, T., and Bechtel, B. 2004. Gall's Legacy Revisited: Decomposition and Lo-
calization in Cognitive Neuroscience. In C. E. Erneling and D. M. Johnson (eds.),
Mind as a Scientific Object: Between Brain and Culture (pp. 293–316). Oxford:
Oxford University Press.

Comment: Taming Causal Complexity
Sandra D. Mitchell, Ph.D.

Dominic Murphy's chapter investigates the crucial question of how to
manage the complexity of factors and entities involved in generating psychiatric disorders. His strategy is to use cognitive neuroscience as the
model, present an account of how explanation works in that field, and
then see whether and when a transfer of the same types of explanatory
strategies might work in psychiatry.

The basic approach to finding explanations of how cognitive states (for
example, beliefs, perceptions, desires, and so forth) are related to the biology of the brain is by means of decomposition and localization. "Decom-
posing an empirical system into a set of hypothetical related components,
and then validating this decomposition through experiments is part of the
goal of cognitive science" (Bower and Clapper 1989, p. 255). The decomposition can be done functionally (such as, in the late 1950s experiments
were interpreted to suggest that remembering and forgetting were the result
not of a single system but of two subsystems: short-term and long-term
memory [Petersen and Petersen 1959]). Cognitive neuroscience attempts
to both decompose complex cognition into computational subcompo-
nents and localize the behavior in specific areas of the brain. A simple example of localization is that of Broca's area, the frontal cortex that Broca,
in the late nineteenth century, identified as the location for articulate
speech. Most attempts to physically locate the part of the brain involved
in complex cognition and behavior are much less straightforward.

Murphy considers a series of alternative ways to approach explanation in cognitive science, including Marr's epistemic levels of cognition as akin to information processing (computation, algorithm, and implementation), and ontological conceptions of the compositional relationship between levels of organization in the thinking and behaving organism. He finds both of these inadequate ways of locating explanations for psychiatry. Murphy suggests the first, Marr's alternative ways of looking at the same process, fails to address the different processes that are operating at different levels of actual biological organization. The latter, the nested part-whole relationships characterizing hierarchical organization (for example, gene, neuron, cell, brain, organism), fails to recognize the interactions among levels. Explanation in psychiatry, Murphy argues, requires real levels and interaction across them.

The explanatory strategy for cognitive neuroscience is methodologically reductionistic in that decomposition investigates a complex system by looking at the subsystems or parts of that system that are compositionally at a lower level. Investigation is top-down, but explanation of behavior of the system is bottom-up. Indeed, only when the ways in which the "cognitive parts" are related is aggregative or composite will such a strategy alone yield satisfactory accounts (see Mitchell, this volume). If the properties and behavior of the parts themselves depend on properties of the entire system (that is, its composition is integrative), however, decomposition and localization will give only partial information about how a complex behavior is generated.

Murphy argues that the investigation of multiple levels of organization need not be reductionistic in the sense that the final explanation will not privilege a particular level, say, the genetic level. The method might be top-down, but explanations may not be purely bottom-up. Multiple levels will be involved in the final explanation. Indeed, Murphy suggests that because environmental causal factors outside the cognitive agent may influence the behavior of the agent, there could be no adequate reductive explanation purely in terms of molecular level descriptions. I find I agree with Murphy's conclusion (that is, that multiple levels are required), but not with the argument that seems to lie behind it (namely, that external or contextual factors inevitably entail a multilevel approach).

One example Murphy discusses in defending antireductionist multilevel explanation as due to the role of environment is David Lykken's work attributing a genomic basis for psychopathy. According to Lykken some genomes have the phenotype of "hard-to-socialize," which typically leads to psychopathy being expressed in the adult. But, as Murphy tells us, the disorder phenotype can be avoided by environmental factors (that is, a particularly lucky combination of countervailing socialization factors). Thus, knowing the properties of the genetic level alone will not be sufficient to predict or explain the incidence of adult psychopathy. Whether the genes will result in psychopathy depends on the environment as well. Murphy concludes, "Molecular biology cannot aim at replacing generalizations about environmental factors like a socialization process with generalizations about the molecular basis of those environmental factors. Most of the causal relations that psychiatry will need to understand will be these organism-environment interactions that cross levels" (p. 109).

There are two ways to interpret Murphy's claim, only one of which entails the necessity of a multilevel explanation. The weaker claim invokes only the *fact* that components besides the genetic ones contribute to the final outcome, but there are different ways in which environmental factors contribute to an outcome, not all of which require a nonreductive explanation. It is in the specific *way* in which the nongenetic factors contribute that an argument for multiple levels can be justified.

Any explanation that appeals to the cause of an effect has to specify the conditions under which that causal relationship will be realized. The other background factors besides the targeted causal agent will contribute to the final outcome. One says that striking the match causes the flame, even though oxygen is a required background condition. One says that the autosomal recessive genetic mutation on chromosome 12 causes PKU disease (that is, a failure of the normal enzyme development required to convert phenylalanine to tyrosine), although it is in conjunction with standard background conditions that the etiology produces mental retardation. Clearly in other environmental conditions, contrived nonstandard ones, the final effect—mental retardation—can be counterbalanced. Indeed, that is why there is neonatal screening for PKU, so the nonstandard background conditions can constitute treatment to avoid the more dire effects of the genetic structure. In any of these environments, the gene still causes the disease and explains why it occurs, even when there are special conditions that confound the normal final outcome on neuronal development. This is the classic genetic disease, a molecular explanation *par excellence*. Yet its outcome varies with different background conditions.

The mere fact of environmental contributions does not require multiple level explanations of psychiatric disorders. What does make the molecular level explanation insufficient is when the type of interaction of contributing causes is nonadditive or not simply interactive, but mutually determining. This will occur when the environment or nongenetic levels change the genetics or the gene expression within the organism. There are systems in which heritable change in gene expression can be induced by changing the environment during development (for an example for maize, see Mikula 1995). There are two different diseases with the same molecular signature but whose expression is determined by whether the gene was inherited from the mother or father. Angelman syndrome is associated with intellectual and developmental delay, speech impediment, sleep disturbance, unstable jerky gait, seizures, hand flapping movements, frequent laughter/smiling, and usually a happy demeanor. Prader-Willi syndrome is identified by extreme and insatiable appetite. Both are caused by the same molecular structure, the same genetic segment deletion on chromosome 15. However, whether the molecular structure causes one or the other syndrome depends on whether the genes were inherited from the mother or father, respectively. The causal properties of the same molecular level structure are themselves determined by other contextual factors. In this case knowing the molecular level, reductionist description alone doesn't tell you the causal upshot. The role of external environment in mediating some distal phenotype may still contribute or not, but in the case described another level of organization is required to determine the causal properties of the gene. The type of interaction of causal components, not just the fact that there are other causal components, is what, I believe, entails the need for multiple levels in giving a causal explanation. As Murphy succinctly puts it, "Nothing is fundamental."

Both situations of environmental component contribution or of environmental transformation of the molecular level draw attention to the inadequacy of a standard reductionist approach to causal explanation. Typically a causal narrative is a monologue. There is the main actor (who, for example, is responsible for the effect of interest), and the other factors we relegate to a kind of undistinguished chorus in the shadows in the back of the stage. There is a "gene for" schizophrenia, Bipolar Disorder, and autism (Cloninger 2002; Kendler 2006). Indeed, there is something going on at the genetic level that is relevant to the etiology of these disorders, but the language of "gene for" falls into the trap of the causal monologue, backgrounding the other factors that play an equally contributing causal role in the generation of an effect and whose explanatory status may be as significant as that of the gene. When the organization of the multiple causes involved in producing a complex effect fail, to be aggregative, then reductive approaches are bound to fails and "gene-for" attributions are misleading. As Wimsatt (2000) argued, there are many ways in which a system can fail to be aggregative, and these will correspond to different causal architectures for locating the role of genes.

That psychiatric disease almost invariably involves multiple component causes, complex interactions among the components, variant histories, and large natural variation impels Murphy to endorse explanation by means of exemplars, rather than regularities. The exemplar is an idealized model of an individual experience of a psychiatric disorder with only some features and not the full-detailed idiosyncratic features of the individual represented. The exemplar has only one disorder and the aim is to discover robust features of the individual case that can be exported to explain a class of individuals. "Exemplar explanation works by displaying the causal relations among pathogenic processes that produce the symptoms and cause them to occur when they do and unfold as they do" (p. 116).

The exemplar approach has much to recommend it. My own work on idealized causal models (see Mitchell 2002, 2003) argued that scientific approaches often isolate individual causes to determine what contribution they can make to an effect which is most likely the result of a complex constellation of causes acting in nature. The example I considered was different factors subject to self-organization processes in contributing to the presence of division of labor in social insect colonies. Genetic variation among individuals in response-time to a foraging stimulus, different learned information among individuals, and staggered timing of emergence into the architecturally stratified hive have all been modeled individually, and each predicts colony-level division of labor. The theoretically idealized models described what does not happen in nature, namely that the three causes would act singly in the absence of the others. What I then counseled was for an integrative pluralistic approach to generating explanations. Namely, that modeling individual causes was a useful and tractable enterprise, but that explanation of actual situations in nature required the accounts of the individual causes to be integrated.

I believe explanatory integration is more appropriate than theoretical unification because natural variation is not only found in biological systems but is expected based on historical contingency and evolutionary opportunism. For example, both euosocial ants and bees display division of labor, yet most ants have little genetic diversity whereas honeybees have a great deal of genetic diversity, Hence the role or even presence of a genetic causal component in generating division of labor would differ in the two cases.

Murphy's exemplar approach is importantly different from integrative pluralism. He suggests than an individual, though ideal, case with multiple causes be modeled to determine how all the component causes contribute to bringing about the effect of interest. Multiple levels of organization—genes, neuronal behavior, brain anatomy, childhood experiences, and wider environmental factors—would all be included in a single integrated model of the etiology of schizophrenia or depression. Exemplars let the scientist explore the space of causal interaction among levels of organization as well as what might be multiple causes within a level. How levels and causes work together to produce the disorder in a single idealized case is the goal of exemplar explanation. In my account of integrative pluralism, the theoretical work was directed to determining how each level or cause could contribute alone, and the integrative work of putting them together was left for the application of multiple models simultaneously to a specific concrete case.

There are advantages and disadvantages to each of these approaches to managing the causal complexity ubiquitous in biology in general and characteristic of human psychiatric disorders in particular. Both exemplars and integrative pluralism are approaches that acknowledge the multiplicity of causal components, the significance of their interaction and the variability in the individual realizations of some complex effect. Exemplar models tell us how a disorder could causally come about, but the variability of patients in the clinical environment may mean that the constellation of factors and their interaction modeled in the exemplar does not map directly onto the actual factors and histories experienced by this or that patient. Thus, the issue of how similar the exemplar is to the variety of actual cases becomes important to investigate to know how useable the exemplar is for explanation of the disorder generally. Integrative pluralism models tell us what the causal potential is of each cause in isolation, but it does not say how they jointly contribute and modify and mediate each other in any actual case. For explaining particular actual cases of a complex effect like major depression, which varies from individual to individual, which factors are present and how they can be integrated becomes instrumental to explaining depression.

I suggest that we need both exemplar models and individual models, explanation by similarity and by integration (and probably more) to tame the causal complexity that vexes our understanding of psychiatric disorders. In support I repeat Murphy's closing words, "We should not expect any kind of explanation to be fundamental" nor, I would add, any one kind of investigative strategy to be universal.

REFERENCES

Bower, G. H., and J. P. Clapper. 1989. Experimental Methods and Cognitive Science. In M. I. Posner (ed.), *Foundations of Cognitive Science* (pp. 254–300). Cambridge, MA: MIT Press.

Cloninger, C. R. 2002. The Discovery of Susceptibility Genes for Mental Disorders. *Proceedings of the National Academy of Sciences USA* 99(21):13365–13367.

Kendler, K. S. 2006. "A Gene for . . .": The Nature of Gene Action in Psychiatric Disorders. *Focus* 4:391.

Mikula, B. C. 1995. Environmental Programming of Heritable Epigenetic Changes in Paramutant r-Gene Expression Using Temperature and Light at a Specific Stage of Early Development in Maize Seedlings. *Genetics* 140:1379–1387.

Mitchell, S. D. 2002. Integrative Pluralism. *Biology and Philosophy* 17:55–70.

———. 2003. *Biological Complexity and Integrative Pluralism.* Cambridge: Cambridge University Press.

Peterson, L. R., and M. J. Peterson. 1959. Short-term Retention of Individual Verbal Items. *Journal of Experimental Biology* 58:193–198.

Wimsatt, W. C. 2000. Emergence as Non-Aggregativity and the Biases of Reductionisms. *Foundations of Science* 5:269–297.

Cause and Explanation in Psychiatry

An Interventionist Perspective

JAMES F. WOODWARD, PH.D.

Chapter 4 is the longest and probably the most challenging in this book. In addition to summarizing James Woodward's main points—all of which are about the "nature and structure" of causes in psychiatry—I hope to convince you that this chapter will well repay the effort needed to read it.

As in all biomedical sciences, causal claims are critical in psychiatry because we want to learn how to prevent and treat our disorders, efforts that to be maximally effective must be based on an understanding of the relevant causal pathways. Because of the great diversity of possible causes for psychiatric disorders, however, questions about the fundamental nature of causality are likely to be of special importance for our field. Furthermore, because of ethical and practical constraints, a high proportion of research focusing on understanding the causes of psychiatric illness is observational rather than experimental in nature. Making causal claims from such data, although commonly done, is fraught with hazard.

Woodward begins with an important distinction that will run through his chapter—differences between "upper-level" (or "coarse-grained") and "lower-level" (or "fine-grained") causes. By "upper level," Woodward means more abstract and less physical in nature, as might be found in studies focusing on psychological, social, or cultural variables. By "lower level," he means more physical and concrete, as might be found in molecular or systems neuroscience or genetics. (See Woodward's note about his recognition of possible concerns with the widespread concept of "levels" and see Campbell's chapter in this volume, which directly takes on this issue.) One might also think about upper-level explanations as "emergent" and lower-level explanations as "reductive." In this chapter, Woodward "takes on" a hard reductionist agenda, which he amusingly refers to at one point as *causal fundamentalism,* that would argue that "lower-level" explanations should always be regarded as superior to "upper-level" explanations.

This chapter has four parts. Part 1 provides a lucid discussion of the interventionist model (IM) for causation. I won't attempt to repeat Woodward's argument here except to note that the IM is commonsensical in nature. It is based on the intuitively appealing idea that we learn best about what causes what in the world by trying to fiddle—to go out into the world, change things, and then see what happens. That is, we focus on the fundamental question of "What if things had been different?"

The IM model is also a practical one which is well suited for the field of psychiatry and other parts of medicine or psychology, which after all want to alter the world to prevent and treat illness. Note that the ideal approach to learning about causation is experimental intervention (with the randomized controlled trial as the *gold standard*). However, Woodward is more ecumenical and realizes that, with rigorous thinking, design and statistical analysis, it is possible to extract important causal information from observational studies. The IM is a flexible model whose ability to easily move up and down across levels of complexity is a particularly attractive feature.

Woodward emphasizes the importance of *contrastive focus* in thinking about causation. We have to think of cause as the difference between at least two different states of our causal variable—one does or doesn't have a stressful life event. One does or doesn't have a particular genetic variant. He makes the strong point that understanding the right level to optimize the contrastive focus of an effect often will tell us a lot about what "level" of explanation is going to be maximally efficient for understanding and intervening in a complex causal system.

Woodward also addresses the fundamental issue of how to judge the quality of an "explanation" or causal claim about the treatment or etiology of a psychiatric disorder: what makes one explanation superior to another? Think of a controlled trial—drug x is superior to placebo—is this a general law? Well, it was only in adults and only in residents of North America and only in individuals without active drug abuse or mental retardation or schizophrenia, etc. Everything we study has constraints.

Woodward argues that the more general or stable the explanation— the broader the set of conditions under which it operates—the better it is. More general laws just explain more. This is certainly sensible but there is likely to be a relationship between explanatory depth and causal potency for at least some interesting variables in psychiatry. That is, we might find an environmental risk factor that operates in only one particular cultural or sociological context but in that context has a strong impact regardless of any background factors. How would the utility of this compare to a weaker effect that generalized across cultural and sociological contexts?

This idea of generalizability has one attractive feature: it is a "quantitative-like" variable, which is something you can have to a variable degree. This provides a more useful and realistic idea of the explanatory reach of scientific propositions than the dichotomy, popular in some philosophies of science, between laws and accidents. Many important advances in science, and especially in complex areas like psychiatry, fall in between these two extremes.

In the second section of his chapter, Woodward turns to the problem of whether mental states can be true causes—a question of obvious import for the field of psychiatry. He begins this section by noting that from the perspective of the IM model, based on both common human experience (You promise to pay someone to paint your house and darn if he doesn't go off and paint it on the basis of your promise). and science (controlled trials of psychotherapy), mental causation seems to work.

He then goes on, in his third section, to what is probably the most important (and incisive) point of the chapter. He illustrates this point with several examples involving pigeons pecking and monkeys reaching, which deserve careful reading. (I will predict that a focused reading of his section on Andersen's efforts to detect a monkey's motoric intentions from patterns of cortical neuronal firing will produce a satisfying "ah-ha!" experience as readers get his point about why upper-level patterns of activity are more incisively causal than any specific implementation of that pattern.) Here, however, I will try to get to the essence of his argument with a different example. Assume we are trying to predict a particular event—say, suicide attempts. We have one "higher-order" explanatory variable—self-derogatory ideation—proposed by a psychologist and a dozen or more biological explanations (for example, active lateral nucleus of the accumbens, elevated cortisol levels, reduced serotonin metabolism, and so forth) proposed by neuroscientists. Now, let's assume that all the biological explanations truly influence the risk of suicidal ideation but they all "flow through" self-derogatory ideation so that there are many different ways one's brain can get to the state of having self-derogatory ideation. That is, the causal chain goes from many biological explanations to one psychological construct to suicide attempt. What would happen if we analyzed this situation from an IM perspective? We would find that, if we intervened on each biological variable, the effect would be highly dependent (or nongeneralizable) because of the state of all the other complex biological causes. By contrast, if we intervened on self-derogatory ideation (for example, by cognitive therapy) the impact would be more consistent and generalizable. In this artificial case, we can see that if the web of causation is such that a complex and inter-acting set of lower-order causes flows through a simple set of higher-order causes, intervening at the higher level will likely be more effec-tive, generalizable, and just plain "better."

In his fourth section, Woodward turns somewhat more briefly to a related and critical set of topics. Whereas his previous arguments have tended to support the causal effectiveness of upper level processes like the mental, these last set of points raises important concerns about that claim. I would like to emphasize two of his major points here. The first is that many variables that we deal with in psychiatry (think about such constructs as "self-esteem," "depressive cognitions," or "social support") are multifaceted constructs that are unlikely to be causally homogeneous. When we say that high levels of social support reduce risk for depression, how sure are we that all the subcompo-nents of social support (such as social integration [for example, mem-bership in clubs and church groups], the presence of positive emo-tional relationships, the absence of negative, critical relationships, and the presence of instrumental support [for example, someone to come get you if you car breaks down]) are acting in concert on the risk for depression? A priori this is unlikely. That is, to use Woodward's termi-nology, social support may be *causally heterogeneous*. It seems highly likely that Woodward is correct here. However, in some sense, this is the "price of doing business" in the psychological sciences. It is some-thing that we need to get better at but does not in and of itself pose deep problems for causal inference. We just need to get better at de-fining our constructs and using them precisely.

His second point in this fourth section strikes deeper. Recall that a key element in the entire IM is the ability to make "surgical interven-tions" in causal processes—that is, to just change one variable, leaving all the surrounding processes unaltered. He asks whether it is even possible to do this with mental states like beliefs or desires. Could it be that our beliefs and desires are so intertwined that changing one will inevitably change others? While far from a fully satisfactory re-sponse, it is worth considering that behavioral therapies for phobias can be very specific, focusing on altering the fearful response to one stimulus—such as rats or heights or flying. Cognitive therapists also claim to be able to target one relatively specific belief for change. Fi-nally, although this argument has force for the mental world, it also almost certainly describes the neural (or "brain") world as well. In the brain, one cannot easily (especially in humans) change the function of one cell or one subsystem without changing many others as everything is interconnected. It is worth pondering the implications for this high level of interconnectedness (in both mind and brain) for the concept of "surgical" interventions that lies at the heart of the IM of causality.

Those who are interested in following up in greater detail many of the points Woodward raises in this chapter would profit by consulting his recent *Making Things Happen* (2003).

Kenneth S. Kendler, M.D.

REFERENCE

Woodward, J. 2003. *Making Things Happen.* New York: Oxford University Press.

* * *

Issues about the nature and structure of causal explanation in psychiatry and psychology play a central role in methodological discussions in these disciplines. What is involved in discovering "causes" and "causal explanations" in these contexts? To what extent do candidate causal explanations involving "upper-level" or relatively coarse-grained or macroscopic variables such as mental or psychological states (for example, highly self-critical beliefs or low self-esteem) or environmental factors (such as parental abuse) compete with explanations that instead appeal to underlying, "lower-level" or more fine-gained neural, genetic, or biochemical mechanisms?[1] When, if ever, is it more appropriate to frame causal explanations in terms of the former, and when in terms of the latter?

In this chapter, I examine these issues within the framework of the account of causation and causal explanation worked out in my recent book, *Making Things Happen (MTH)(Woodward 2003a).* One of my themes will be that a great deal of philosophical discussion of these issues rests on mistaken assumptions about what it is for a relationship to be causal, about what is involved in providing a causal explanation, and about the role of generalizations in causal explanation. These mistaken assumptions involve an interrelated complex of ideas, described below: a deductive-nomological (*DN*) conception of explanation according to which explaining an outcome is simply a matter of exhibiting a nomologically (or lawfully) sufficient condition for it (that is, deriving a description of the outcome from a "law" and a statement of antecedent conditions), an associated conception of causation according to which a cause is simply a condition (or a nonredundant conjunct in a condition) that is nomologically sufficient for its effect, and the assumption that the contrast between laws and nonlaws is crucial to understanding causation and explanation. By replacing these assumptions with more acceptable alternatives, we will gain a more adequate understanding of the empirical issues that surround the choice of levels of explanation in psychiatry.

My discussion is organized as follows: section 1 sets out my general framework for understanding causation and causal explanation. Sections 2 and 3 then discuss and criticize several arguments that attempt to show that upper-level causal claims (for example, claims that attribute causal efficacy to mental or psychological states) and lower-level causal claims involving neural or physical mechanisms are always in competition with each other, with the former automatically being undercut and rendered false by the latter. The conclusion of this section is that these arguments are misguided: causal claims at different levels do not automatically compete and when they do, there are cases in which upper-level causal claims provide better explanations than lower-level claims; however, as section 4 suggests, there are also cases with the opposite profile, in which lower-level causal claims provide superior explanations. What level of explanation is most appropriate is an empirical matter, dependent, in ways that I will attempt to describe, on the details of particular cases.

1. Interventionism and Its Implications
An Interventionist Conception of Causation

MTH defends a *manipulationist* or *interventionist* account of causation: causal (as opposed to merely correlational) relationships describe what will happen to some variables (effects) when we manipulate or intervene on others (causes). To say that a relationship is causal is to say that it is exploitable for purposes of manipulation and control in a way that merely correlational relationships are not. In view of the goal of finding interventions that will improve patient's mental health, there is an obvious reason why psychiatrists (and others) should care about identifying causal relationships in this sense.

Consider an illustration from Blair, Mitchell, and Blair (2005). These authors note that there is an association between damage to dorsolateral prefrontal cortex D (with accompanying impairment of executive function) and antisocial behavior A but raise the possibility that this may occur not because damage to the dorsolateral prefrontal cortex causes antisocial behavior but because whatever insult I causes damage to the cortex is also likely to cause damage to ventromedial and/or orbitofrontal cortex V, with only the damage to the ventromedial and/or orbitofrontal cortex causing antisocial behavior. If so, Blair et al. remark, the "association between impairment of executive function thought to rely on the dorsolateral prefrontal cortex and anti-social behavior is correlational rather than causal" (2005a, p. 86). This suggestion may be represented graphically as in Figure 4.1.

This causal structure has a natural interpretation in terms of claims about what would happen if certain manipulations were performed. For example, an appropriate manipulation that alters D alone (for example, by damaging it in a normal subject) while leaving V undisturbed should not alter whether the subject exhibits antisocial behavior. By contrast, a manipulation that damages V alone in a normal subject while leaving D intact should change subject's tendency toward antisocial behavior.

Note that it is crucial to the logic of these claims that when we consider, for example, a manipulation of V, the manipulation must not itself cause or be correlated with other causes (such as D) of the putative effect A that are independent of V. Suppose, for example, that Figure 4.1 is correct but that we don't know this and wish to learn whether D causes A—that is, on the interventionist account, whether A will change under an appropriate manipulation of D. One way of manipulating D would be to manipulate I. This would change the value of D in the population, but it would (obviously) not be a good experimental design for determining whether D causes A because this manipulation will also change V and hence confound any effect of D on A with the effect on A of changing V. Instead, we want the manipulation to be such that the variation in D it introduces should be uncorrelated with or independent of other possible causes (such as V) of the putative effect A that are not themselves caused by D. In other words, we want the manipulation of D to be "surgical" in the sense that it affects only D and what is caused by D and does not at the same time change other possibly confounding variables. In the philosophical and statistical literature, a manipulation having these sorts of characteristics is called an *intervention* (see Spirtes, Glymour, and Scheines 2000; Wood-

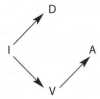

Figure 4.1. Correlational relationship between impairment
of executive function and antisocial behavior.

ward 2003a). If the structure in Figure 4.1 is correct, a genuine intervention on *V* will lead to changes in *A* but an intervention on *D* will not.

Interventions

Giving a precise characterization of the notion of an intervention turns
out to be nontrivial, and the reader is referred to chapter 3 of *MTH* for details. For our purposes, it will be enough to stick with the intuitive conception just illustrated: think of an intervention on one variable *X* with respect to a second variable *Y* as an idealized experimental manipulation of
X which is well designed for the purpose of determining whether *X* causes
Y, in the sense that it excludes various confounding possibilities such as
those described above. In general, an intervention *I* on *X* with respect to *Y*
will be such that *I* causes a change in *X*, *I* does not cause a change in *Y* via
some route that does not go through *X*, and *I* is exogenous in the sense of
not itself having a cause that affects *Y* via a route that does not go through
X. Depending on the system of interest, there are many different ways of
carrying out interventions—in biological/psychiatric contexts, these may
include randomized experiments, the use of gene knockouts in genetics,
and precisely targeted surgical ablations (or other sorts of incapacitations
such as those produced by transcranial magnetic stimulation) of neural
areas in animal models.

Given the notion of an intervention, it is straightforward to give a characterization of what it is for *X* to cause *Y* (or be causally relevant to *Y*). I
will use these notions interchangeably:

(M) *X* causes *Y* if and only if were some intervention (where the notion of an
intervention is understood as above) that changes the value of *X* to occur, *Y*
or the probability distribution of *Y* would change in some regular, stable way,
in some range of background circumstances *B*.

As a further illustration of M, consider the correlation between socioeconomic status (*SES*) and various forms of mental illness: subjects with lower *SES* tend to have a greater prevalence of many forms of mental illness, including schizophrenia and depression (compare Dohrenwend et al. 1992). The existence of these correlations raises obvious causal questions: (1) does lower *SES* cause (some particular form of) mental illness but not vice versa (the "social causation" hypothesis), (2) does mental illness cause lower *SES* but not vice versa ("social selection"), or (3) is it perhaps true both that various forms of mental illness causally influence SES and vice versa?[2] Within an interventionist framework, these possibilities correspond to different claims about the outcomes that would occur if various hypothetical experiments were to be performed. Statement (1) suggests that, if an intervention were to be performed that changes subjects' *SES* (for example, perhaps by provision of additional income, but see below), there would be a corresponding change in the prevalence of mental illness among those subjects but that if we were to perform an intervention that changes the incidence of mental illness (such as by successfully treating these by various drugs or other therapies) there would be no change in subjects' *SES*. (Note that if these manipulations are to count as interventions, the additional income should not affect mental health directly but only through *SES,* and so on.) Statement (2) suggests the opposite profile, whereas statement (3) suggests that interventions on *SES* will be associated with changes in the prevalence of mental illness and that interventions that change the incidence of mental illness will be associated with changes in *SES*.[3] (In fact, according to Dohrenwald et al. [1992], the dominant direction of causation seems to be different for different illnesses.) Low *SES* seems to play an important role in the etiology of depression, while schizophrenia causes a downward drift in *SES*. Obviously, the question of which of these claims about the direction of causation between various forms of mental illness and *SES* is correct has important policy implications. As the authors of a recent study put it, in a way that directly underscores the relationship between causal claims and claims about what will happen under interventions that is embodied in M,

> In terms of policy, the question is important in determining whether intervention and prevention efforts should target socially based adversities that foster depression (e.g., poverty) or focus on protecting persons with mental illness from downward social mobility (e.g., by increasing access to treat-

ment and services, reducing employment discrimination and social stigma, and favoring community integration). (Muntaner et al. 2004, p. 55)

Implications of M

Returning now to statement (M) above, it has several features that will be important to our subsequent discussion. First, it is important to recognize that statement (M) is intended as a characterization of what it *is* for X to cause Y. It is not claimed (indeed, it is obviously false) that the only way to *tell* whether X causes Y is to experimentally intervene on X and see what happens to Y. It is clear that one can sometimes learn about casual relationships by means of inference from passive, nonexperimental observations (for example, by use of various sorts of causal modeling techniques). An illustration is provided by the path diagram in Kendler (2006) (see the introduction to this volume), which is a proposal about the etiology of major depression, arrived at on the basis of structural equation modeling with passive observational data, rather than by carrying out active experimental manipulations of the variables occurring in the model and observing how other variables change. Nonetheless, this path model certainly makes claims about causal relationships. What statement (M) claims is that, to the extent that the relationships posited in the model are correct, they should accurately describe how variables will respond to hypothetical experiments in which interventions occur on the variables that are represented as their causes. Thus, for example, the presence of an arrow in figure I.1 from "dependent stressful life events in the last year" to "episode of major depression in the last year" amounts to the claim that an intervention that changes the incidence of the former variable will alter the incidence of the latter, with the magnitude of this change in standardized units being given by the associated path coefficient—the path diagram is correct to the extent that this claim about what would happen under an intervention is correct.[4] By contrast, the double-headed arrows (which are intended in this context to represent correlation coefficients) carry no such implication: they are claims about "mere correlations." Thus, the double-headed arrow connecting "genetic risk for major depression" to "childhood parental loss" does not imply that intervening to manipulate features of the subject's genotype that increase the risk of depression will alter whether subject is likely to lose a parent.

Well-Defined Variables

A second implication of statement (M) is that for a variable to qualify as a legitimate causal variable within an interventionist framework, the notion of manipulating it must be well defined: it must be the sort of thing that it makes sense to think of as a target for an intervention and there must be a well-defined, unambiguous answer to the question of what will happen to other variables of interest under this intervention. That is, these other variables must exhibit a (somewhat) stable response to the intervention. Some variables that occur in candidate causal claims of interest to psychiatrists and psychologists may not meet this condition. Consider, again, the notion of an intervention on *SES* in connection with the mental illness example. Although income or wealth is one of the variables that usually goes into an index of *SES,* it is far from obvious (as I assumed in passing above) that merely providing subjects with a sizable (even permanent) income supplement will raise their *SES* in the relevant sense, in the absence of other sorts of changes in, for example, occupation, education, social network, and so forth, that are also relevant to *SES*. Relatedly, one may wonder whether alternative ways of intervening to set *SES* to some new level (such as changing income versus changing occupation) are likely to have the same effect on other variables of interest like the prevalence of mental illness. (In fact, there is considerable evidence that income or wealth has a different effect on health, including mental health, than variables associated with occupational position.)[5] To the extent that we are unsure what counts as an intervention on *SES* or the results of such interventions seem to vary depending on whether it is income or occupation that we manipulate, *SES* will be not a well-defined (or at least an entirely well-defined) causal variable from the point of view of an interventionist approach to causation.

I will return below to the question of what makes a variable "well defined," but let me note at this point that one obvious response to the presence of an ill-defined variable is to disaggregate or disambiguate it into more specific, fine-grained variables. Thus, if changing *SES* by changing income is thought to have different effects from changing *SES* by changing occupation, this may mean that we should replace *SES* with two more specific variables, one measuring income and the other some aspect of occupation. As we shall see, this is a consideration that *sometimes* (but not always or automatically) provides a motivation for preferring theories with more fine-grained ("lower-level") variables to theories with more macroscopic, coarse-grained variables—depending on the details of the case, the former variables may have a more well-defined notion of intervention associated with them. To turn to a different illustration, there may be better-defined notions of intervention associated with genetic, molecular, or biochemical mechanisms than with coarse-grained psychological variables such as low self-esteem. To the extent this is so, an interventionist account will regard causal and explanatory claims formulated in terms of the former variables as more satisfactory.

Contrastive Focus

A third point to note about statement (M) is that it relates *changes* in the value of X to *changes* in the value of Y. Statement (M) thus implies that for X to count as a cause of Y, there must be at least two different values of X, x and x', and two different values of Y, such that under an intervention that changes x to x', the value of Y changes from y to y'. This captures the intuition that, whatever else a cause is, it must *make a difference* to its effect: to say that a cause makes a difference to its effect implies that there must be at least two possible states, corresponding to the cause being present or the cause being absent or to the cause being in one state rather than another such that which of these is realized is associated with some change or difference in the state of the effect (the difference between the effect being present or absent, et cetera). Causal claims thus have built into them the feature that philosophers call *contrastive focus* or "rather than" structure: when we make the structure of a causal claim explicit, we see that the real content of the claim is something like this: it is the contrast between X's taking some value x and taking some different value x' that causes the contrast between Y's taking value y and taking some different value y'.

As an illustration, suppose that the display of a red cape (of any shade of red) will cause a bull to charge. This is naturally glossed in contrastive language as the claim that the contrast between the cape's being red rather than not red causes the contrast between the bull's charging rather than not charging. Note, however, that as we vary the contrast within a causal claim, we may change both the meaning and truth-value of the claim. For example, in the example given above it is not true that the contrast between the cape's being one particular shade of red rather than some other, different shade of red causes the bull to charge rather than not charge. This second claim involves a different contrast from the contrast implicit in the original causal claim. More generally, the causal claim that it is the contrast between $X = x$ rather than $X = x'$ that causes the contrast between $Y = y$ rather than $Y = y'$ will be a different causal claim, with a different meaning, from the causal claim that $X = x$ rather than $X = x''$ (where x' x') accounts for this contrast. This is important because in many cases, some changes in the value of a variable will be associated with changes in the value of a second variable and other changes will not be—again, we make the content of the causal claim explicit by spelling this out.

When the contrastive focus of a causal claim is not made explicit, the usual, default convention is to interpret it as claiming that it is the contrast between the presence of the cause and any condition in which the cause is absent (and no other potential cause of the effect is present) that causes the contrast between the occurrence of the effect and its absence. Some examples will help illustrate this point.

As a simple physical illustration, suppose platform will collapse if and only if a weight greater than 1000 kilograms is placed on it. Consider the claim that

(1.1) The fact that the weight on the platform was greater than 1000 kilograms caused the platform to collapse.

Statement (1.1) is naturally interpreted as the claim that the contrast between the weight's being greater than rather than less than 1000 kilograms caused the platform to collapse, a claim that is correct in the specified circumstances. Suppose that, under these same circumstances, it was instead claimed that

(1.2) The weight's being 1600 kilograms caused the collapse.

Statement (1.2) is potentially misleading because it is naturally interpreted as suggesting that the contrast between the weight's being 1600 kilograms rather than some different (presumably lesser) weight accounts for the collapse. Once we recognize the contrastive character of causal claims, we see that, at the very least, statement (1.2) is deficient, in comparison with statement (1.1), in failing to communicate information about the conditions under which the platform would not have collapsed.

Understanding the significance of contrastive focus is important in connection with many causal claims in biomedicine—for example, those that involve threshold effects or systems that respond in a uniform way to stimuli in a certain range but not others. Suppose that an axon will discharge when and only when a stimulus S exceeds a certain threshold k^*. If on some specific occasion or series of occasions, the stimulus takes the specific value k where $k > k^*$, it will be (at best) misleading to cite this specific value as the cause of the axon's discharging, for the same reason that the analogous claim is misleading in the platform example. Instead, it is more perspicuous and accurate to cite the fact that the stimuli are above the threshold (rather than below it) as the cause of the axon's discharging rather than not discharging, thus making the correct contrastive focus of the claim explicit. Similarly, for a neuron or neural region (if there are such) that responds to human faces in an upright position (that is, any human face) and no other stimuli. In this case, it is the contrast between the stimulus being a human face rather than not being a human face that causes the contrast between the response and the absence of any response at all. In such a case, it is misleading to cite the particular face that may have been presented (for example, Bill Clinton's) as the cause of the firing because this suggests that it is the fact that the stimulus was Clinton's face rather than some other face that is relevant to whether the region responds, and we are assuming that this is not the case. Put slightly differently, the claim that it is Clinton's face rather than some other human face that causes the response is a different causal claim that makes a different (and competing) claim about what would happen in a hypothetical experiment from the original causal claim. If we want to learn which of these claims is correct, we can do the relevant experiments—present a non-Clinton but human face and see if the region responds.

I noted above that the demand that variables be well behaved under interventions can sometimes generate a preference for causal claims involving more fine-grained variables. We will see below that respect for the contrastive features of causal claims can sometimes generate an "opposite" (or at least different preference) for claims that involve variables that are more coarse grained and less specific (variables that take values such as "human face" versus "not a human face," rather than more specific values such as "Bill Clinton" or "George Bush"). More generally, one of the reasons why an appreciation of contrastive structure is so important is that it often has important implications for the choice of "level" of explanation.

Pluralism about Levels

How these different considerations (some favoring the fine grained, some the coarse grained) interact and the methodological recommendations they yield will depend on the details of specific cases. This leads to the final point I want to note in connection with statement (M): it does not give automatic or a priori preference to any particular grain or "level" of causal description over any other. In particular, according to M, there is no barrier in principle to relatively upper-level or coarse-grained variables being bona fide causes as long as it is true that interventions that change their values are reliably and stably correlated with changes in their putative effects. Thus, if there is a well-defined notion of manipulating "humiliation" (H) and this is associated in a stable way with changes in depression D (at least for subjects with certain genotypes [see below]), H will count as a legitimate cause of D, despite the fact that these are both relatively coarse-grained or upper-level variables. The interventionist account thus rejects the claim (which we might call *causal fundamentalism*) that we somehow know a priori, as a matter of principle, that variables like H are always causally epiphenomenal, with all of the "real causal action" going on at some lower, more fundamental level that needs to be specified in a much more fine-grained way.

For similar reasons, on an interventionist account, there is, in principle, no bar to mixing variables that are at what might seem to be different "levels" in causal claims. Macrovariables can count as causes of microvariables and vice versa, as long as the right sorts of stable manipulability relationship are present. Thus, if it is true, as it apparently is, that manipulating a monkey's position in a dominance hierarchy (for example, by removing higher-ranking animals) will change its serotonin levels, this will count as a case in which a "social" or environmental variable causally influences a "physiological" variable. Similarly, if interventions on serotonin levels are associated with changes in the monkey's social behavior, this will count as a case in which a physiological variable causally affects a variable describing molar behavior. More generally, on a interventionist conception, relatively coarse-grained environmental events (such as maternal nurturing) can causally influence fine-grained patterns of gene expression, which in turn can influence more macroscopic neural processes (for example, heightened activity in the amygdala), which in turn alter macroscopic mental or behavioral patterns (such as fearful behavior or depression). I emphasize these points because, as we shall see, alternative accounts of causation in the philosophical literature make it much more difficult to make sense of causal claims involving variables at more macrolevels and also to make sense of interlevel causal claims.

Laws, Generalizations, and Stability

I said above that for X to count as a cause of Y on the interventionist account, there must be a "stable" or regular response of Y (or the probability distribution of Y) to some interventions on X, at least in some background circumstances. Some candidate causal claims will fail to satisfy this condition at all, for any interventions or background circumstances. To return to the earlier example, suppose that D and V are correlated, but only because they are joint effects of the common cause I. Then any intervention (in any background circumstances) on D will disrupt this correlation, making D and V independent—in other words, the association between D and V is not stable under *any* intervention on D. This sort of instability (or, alternatively, noninvariance) is thus the mark of an accidental or merely correlational relationship, as opposed to a casual relationship.

Turning now to those relationships among variables that are stable under at least some interventions, in some background circumstances, we see that these may differ with respect to their degree of stability: Some relationships (and the generalizations that describe them) are stable under a wider range of interventions and under a wider range of background conditions than others. At one extreme are relationships that hold under some interventions but only under a restricted set of all possible interventions or only in specialized background circumstances. These relationships (and the generalizations that describe them) count as causal (rather than merely correlational) on the interventionist conception because they can be exploited for purposes of manipulation and control, but they are highly sensitive or fragile: everything has to be "just right" if we are to use them to manipulate. A mechanical example of such a relationship is the input/output relation instantiated by a complicated Rube Goldberg–type machine, the successful operation of which is extremely sensitive to environmental and other sorts of contingencies: if you intervene to pull on the cat's tail with a force of just the right magnitude (neither too hard nor too softly), it will produce a screech, which is picked up by a microphone, which on activation transmits an electrical signal, which (here many intermediate steps) . . . with the end result that a cigarette is lit.[6] Suppose that the nature of the apparatus is such that the cigarette will be lit only if the apparatus is within a narrow range of temperatures, there are no background wind currents, the cat is in some appropriate physiological state, the tail pulling is just the right magnitude, and so on. The relationship between pulling on the cat's tail and the lighting of the cigarette that is instantiated by the apparatus is a genuinely causal (as opposed to merely correlational) relationship because under the right conditions, intervening to pull on the cat's tail is a way of manipulating whether the cigarette is lit, but it is also a highly unstable or sensitive relationship.

As a biological illustration of a relationship that is causal but relatively unstable, consider a particular response pattern acquired through instrumental conditioning, as when a pigeon is trained to peck at all red targets and only at such targets. The pattern of behavior so acquired—call it PECK—is such that we can use it to manipulate whether the pigeon will peck by intervening to present a red or alternatively nonred target. It thus is correct, on an interventionist account of causation, to think of the presentation of the red target as causing the pigeon to peck. Nonetheless, the relationship PECK is obviously relatively fragile in the sense that it would not continue to hold if various background conditions were present—to take only the most obvious possibility, the pigeon might be conditioned to behave differently.

As another biological example, consider a gene Z with the following characteristics: when subjects possess a defective form they are unable to learn to read, when they possess the normal form (and when many other conditions, both genetic and environmental, are satisfied, including exposure to a culture in which there is writing, availability of appropriate instruction, and so forth) they do learn to read. Richard Dawkins (1982), from whom this example is taken, claims that it is appropriate to think of the normal form of Z as "causing" reading. My remarks above suggest that there is something both correct and misleading about this claim. Dawkins is correct in the sense that the relationship between gene Z and reading is, so to speak, minimally causal rather than merely correlational—if all of the other necessary background conditions for acquisition of the ability to read are present, it is true that manipulating whether someone possesses the normal or defective form of the gene is associated with a change in whether that person learns to read or not. On the other hand, the gene $Z \rightarrow$ reading relationship is relatively unstable in the sense that it is exploitable for purposes of manipulation and control only in relatively specialized background conditions; change these very much and the relationship will break down. In particular, the gene $Z \rightarrow$ reading relationship will break down not just under various changes that are internal to the subject such as changes elsewhere in the subject's genome but also under various environmental changes such as changes in whether the subject is exposed to writing, receives certain training, and so on. In this respect, the gene $Z \rightarrow$ reading relationship contrasts with other gene $\rightarrow$ phenotype relationships (such as the relationship between possession of an X rather than a Y chromosome and possession of various secondary sex characteristics), which are comparatively more stable.

Generalizations such as gene $Z \rightarrow$ reading contrast, in the extent of their domains of stability, with the sorts of generalizations we naturally regard as paradigmatic laws of nature. Consider, for example, the field equations of general relativity. It is possible that these will be found to break down under certain special conditions—at very small length scales at which quantum gravitational effects become important—but the current evidence is that they are stable under all other possible interventions and changes in background conditions. They thus have a much wider range of stability/ invariance than generalizations like gene $Z \rightarrow$ reading. A similar point holds for other paradigmatic laws like the Newtonian laws of motion, Maxwell's equations, the Schrodinger equation, and so on.

Other things being equal, explanations that appeal to more stable causal relationships both provide more extensive possibilities for manipulation and control and often at least seem to provide better or deeper explanations—for one thing, such generalizations will often contribute information about more extensive patterns of dependence linking explanans and explanandum[7] variables (than what is contributed by less-stable generalizations). They are thus able to figure in the answers to a wider range of "what if things had been different?" questions (see below). Thus, a generalization like gene $Z \rightarrow$ reading strikes us as explanatorily shallow: we get little or insight into why or how subjects come to read if we are told merely that they have the gene Z for reading. By contrast, more stable generalizations strike us as providing much deeper understanding and, of course, much more information relevant to manipulation.

We may think of generalizations such as gene $Z \rightarrow$ reading and laws of nature as, so to speak, at (nearly) opposite ends of a continuum of stability. Where do typical causal generalizations (or at least the sorts of generalizations we might reasonably hope to discover) in psychology, psychiatry, and biomedicine lie on this continuum? I suggest they lie somewhere between the two extremes described above. On the one hand, it seems clear that most if not all such generalizations are contingent on *some* specialized background conditions and will break down or have exceptions if these conditions are not satisfied. Even causal processes and relationships that are of fundamental importance in biological contexts such as the mechanisms of DNA replication, or the mechanisms underlying the generation of the action potential, obviously require the presence of various sorts of background machinery and conditions and will break down when these are no longer operative. This is reflected in the tendency of biologists, psychologists, and others to eschew or downplay references to "laws" and instead use words such as "cause" (or more specific versions of this word, such as "inhibits," "excites," and so on), "mechanism," "principles" (when referring to causal generalizations), and so on. I take these linguistic practices to be an acknowledgment that, although these disciplines claim to discover causal relationships, these relationships typically lack the sort of universality, near exceptionlessness, and unconditionality we associate with fundamental laws of nature.

On the other hand, it seems a reasonable (and achievable) goal in psychiatry and psychology to aim at the formulation of generalizations and causal relationships that (while they inevitably have some exceptions) are not as highly unstable as generalizations like gene $Z \to$ reading and PECK. In other words, one may hope to find generalizations at, so to speak, an intermediate level of stability. As a first illustration of what this might involve, consider a generalization such as the Rescorla-Wagner rule that describes the conditions under which and the rate at which classical conditioning will occur. In contrast to PECK, which may be disrupted simply by a change in training history, generalizations like Rescola-Wagner are stable under a range of different training histories, even if they are far from exceptionless: they are thus more fundamental than generalizations such as PECK or gene $Z \to$ reading.

As a second illustration, consider the generalization describing the genetic basis for Huntington disease.[8] This disease is caused by abnormalities in a gene (called Huntingtin) on the short arm of chromosome 4—those who develop the disease have a form of the gene with an abnormally large number of CAG repeats. The probability of developing the disease is linked to the number of repeats, with those who have more than 40 repeats having a virtual certainty (or at least an extremely high probability) of developing Huntington disease (provided, of course, that the possessor does not die of something else prior to the onset of the disease). The relationship between, on the one hand, possession of an abnormal form of the Huntingtin gene in which there are more than 40 CAG repeats and, on the other, development of Huntington disease is stable in the sense that if you have this abnormal form of the gene, one has a high probability of getting Huntington disease no matter what else is true—it doesn't matter what else is in one's genotype, or what one's environment is. In my view, this relationship thus furnishes more satisfactory explanations than the gene $Z \rightarrow$ reading relationship.

It may help deepen our understanding of the notion of stability to distinguish it from the notion of the *scope* or *breadth* of a generalization. The scope of a generalization has to do with whether it applies to a wide range of different kinds of systems—that is, with how *widely* or *broadly* it applies. Newton's gravitational inverse square law has, intuitively, very wide scope because it applies at least approximately to any system of masses anywhere in the universe. Darwinian natural selection is a theory that has relatively large scope in the biological realm because it applies in principle to all living things with heritable variation in fitness. By contrast, a generalization has relatively narrow scope if it applies to only some special or specific set of systems rather than generally. The generalization describing the genetic causes of Huntington disease has relatively narrow scope in this sense because it concerns the role of abnormalities in a specific gene in producing a particular form of illness. Note, though, that this relative narrowness of scope is compatible with this generalization being stable; the generalization may apply to only a specific sort of system, but it holds over all sorts of changes or variations in the background circumstances in which that system may be found.

Suppose that, as I think plausible, many of the generalizations that we are able to frame in psychiatry turn out to have relatively narrow scope. One reason why the distinction between stability and scope matters is that this scenario is consistent with those generalizations being relatively stable and thus having, on my view, significant explanatory power. Put slightly differently, whereas generality of scope is unquestionably a desideratum in theory construction, on the interventionist view this is *not* the only desideratum; sometimes it will make sense to prefer generalizations that are relatively narrow in scope but highly stable to generalizations of greater breadth and scope that are less stable.[9]

As a final illustration of the notion of stability, consider the relationship between stressful life experiences, particularly those that have a social dimension and involve humiliation, and depression. As John Campbell (chapter 5 in this volume) notes, it is widely believed that genetic differences cause different people to have different propensities to develop depression in response to stressful experiences. Although several articles have reported a failure to replicate one of the best-known specific proposals about the genetic basis for this difference (that it is due to a polymorphism in the promoter regions of the serotonin transporter 5-HTT gene),[10] let us assume, for the purposes of illustration, that there is some genetic factor that influences the relationship between stress and depression, in the sense that those with genotype G are much more likely to develop depression D in response to certain kinds of stress S than those with a different genotype G'. Although the relationship $S \rightarrow D$ between stress and depression is not stable under variations in genotype, it may well be that for both those with genotype G and those with genotype G', the $S \rightarrow D$ relationship is stable (at least qualitatively) under many *other* sorts of alterations in background conditions (for example, it holds for people of different ethnicities and backgrounds, living in different circumstances, and so on). To the extent this is so, the $S \rightarrow D$ relationship will at least be more stable than the gene $Z \rightarrow$ reading relationship even if it is less stable than the relationship describing the genetic basis for Huntington disease.[11]

Stability versus Laws

This view (that generalizations can differ in degree of stability and that this matters for the quality of the explanations in which the generalizations figure) differs sharply from what might be described as the received view in philosophy about the role of generalizations in explanation. According to the received view, there are just two, mutually exclusive possibilities: a true generalization is a "law of nature" or it is "accidental" and describes a mere correlation. Thus, to the extent that generalizations in psychiatry are not merely correlational and do seem to describe casual relationships, they must be regarded as laws. A similar conclusion holds for generalizations like gene $\rightarrow$ reading and PECK above.

It is widely recognized that this way of thinking about causal generalizations creates some serious dialectical difficulties. For one thing, philosophers have generally supposed that paradigmatic laws are exceptionless
(or, as they are often called in the literature, "strict"). It is also generally
agreed that in what philosophers call the "special sciences" (roughly every
area of science outside of physics and chemistry, including the biological
sciences, psychiatry, psychology, and the social sciences) typical causal
generalizations are far from being exceptionless and lack many other characteristics commonly assigned to laws. How then can these generalizations qualify as laws? The standard response is to claim that such generalizations are laws of a special kind, called "ceteris paribus" laws, which
describe relationships that hold, "other things being equal." On this view,
the proper way of thinking about the generalization "Humiliation causes
depression" is to construe it as the "law" that, "other things being equal,
humiliation is followed by depression."

There is, however, an obvious problem with this proposal: some further
explication of the "other things being equal" clause is required if ceteris
paribus laws are to avoid the charge of vacuity. (The worry is that without
such an explication, the proposed ceteris paribus law amounts to nothing
more than the claim that As are followed by Bs except when they aren't.)
There have been many attempts to provide such an explication, but for
various reasons (see Earman et al. 2002; Woodward 2003a, 2003b) they
have been unsuccessful. Even if this difficulty could be overcome, there is
a more fundamental objection to this proposal. It does not allow us draw
the kinds of distinction (with respect to degree of stability and so forth)
among true causal generalizations that have exceptions that we need to be
able to draw—all end up in the catch-all category of ceteris paribus laws.
For example, on this approach, the generalizations gene $Z \rightarrow$ reading and
PECK as well as more stable relationships like Rescorla-Wagner and the
generalization describing the genetic basis of Huntington disease all are
classified together as ceteris paribus laws, despite the important differences among these generalizations. In other words, the "ceteris paribus
laws" approach does not have the resources to distinguish between causal
generalizations that are shallow and superficial and those that are of more
fundamental interest, as long as both have exceptions (and, to repeat, all
generalizations in the special sciences will).[12]

At this point the reader (especially if he or she is not a professional
philosopher) may well wonder what the motivation is in the first place for

trying to construe causal generalizations in the special sciences as laws of any kind, whether strict or ceteris paribus. Why try to shoehorn such generalizations into a category that they don't seem to fit? Several factors are at work. Until recently, the law versus accidental generalization dichotomy has been the only framework philosophers have had for thinking about the status of generalizations that describe true causal relationships but that also seem to have exceptions. Because such generalizations do not describe mere correlations, philosophers have thought that treating them as laws of some kind is the only alternative.

Another strong motivation has been a widespread commitment to philosophical theories that take the notion of law to be crucial to understanding causation and explanation. It is widely believed that all true causal claims must "instantiate," or be backed by laws—this is often described as the thesis of the nomological character of causation, "nomological" being a philosophers term of art for "lawful." On this view, a cause is just an event or property that is a nomologically sufficient condition (or a part or conjunct in such a condition) for its effect: C causes E if and only if there is a law stating that when C occurs (and perhaps certain other conditions are met) E always follows. Explanation is understood along similar lines: explanation of an outcome consists in the exhibition of a nomologically sufficient condition for the outcome. This is the heart of the DN model of explanation, which is discussed briefly below. On such law-based accounts of causation and explanation, it again seems natural (even unavoidable) to insist that if a generalization describes a genuine causal relationship and figures in explanations it must be regarded as a law.

The interventionist account of causation and causal explanation undercuts this motivation by insisting that we should think of causal relationships as connected to the notion of stable or invariant relationships rather than laws. Causal explanation requires not laws or the identification of nomologically sufficient conditions but simply generalizations that describe relationships that are stable under some appropriate range of interventions and changes and that allow us to see how changes in the explanandum[13] are systematically connected to changes in the explanans.

More specifically, according to the interventionist conception, we provide a causal explanation of an outcome by citing causal information that can be used to answer "what if things had been different?" questions: we identify conditions under which the explanandum-outcome would have been different, that is, information about changes that might be used to manipulate or control the outcome. Ideally an explanation should cite all and only those factors, such that changes in them change or make a difference to the explanandum; it is exactly these factors that are casually or explanatorily relevant to the explanandum.

We have already noted that one way in which the interventionist account differs from the *DN* model is that it does not require that a successful explanation cite laws. A second difference is that the *DN* model does *not* impose the requirement that a successful explanation answer "what if things had been different?" questions. As a result, the *DN* model allows pseudo-explanations that cite factors that are explanatorily irrelevant to their explananda in the sense that changes in these factors are not associated with and make no difference to changes in their explananda. Thus, in a well-known example from Wesley Salmon, citing the fact that Jones, a male, has taken birth control pills and the "law" that all men who take birth control pills fail to get pregnant provides a nomologically sufficient condition (and a *DN* style derivation) of Jones's failure to get pregnant but is intuitively no explanation. The interventionist model identifies the crucial factor that is missing: Jones's taking birth control pills is causally and explanatorily irrelevant to his failure to get pregnant because changes in this factor are not associated with (make no difference for) changes in whether he gets pregnant. As this example illustrates, citing a nomologically sufficient condition is *not* the same thing as answering a "what if things had been different" question or identifying a factor that is causally relevant to an outcome. This observation will turn out to be crucial to understanding how explanations at some levels can be more powerful or appropriate than explanations at other levels.

2. Mental Causation
Interventionism and the Mental

I turn now to a closer look at the implications of the framework described in section 1 for how one should think about causation and explanation in psychiatry and psychology. I will focus particularly on the question of whether it is appropriate to think of "mental" or psychological states as genuine causes (of either other mental states or behavior), although many of my conclusions will be applicable to the reality of "upper-level" causation more generally. A number of philosophers have argued for a negative answer to this question, claiming instead that all the causation apparently associated with mental states "really" occurs at some "lower" level (such as physical, biochemical, neural) and must be understood in terms of mechanisms specified at these levels. Although there may *appear* to be causal relationships between mental states, these turn out on more careful analysis to involve mere correlations between causally inert or epiphenomenal items, where these correlations are produced by causal actors at a more fundamental level.

Jagewon Kim gives a clear statement of this view in the following description of the relationship between mental states (M, M*) and the physical states (P, P*) that underlie them or on which they "supervene":[14]

> P is a cause of P*, with M and M* supervening respectively on P and P*. There is a single underlying causal process in this picture, and this process connects two physical properties, P and P*. The correlations between M and M* and between M and P* are . . . regularities arising out of M's and M*'s supervenience on the causally linked P and P*. These observed correlations give us an impression of causation; however, that is only an appearance, and there is no more causation here than between two successive shadows cast by a moving ear or two succession symptoms of a developing pathology. There is a simple and elegant picture, metaphysically speaking, but it will prompt howls of protest from those who think that it has given away something very special and precious, namely the causal efficacy of our minds. Thus is born the problem of mental causation. (2005, p. 21)

To clarify what is being suggested in this passage, it may be helpful to consider Figure 4.2. The vertical arrows from P to M and from P* to M* represent the fact that M supervenes on P and M* supervenes on P*. The ordinary horizontal arrow from P to P* represents the fact that P causes P*. The absence of such an arrow from M to M* corresponds the fact that there is no causal relationship between these two mental states: M and M* are correlated but, as Kim says, only because both supervene on the physical states P and P*, which is where the real causal action resides.

I noted above that the interventionist conception allows "upper-level" factors or variables to be causally efficacious under the right conditions. It similarly seems to provide prima facie support for the claim that "mental" or psychological states can be bona fide causes, both of behavior and other mental states, including states that we associate with mental illness. It certainly seems as though we sometimes intervene on both the mental states

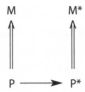

Figure 4.2. Supervenience of mental on physical without mental causation.

of others and perhaps our own mental states as well, and in many circumstances these interventions in turn seem to be stably associated with changes in other mental states and in behavior. If these appearances are correct, then, on an interventionist conception, this is all that is required for genuine mental causation.

Examples of Mental Causation

Apparent examples of mental or psychological causation in this interventionist sense seem ubiquitous in commonsense contexts. Suppose that I promise you aloud that I will pay you $1,000 to paint my house. Then I seem to be trying to manipulate your beliefs—to induce you to believe that I will pay you for performing this service in circumstances in which at least typically you had no such belief before my promise. Furthermore, I hope that this change in belief will cause changes in other beliefs of yours and in your behavior (for example, I hope that this change in belief will [help to] cause you to begin painting the house). If you do paint the house, why should we not think of this behavior as caused, in part, by the new belief that I induced in you? Similarly, suppose that I successfully deceive you so that you act in a way that is to my financial advantage. Is this not a matter of causing you to hold some false belief that, in turn, causes you to behave in certain ways?

These are everyday, commonsense cases but mental causation in the interventionist sense doesn't seem confined to such contexts. Certain kinds of psychotherapy of a relatively cognitivist variety seek to alter patients' behavior and affect in part by altering their beliefs. For example, patients who are depressed are encouraged to think positive, self-affirming thoughts about themselves and to avoid thoughts that present themselves in a negative, self-belittling light. It is an empirical fact, revealed in numerous randomized experimental trials, that in some patients such therapy can be effective in alleviating depression (and significantly superior to "placebo" conditions such as being on a "waiting" list), even in the absence of medication. It seems natural to think of this as a case in which changes in a patient's beliefs or thoughts about themselves (whether induced by the therapist or the patient themselves) cause changes in emotional experience. For purposes of comparison, consider other mental illnesses and disorders such as schizophrenia. In this case, in most randomized studies, there appears to be no stable difference in the alleviation of core symptoms between subjects with schizophrenia who are exposed to psychotherapy and other schizophrenics who are not. Those holding an interventionist conception of causation will take such results to suggest that psychotherapy does not cause changes in the mental states and behavior associated with this illness. In both cases, however, on an interventionist conception, it is an empirical question, to be decided by experimentation or some other means, whether exposure to psychotherapy causes changes in subjects' thought patterns that, in turn, cause changes in behavior. This question cannot be answered in the negative on the a priori grounds that beliefs and thoughts can never be causes of anything.

3. Arguments against Mental Causation

Although the notion of mental causation thus seems, at least on the surface, unproblematic from an interventionist perspective, the philosophical literature, as I have already noted, is full of arguments to the contrary—arguments that purport to show that mental states or properties cannot (ever) cause other mental states or behavior. Some of these arguments are intricate and likely to be of interest only to professional philosophers. In what follows, I will try to eschew technicalities and just give the reader a general sense of some of the considerations that have been taken to support the this conclusion and why in my view they are unconvincing.

Multiple Realizability

Some brief stage setting is necessary. The current orthodoxy in philosophy about the relationship between the mental or psychological and the neural or physical (I will use these terms interchangeably) is that mental states are "multiply realized." This means that a number of different physical states and/or neural states may and typically do correspond to or realize or serve as the substrate for the same mental state. Different philosophers have different expectations about how much (or what sort of) variability of this sort should be expected. One relevant possibility is variability of realization of the same (type of) mental state within a single person over time or on different occasions. It may be, for example, that my intention I to reach for a grape at time t is realized by some physical or neural state P_1 and that same intention I, formed at some later time t', is realized by some somewhat different physical state P_2. (See below for why I have chosen this particular example.) Similarly, there may be variability of realization across people—the neural state that realizes the intention to reach for a grape in you (on a particular occasion or more generally) may be different from than the neural state or states that realize this intention in me. Finally, and more radically, many philosophers are prepared to countenance the possibility that, if there should exist sufficiently cognitively sophisticated creatures or machines with a different biology or material composition from humans, then the "same" beliefs and other mental states might be realized in them in different ways from in humans.

It is usually supposed that, if mental states are multiply realizable, then this rules out the possibility of any theory according to which types of mental state or mental property are identical with types of physical state or property. If the belief that the Pythagorean theorem is true is realized one way (in a certain neural structure or class of such structures) in humans and a different way in silicon-based Martians, then (it is supposed) there will be no common physical structure or property holding across these two set of creatures to identify with this belief.[15]

What is the bearing of the doctrine of multiple realizability (hereafter MRT) on issues of mental causation? The doctrine was seen by its original proponents, like Fodor and Putnam, as a way of preserving the autonomy (and causal efficacy) of the mental,[16] but more recently a number of philosophers (for example, Kim 2005) have argued that MRT undercuts or at least is in considerable tension with the idea that there is such a thing as mental or psychological causation. In what follows I explore some of these arguments.

The Preference for Fine-Grained Causal Explanations

One motivation for skepticism about assigning any causal role to the mental derives from the assumption of MRT combined with the thought that there is a general preference for detailed or fine-grained or more microlevel causal claims (or explanations) over less-detailed, more macrolevel claims. Suppose that my intention I to reach for a grape on some particular occasion is followed by my reaching for that grape (call this behavior R). The intention I is described in a commonsense psychological way, but, according to the doctrine of multiple realizability, I will be realized in the brain on any particular occasion by some complex neural/physical structure P. Suppose, furthermore, that P is by itself "nomologically sufficient" for the occurrence of R, given the rest of the condition of my brain—that is, it follows, as a matter of law, from the occurrence of P and the rest of the condition of my brain that R must occur. (This assumption will be plausible if the brain is (or is nearly) a deterministic system.) Then, one argument goes, given the greater detail of P, why isn't it at least preferable and perhaps mandatory to explain R in terms of P rather than I? Or, as an alternative route to the same conclusion, why can't we argue as follows: because, given the condition of the rest of the brain, P is nomologically sufficient for R, why do we need to bring I into the picture at all? If P by itself is "enough" for R (in the sense of being sufficient for it), it looks as though there is "no causal work" left over for I to do and that I is redundant or causally idle.[17] (This is a version of the so-called *causal exclusion argument*, according to which the causal role of P in bringing about R *excludes* any causal role for I.)

To explore the cogency of this reasoning, consider some other examples involving a choice between more or less fine-grained causal information. Stephen Yablo (1992) describes the case (already briefly encountered in section 1) of a pigeon that been trained to peck at a target when and only when presented with a red stimulus (that is, a stimulus of any shade of red). Suppose that on some particular occasion, the pigeon is presented with a particular shade of scarlet and pecks at the target. Consider the following two causal claims/causal explanations:

(3.1) The presentation of a scarlet target caused the pigeon to peck.

(3.2) The presentation of a red target caused the pigeon to peck.

There is an obvious sense in which explanation (3.1) seems inappropriately specific or insufficiently general, in comparison with explanation (3.2). Or, at least, to make a much weaker claim, it does not seem plausible that explanation (3.1) should be judged superior to explanation (3.2) just on the grounds of its greater specificity. (It is true, as noted, that the red target → pecking relationship is relatively unstable but the pecking → scarlet relationship is equally unstable, so considerations of stability provide no grounds for preferring the one to the other.) Moreover, even if we accept explanation (3.1) as a true causal claim, it seems misguided to regard it as in competition with explanation (3.2) in the sense that acceptance of the former requires us to regard the latter as false or that the truth of the former "excludes" the latter. The basis for these assessments falls naturally out of the interventionist account of section 1. What we are usually interested in when we ask for a cause or causal explanation of the pigeon's pecking is something that accounts for the contrast between the pigeon's pecking rather than not pecking at all. There is relevant information about this contrast—about the conditions under which both pecking and not pecking will occur—that is conveyed by explanation (3.2) but not by explanation (3.1). The default reading of explanation (3.2) with its contrastive focus made explicit is:

> (3.2) The contrast between the target's being red rather than not red causes the contrast between the pigeon's pecking rather than not pecking.

Explanation (3.2) thus tells us, for example, that if the target had been some other shade of red besides scarlet the pigeon still would have pecked and that for the pigeon not to peck we must produce a target that is not red at all. (Note also that this has a straightforward interventionist interpretation in terms of what will happen under interventions that change the color of the target from red to not red.) By contrast, the default reading of explanation (3.1) is:

> (3.1) The contrast between the targets being scarlet rather than not scarlet causes the contrast between the pigeon's pecking rather than not pecking.

Interpreted as claiming that the pigeon will not peck if the target is not scarlet (but still red), explanation (3.1) is false. Even if we find this default interpretation uncharitable, it remains true that explanation (3.1) tells us less than we would like to know about the full range of conditions under which the pigeon will peck or not peck. In this sense, explanation (3.1) conveys less causally and explanatorily relevant information than explanation (3.2), despite invoking a causal factor (the target's being scarlet) that is in some obvious sense "more specific" that the causal factor to which explanation (3.2) appeals.

How is it possible for explanation (3.1) to convey more specific information and yet be a less good or accurate explanation than explanation (3.2)? The broad outlines of the answer to this question were given by Wesley Salmon years ago (see, for example, Salmon 1984, pp. 92ff) when he observed that citing factors that are relevant to the explanandum is at the heart of successful explanation and that the addition of causally irrelevant information to an explanation can make it a less good explanation (or even no explanation at all), even though this also may make the explanation more specific and detailed. In other words, when it comes to explanation, what matters is not detail and specificity per se but *relevant* detail and specificity. Recall that within the interventionist framework, (1) a factor is causally and explanatorily irrelevant if variations in its values (when produced by interventions) are not associated with any changes in the value of the explanandum-phenomenon. In addition, (2) we want to cite explanans factors variations in the value of which (when produced by interventions) are associated with the full range of variation in the explanandum outcome and do not misleadingly suggest that certain variations will be associated with changes in the explanandum outcome when this is not the case. The possibility of complete irrelevance (1) is illustrated by the birth control pills example described in section 1. Causal claims/explanations like explanation (3.1) illustrate the importance of desideratum (2), which can also be thought of as requirement that excludes causally irrelevant information (in this case, information that is overly specific in the sense illustrated by explanation [3.1]). Both 1 and 2 are at the heart of the "what if things had been different?" conception of explanation: a good explanation should cite factors variations in the value of which (when produced by interventions) are associated with the full range of variation in the explanandum phenomenon that we are trying to account for and it should cite only such factors.

Returning to the pigeon example, note that, under the imagined conditions, the presentation of the scarlet target is nomologically sufficient (or at least part of a nomologically sufficient condition) for the pigeon to peck, given the way that the philosophical literature understands the notion of "law." This again illustrates the point that there is more to successful explanation or informative casual claims than the provision of nomologically sufficient conditions or the construction of *DN* explanations.

Note also that under a different experimental set-up in which the pigeon was instead trained to peck only in response to the target's being scarlet, it would be natural to regard explanation (3.1) as true and explanation (3.2) as false. This again underscores the point that we should think of explanation (3.1) and explanation (3.2) as *different* causal claims, having different implications about the manipulability relationships or the patterns of dependency that hold in the situation of interest: explanation (3.1) claims that we can manipulate whether the pigeon pecks by changing the target from red to not-red, whereas explanation (3.2) claims that merely changing whether the target is scarlet will do this. If this is correct, there can be no general preference for explanation (3.2) over explanation (3.1) simply on grounds of its greater specificity—the appropriateness of each will depend on such facts as whether the pigeon pecks in response to nonscarlet shades of red.

What does this have to do with mental causation? My contention is that, at least sometimes, claims about mental causation and its relationship to underlying physical or neural states are relevantly like the red/scarlet example. Consider some research concerning the neural coding of intention to reach carried out by Richard Andersen and colleagues at Caltech (Mussalam et al. 2004).[18] They recorded from individual neurons using arrays of electrodes implanted in the parietal reach region (PRR) of the posterior parietal cortex in macaque monkeys. Previous research had suggested that this region encodes what Andersen et al. call "intentions" to reach for specific targets—that is, higher-order plans or goals to reach toward one target or goal rather than another (for example, an apple at a specific location rather than an orange at some other location) rather than more specific instructions concerning the exact limb trajectory to be followed in reaching toward the target, the latter information being represented elsewhere in motor areas. Andersen used a data-mining program to learn how variations in the recorded signals were systematically associated with variations in intentions to reach for specific goals, as revealed in reaching movements. After several months, this program was able to forecast accurately where the monkeys would reach toward one of eight positions at which an icon was located some 67 percent of the time as opposed to the 12 percent prediction rate that would be obtainable by chance.

One of Andersen's goals is to enable paralyzed subjects to use the neural signals encoding intentions to direct a prosthetic limb toward one or another goal. That is, his hope is that such subjects could control the goals toward which a prosthetic limb would be directed by forming different intentions, which would then be decoded, the resulting neural signals directing the limb. From an interventionist perspective, this is as about as clear a case of mental causation as one could imagine: the subject's having intention I_1 to reach for some goal rather than the different intention I_2 to reach for a different goal causes movement of the limb toward the first goal rather than another—the subject uses her intentions to manipulate the position of the limb. Presumably one could also in principle run this whole procedure backward—if we were to introduce the right pattern of activation exogenously in the PRR of a normal, nonparalyzed subject, this would cause reaching behavior.

Let us consider the causal structure of this example in a bit more detail. The signals that were recorded in Mussalam et al. (2004) were the firing rates (spikes/second) over a temporal period from a number of individual neurons, which were then aggregated.[19] Suppose that a particular monkey forms the intention to reach for a certain goal on several different occasions. At this point it is not known to what extent the pattern of neural firing down to the behavior of individual neurons varies across these occasions.[20] One extreme possibility is that the pattern of firing at the level of individual neurons (that is, not just firing rate but the exact temporal characteristics of the signal) is exactly the same on each of these occasions. Another, arguably more plausible, possibility is that what matters to the realization of the same intention is some function of the aggregate behavior of many neurons taken together and that sameness of this aggregate profile is consistent with significant variation in the behavior individual neurons on different occasions on which the intention is realized. Note that, to the extent that the (or a) crucial variable in the encoding of intention is firing rate,[21] this seems to open up the theoretical possibility that some variations in the behavior of individual neurons that are consistent with their realizing the same aggregate function of neural firing rates will not be relevant to which intention is represented. To the extent this is so, it will be possible for the same intention to be "multiply realized" on different occasions. In what follows, I will assume that such multiple realization sometimes occurs and will explore some implications of this assumption.

Assume, then, that some particular (individual or token) pattern of firing N_{11} in the relevant set of neurons realizes or encodes the intention I_1 to reach for a particular goal on some particular occasion. Call the latter action $R_1.$ Assume that there are other token patterns of neural firing, $N_{12,}$ $N_{13,}$ and so on, that would have realized the same intention I_1. The preference for micro or fine-grained causation we are considering recommends in this case that we should regard N_{11} as the real cause of R_1 on this occasion. But this seems wrong for the same reason it seems wrong to say that it is the scarlet color of the target that causes the pigeon to peck in circumstances in which the pigeon will peck at any red target. What we are interested in explaining (finding the cause of) is variations in reach toward different goal objects—why the monkey exhibits reaching behavior R_1 rather than different reaching behavior R_2. To explain this explanandum we need to identify states or conditions, variations in which, when produced by interventions, would be stably correlated with changes from R_1 to R_2. Ex hypothesi, merely citing N_{11} does not accomplish this, because it tells us nothing about the conditions under which alternatives to R_1 would be realized. This is because many variations on N_{11} (N_{12}, N_{13}, etc.) are consistent with I_1 and hence will lead to R_1, rather than some alternative to R_1, and the proposed explanation which appeals just to N_{11} does not tell us which of these variations on N_{11} will lead to alternatives to R_1 and which will not. By way of contrast, both appealing to the monkey's intentions *and* appealing to the abstract facts about patterns of neural firing that distinguish the encoding of one intention from the encoding of a distinct intention will accomplish this: it is the fact that the monkey has intention I_1 rather than intention 1_2 that causes behavior R_1 rather than R_2. Similarly, it is the fact that the PRR exhibits the pattern of neural firing P_1 rather than the different pattern of firing P_2 (which encodes a distinct intention) that causes the monkey to exhibit R_1 rather than R_2.[22]

The general form of this solution to the problem of how mental (and other "upper-level") properties can play a causal role is not original with me. Broadly similar proposals have been advanced by Yablo and by Pettit and Jackson (1990),[23] among others. Yablo describes his solution in terms of the requirement that causes fit with or be "proportional" to their effects—that they be just "enough" for their effects, neither omitting too much relevant detail nor containing too much irrelevant detail. In this terminology, I_1 fits with or is proportional to R_1 in a way that N_{11} does (is) not. Similarly, on the assumption that the pigeon responds to all and only red targets, the redness of the target fits with the effect of pecking in a way that the scarlet color does not. Yablo's treatment, however, relies heavily on essentialist metaphysics in explaining what is involved in a cause being proportional to its effect. I think that this essentialist metaphysics is not necessary and that, in explicating the intuition behind the requirement of proportionality, one need only appeal to the framework in section 1—an interventionist account of causation, contrastive focus, and so on.

In the cases considered so far, certain candidates for causes are too detailed or specific for the effects we want explained—in this sense, they are at the wrong "level" for their effects. It is interesting to note that a failure of proportionality (or a mismatch of levels) between cause and effect can occur in other ways as well: another possibility is that the candidate effect is too specific for the cause. An illustration is provided by two thought experiments due to Kendler:

> [Suppose that] defects in gene X produce such profound mental retardation that affected individuals never develop speech. Is X a gene for language?

> [Suppose that] a research group has localized a gene that controls development of perfect pitch. Assuming that individuals with perfect pitch tend to particularly appreciate the music of Mozart, should they declare that they have found a gene for liking Mozart? (Kendler 2005)

In both cases, Kendler's view is that the answers to these questions is "no." I agree. The defects in gene X are better described as causing mental retardation—muteness is an insufficiently general (overly specific) description of what the defects cause. Similarly the gene in scenario 2 is better described as a gene for perfect pitch or for pitch perception—again, "liking Mozart" is a too specific effect.

The interventionist account provides a natural justification for these judgments. In the first scenario, changes in whether gene X is defective or not (that is, changes that replace the normal form of the gene with a defective form and vice versa) are associated not just with changes in the ability to speak but with many other changes as well—in the ability to read, do mathematics, live independently, and so on. In describing the effect of variations in gene X, we prefer a characterization that captures the fact that such variations are associated with all of these other changes as well and that presents such information in a parsimonious way, revealing what all these more specific consequences have in common. Thinking of the defects in the gene as causing mental retardation provides more information regarding the answers to "what if things had been different?" questions than if we think of the defect in the gene as causing muteness. Similarly for the gene that influences pitch perception—indeed, in this case the fit between the gene and the "effect" of liking Mozart is even more imperfect than in the previous case. Even assuming that those with the gene are more likely to like Mozart, whether they do so will depend on much else besides possession of the gene (for example, on the sort of music to which they are exposed). In this sense the gene → liking Mozart relationship is like Dawkins' gene → reading relationship in being comparatively unstable or noninvariant. The relationship between lacking the gene and not liking Mozart, moreover, is also unstable in that many people who lack the gene will still like Mozart.

Note again that it is crucial to this whole line of argument that we not think of causes simply as nomologically sufficient conditions or as conjuncts in such conditions and that we *not* think of causal explanation as simply *DN* explanation. The defect in gene X in the first scenario is nomologically sufficient for muteness, and we can construct a *DN* explanation for a subject's muteness by appealing to this generalization. The insight that there is nonetheless something misleading about the claim that defects in gene X cause muteness requires for its motivation the different way of thinking about causation and causal explanation outlined in section 1, according to which causal explanation has to do with the accurate exhibition of systematic patterns of dependency between explanans and explanandum. It is the limitations of "defects in gene X cause muteness" along this last dimension that explain its inadequacy as an explanation.

We can bring out this point in a slightly different way by returning to the research conducted by Andersen et al. and asking what it would look like if its focus or goal were simply the identification of conditions that are nomologically sufficient for the production of reaching behavior. If this were the goal, it would be acceptable to cite the entire state of the whole brain (or any part of it that includes the PRR as a proper part) during the time immediately preceding the behavior of interest, for this will assuredly be a nomologically sufficient condition for the behavior, if anything is. Of course, neither Andersen nor any other neuroscientist does this. Andersen's goal, as he puts it, is to identify "intention specific" neurons—that is, to identify the specific neurons or collections of neurons variations in the state of which correlate with the monkey's intentions and hence are responsible for or make a difference for the monkey's behavior. Then, among these neurons, he wants to identify those specific features of their behavior (whether this has to do with some aggregate function of spike rate or whatever) that encode different intentions. Other states of the monkey's brain in, for example, the occipital cortex that don't covary with changes in the monkey's intentions are irrelevant to this task and hence are ignored. This concern with neural specificity falls naturally out of a concern with causal relevance or with the identification of conditions that make a difference for the behavior of interest but is lost if we focus just on the identification of nomologically sufficient conditions for that behavior.

4. When Micro Is Better

In my discussion so far, I have rejected various arguments designed to show that mental and other upper-level properties are casually inert. In the remainder of this chapter, I want to shift perspective somewhat and explore some other considerations, less discussed in the philosophical literature, that bear on the causal role of upper-level properties, but that in contrast to the arguments surveyed in section 3 do sometimes provide reasons for preferring lower-level or more microlevel causal explanations. Again, many of my examples will concern mental properties, but my discussion will have implications for other sorts of macroproperties as well. The considerations on which I will focus do not undercut *any* possible causal role for the mental in the way that the arguments surveyed in section 3 (if correct) would. They do, however, suggest various ways in which, depending on the empirical details of the case, mental (and certain other upper-level) causal claims may turn out to be less illuminating or satisfactory from the point of achieving scientific understanding than causal claims involving lower-level relationships.

Causal Heterogeneity

The first possibility I want to explore can be introduced by means of an example, recently discussed by Sheines and Spirtes (2004). Before the discovery of the difference between HDL cholesterol and LDL cholesterol, investigators thought in terms of a category which we would now describe as total cholesterol (TC), understood as the sum of HDL (H) and LDL (L) cholesterol levels. Investigators were interested in the causal effect of TC on heart disease D and concluded that higher TC levels caused higher probability of D. Only later was it recognized that H and L have different causal influences on D, with the latter increasing the probability of D and former acting as a preventive of heart disease. Consider an experimental manipulation that increases TC to some new value $TC = c$. There are many different ways of increasing the value of TC—by holding H constant and increasing L, by increasing H and holding L constant, and so on. These different manipulations will have different effects on D, even though they involve the same level of TC, depending on the mix of H and L involved. TC thus might be described as a *causally heterogeneous* variable with respect to D; the effect of a given level of TC on D will depend on how TC is realized. (Spirtes and Scheines say that this is a case in which manipulations of TC are "ambiguous.") To the extent that in different experimental manipulations the same level of TC is achieved by different mixtures of H and L, this ambiguity/heterogeneity will show up in an instability in the relationship between TC and D.

The possibility that I want to consider is that this sort of phenomenon may be common in connection with many macrolevel variables in the social and psychological realms, including mental variables. We have already encountered one possible instance in section 1, where we considered the possibility that different realizations of the SES variable might have different effects on mental illness. As another illustration, consider a causal model in which one attempts to determine the effect of the subject's educational level or whether the subject is divorced on some other macroscopic variable (for example, delinquency of children or depression). If educational level E is measured by, for example, years of schooling, it is plausible that this variable may have a different effect on other behavioral variables, depending on how E is realized—the same number of years in school may involve educations of different quality and so on, and these may have different effects. Similarly, "divorce" may have a different causal effect on other variables, depending on how the divorce is "realized"—acrimonious divorces may have different consequences for childhood delinquency than more amiable divorces.

It seems entirely possible that a similar pattern will sometimes hold for causal claims involving mental states. Suppose, for example, that the same belief B_1 is sometimes realized by neural structure N_{11} and sometimes by neural structure N_{12}. B_1 is the same belief under these two realizations in the sense that whatever procedures we have for attributing and individuating beliefs don't in themselves lead us to make any distinctions among beliefs that are realized in these different ways. If N_{11} tends to cause behavior R_{11} and N_{12} causes behavior R_{12}, where R_{11} and R_{12} are mutually exclusive, B_1 will have a different casual effect on behavior depending on how it is realized neurally. B_1 may either encourage or discourage behavior R_{11}, depending on how B_1 is realized neurally.

Note that these possibilities are different from the possibilities that concerned us in section 3. There it was assumed that (a) some mental state B_1 has disparate neural realizations but (b) all of them are associated with or followed by the same second mental state or behavior B_2—the question was whether the sorts of considerations that underlie the exclusion and related arguments show that B_1 cannot cause B_2. Now we are considering the possibility that although assumption (a) is true, assumption (b) is false—the different realizations of B_1 cause different subsequent mental states or behaviors.

It seems plausible that this sometimes happens in the psychological realm. If a mental state can have disparate neural realizations, why should we expect that all of these realizations will have the same causal homogenous effect on some other mental or behavioral variable of interest? Reinforcing this possibility is the commonplace observation that causation in the mental realm often exhibits apparent indeterminism or instability of results. What looks like the same or similar sets of beliefs, desires, emotions, and so forth can lead to different subsequent mental states or behaviors. One (but, as explained below, not the only) possible explanation of this is that these mental states have causally heterogeneous realizers in the way just described.

As a possible[24] real-life illustration, consider the significance of the discovery of distinct, dissociable fear systems for the etiology of psychopathy. The background is the so-called fear modulation hypothesis (Blair et al. 2005) according to which psychopathy is the result of impairment in the systems involved in the learning of appropriate responses to fear-inducing or aversive stimuli: the psychopath fails to acquire normal patterns of prosocial behavior because he lacks the fearful response to the threat of punishment on which the acquisition of such behavior depends. This hypothesis comports with the observation that psychopaths seem to be much less fearful than normals but fits much less well with other data: for example, there is considerable evidence that successful moral socialization in normal individuals is not based on the threat of punishment as the fear modulation hypothesis apparently requires but instead on the learning of empathetic responses toward potential victims. Moreover, the fear modulation hypothesis has no obvious explanation for the empathy deficits and poor emotional learning that psychopaths exhibit. Finally, and most crucially for our purposes, the hypothesis in effect assumes that there is a unitary fear system that is impaired in psychopaths. There is, however, considerable evidence that humans possess a number of dissociable neural systems that are involved in fear processing and acquisition of responses to aversive stimuli. Moreover, psychopaths are impaired in some kinds of tasks involving fear based conditioning and learning but not others—in particular, they are impaired on passive avoidance learning (in which subjects must learn to respond to "good" stimuli and avoid responding to "bad" stimuli) and more generally on tasks that involve the formation of associations between conditional stimuli and "affective representations" but not on punishment-based instrumental learning tasks that rely on stimulus response associations. Normal performance in the former tasks but not on the latter is dependent on the integrity of the amygdala and, according to Blair et al., amygdala damage is common in psychopaths.

These observations suggest a more specific hypothesis (called by Blair et al. the "integrated emotional systems model," or IES) about the kinds of fear/aversive stimuli processing that are impaired in psychopaths—that the relevant impairments have to do with learning to associate affect-based representations of the badness of moral transgressions with aversive stimuli connected with victim's distress. Roughly the idea is that an intact amygdala in normal individuals allows them to learn to associate moral trangressions with aversive stimuli in the form of fear, sadness, and other emotions of the person transgressed against and hence to learn to avoid such transgression. In psychopaths amygdala dysfunction prevents the learning of such associations.

My concern here is not whether the IES model is correct but, rather, the general strategy that it implements, which consists of taking the causal factor (a general deficit in the system processing fearful or aversive stimuli F) originally proposed as playing a role in the etiology of psychopathy P and replacing it with a more fine-grained factor F^* involving deficits in just certain specific components in this system but not others. If Blair et al. are correct in their empirical claims, this is a case in which F is a causally heterogeneous variable with respect to P (because some but not all subjects with impairment in fear-based learning exhibit P) and a better explanation is achieved by descending to a more fine-grained level of analysis that requires neuroanatomical information (about dysfunction in certain nuclei in the amygdala) for its specification. As in the total choles-

terol example, the more fine-grained variable F^* has more stable and reproducible effects on P than the more coarse-grained variable F.[25]

In my sketch of an interventionist account of causation in section 1, I
in effect noted (although I did not explicitly put it this way) that causal
claims and explanations are subject to at least two desiderata. On the one
hand, we want causal claims to capture the full range of changes in the
cause that are relevant to the effect. On the other hand, we also want the
relationships between the cause and effect variables to be relatively
stable—to hold under some substantial range of interventions and
changes in background conditions. In the examples in section 3 designed
to illustrate the idea that there is no automatic preference for more fine-
grained or lower-level causal claims, we assumed that the upper-level or
more macrocausal claims were relatively stable and not subject to problems like causal heterogeneity—in other words, we set up the examples
so that these two desiderata were not in conflict. For example, we assumed that the red target → pigeon pecking relationship was no more or
less stable than the scarlet → pecking relationship. Because the former captured a dependency relationship that was omitted by the latter—that the
pigeon would peck in response to nonscarlet shades of red—there was an
obvious motive for preferring "red" to "scarlet" as a cause of pecking.

We now see, however, that many real-life examples involving upper-
level causal claims may have a more complex structure: the upper-level
claim may do a better job of capturing a wider and more general range of
dependency relationships than do more fine-grained causal claims, but it
may also be less stable or invariant than the more fine-grained claims.
Thus, the two desiderata *can* come into conflict or be in tension with one
another, although whether they actually *will* be in conflict depends on the
details of the case before us.

As an illustration, consider again a theory involving a macrolevel variable like "humiliation" as a potential cause of, for example, depression. It
seems uncontroversial that "humiliation" will be multiply realized at a
more fine-grained level—call these realizers $N_1, N_2, \ldots N_i$. If the argument
of section 3 is correct, this multiple realization per se is no bar at all to attributing a causal role to humiliation. Indeed, arguing in parallel with the
examples in section 3, we see that if we insist that the true cause of depression on some specific occasion is the realizer N_1 on that occasion,
rather than "humiliation," we are being misleadingly and overly specific,
as long as it is true that the other ways of realizing humiliation (for ex-

ample, via N_2) would have had the same effect on depression; however, we should also appreciate that the italicized phrase contains a major assumption that may well not be satisfied. It may instead be true that some of the different ways of realizing "humiliation" have different causal effects on depression and mental health. To the extent that "humiliation" behaves like "total cholesterol" or "fear" as a causal variable, we have a motive for fragmenting that variable into more fine-grained subunits or categories that have more stable or uniform effects on mental health. We thus may well find ourselves pulled in two different directions, with our interest in generality (as well as sheer ignorance of the relevant fine-grained realizations) prompting us to employ coarse-grained generalizations involving variables like "humiliation," while our interest in finding generalizations that describe more stable and uniform effects (and the greater possibilities of control these afford) instead pull us in the direction of fine-grained microcategories.[26] In this sort of situation, which I suspect is common in the psychological and social sciences, I see no reason to suppose that there must be some single right way of striking the balance between these two sets of considerations. Instead, it will be more reasonable to construct a plurality of different models or representations of causal relationships, embodying different tradeoffs, and appropriate for different purposes.

Instability Again

So far I have focused on the possibility that variables describing macrolevel causes may be causally heterogeneous in the sense that different realizations of the same value of that variable may have different effects on some macroscopic effect variable, even when those macroscopic variables are realized in the same background circumstances (that is, from the point of view of macroscopic description). There is, however, a second possibility, already encountered, that may also lead to a preference for explanation in terms of "lower-level" variables, especially in the psychological realm. Consider a macroscopic variable C and assume that at least in some appropriate set of background circumstances B_1, the different realizers of C have a uniform effect on some second macroscopic variable E, so that causal heterogeneity, as defined above, is not a problem. Suppose, however, that the relationship between C and E, although genuinely causal in the sense that E changes in a reproducible way under interventions on C, is highly unstable or sensitive in the sense described in section 1: specifically assume that the relationship $C \rightarrow E$ relationship will fail to hold in many other possible background circumstances $B_2, \ldots B_n$, which are alternatives to B_1.

I already considered several examples having this structure in section 1. The possibility that I now want to briefly raise is that some or even many causal generalizations involving mental states or psychological states, including perhaps especially many of those taken to characterize commonsense psychology, may have a similar character—they may describe genuine causal relationships, but it may be that these relationships are rather unstable and hold only under a limited range of interventions and background circumstances. Moreover, it may be that we are unlikely to succeed in making them more stable just by refining them using concepts drawn from common sense psychology or everyday "mentalistic" talk. To the extent that they are relatively unstable, such "mental cause" relationships will strike us as not very deep or illuminating from the point of view of explanation. Again, finding more stable relationships may require descent to a more fine-grained, perhaps neural level. (In saying that I wish to raise this as a possibility, I mean just that—not that we have conclusive reasons to think that most mental cause generalizations are unstable but instead merely that this is an empirical issue that needs to be investigated on a case-by-case basis.)

To illustrate what I have in mind, consider some of the candidates for causal relationships (often, indeed, described as "laws") that philosophers of psychology have proposed

1. If S believes that p and believes that p implies q, then, ceteris paribus, S will believe that q.
2. If S wants that p, and believes that $-p$ unless q, and S believes that it is within his power to bring it about that q, then ceteris paribus S brings it about that q (compare Fodor 1987, p. 13). That is, (in English) if someone wants p and thinks that they won't get p unless they do something else q and they also think they can do q, then, other things being equal, they will do q.

The distinctive feature of these generalizations is not (or not just) that they have some exceptions—as we have noted, this is true as well of many relatively stable generalizations. It is rather that these generalizations seem to be (although arguably causal) unstable: if they are to hold at all, an elaborate and specific set of background conditions has to be in place. These background conditions include both other beliefs and desires and physiological conditions that it may be difficult to specify in psychological terms. Change these background conditions very much and these generalizations will no longer hold. Moreover, we find it hard to specify in a nontrivial way what the background conditions must be like for these generalizations to hold. In the case of generalization (1), for example, one of these conditions is that S must "notice" the connection between his two beliefs and perhaps be motivated to "use them together" as premises in an inference whose conclusion is q. (Needless to say, we do not come to believe all possible conclusions that follow from arbitrary conjunctions of our beliefs.) Another possibility that must somehow be excluded is that S does not come to believe that q is false on other grounds (for example, by inferring this from some independently believed premise r) and then use this fact to reject his belief in p or his belief that p implies q. And so on. In the case of generalization (2), there is the obvious relevance of S's other preferences, which may preclude bringing about q and so forth.

As I have remarked, the fact that generalizations like (1) and (2) have exceptions is not news and is recognized by all; philosophers of psychology acknowledge this point when they formulate these generalizations with ceteris paribus clauses. The issue I want to raise might be framed as follows: where along the continuum of relative stability are generalizations such as (1) and (2) located? This is of course an empirical question, but one might think that to the extent that various mental cause generalizations are located near the unstable end of the continuum (that is, to the extent they are like gene $Z \rightarrow$ reading relationship described above), the prospects of incorporating them into a deep explanatory theory do not look good. Put slightly differently, the problem with generalizations (1) and (2) may be not, as causal exclusion type arguments contend, that beliefs and desires are inevitably causally inert but, rather, that as a matter of contingent, empirical fact, the generalizations in which they figure often turn out to be unstable, with the relatively stable generalizations found only at more fine-grained levels.

The Causal Efficacy of Individual Beliefs

I conclude with a final, related issue, also bearing on the causal role of the mental. As we have seen, within an interventionist framework for a variable to qualify as a well-defined causal variable, it must make sense to think in terms of an intervention that changes the value of that variable in a surgical way. So if we wish to attribute causal efficacy to *individual* beliefs, desires, intentions, and other mental states, there must be a well-defined notion of intervention with respect to these.

Suppose that we are interested in the casual relationship, if any, between your desire D to drink a beer and your action A of opening the refrigerator door or between your belief B that there is beer in the refrigerator and A. Recall that an intervention I on X should not at the same time change the value of other variables that do not lie on the causal route from I to X to its putative cause Y and that may affect Y via some other route. This means that interventions on B and D should not change other beliefs and desires that affect A via some independent route. In light of the apparent holism of mental state ascription, one might well worry that in many realistic cases this will not be possible (or at least that it will be difficult to tell whether this condition is satisfied). Suppose that your belief B changes because (C) I tell you that there is beer in the refrigerator. Almost certainly C will change many of your other beliefs and desires besides B. For example, you will probably also come to believe that I believe that there is beer in refrigerator (unless you think that I am trying to deceive you), you will probably come to believe that I have a refrigerator; in many contexts you will come to believe that I want you to have one of the beers, you may acquire a desire to drink that you did not previously have so as not to appear unsociable and so on. Moreover, these additional beliefs and desires may well affect A via a route that does not go through B or, alternatively, the whole issue of what the independent routes are by which C affects A (and a fortiori whether these routes include B) may seem ill defined. In other words, it may be simply unclear whether we are faced with a situation with the structure shown in Figure 4.3. Put slightly differently, it appears that there will be a number of cases in which it is not clear that it makes sense, even as a thought experiment, to imagine changing only a single belief or desire and only what lies causally downstream from it. Moreover, our understanding of the causal relationships among our beliefs, desires, and actions often does not seem precise or articulated enough to go about determining whether changes in some of these variables do or do not affect other variables via independent routes in a way that is inconsistent with the requirements on interventions.

If correct, I do not think these considerations (by themselves) under-

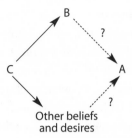

Figure 4.3. Hypothetical relationship between belief and action.

mine the claim that mental or psychological states can be causally efficacious. I do think, however, that they suggest (even if they do not con-
clusively establish) that a certain popular philosophical picture of how
common sense psychological explanation works is misguided. According
to this picture, associated with philosophers like Fodor, it makes sense
to talk of the causal role or effect of individual beliefs and desires, taken
in isolation—causal explanation in folk psychology consists in tracing
changes in mental states and behavior back to the specific individual
beliefs and desires that were efficacious in producing these outcomes. An
interventionist account of causation seems to suggest instead that, to the
extent that there is such a thing as psychological causation at all, often a
rather different picture will be more appropriate, according to which it is
whole clumps or groups of beliefs and desires, taken together that do the
causing, with no possibility of making further distinctions among these as
to the exact details of their causal contribution. On this sort of picture it
still makes sense to suppose, for example, that if patients change their
thought patterns so that they entertain fewer self-critical thoughts, this
can cause changes in mood and the alleviation in depression, but the
causal actor, so to speak, in this (and what is changed by the therapist's or
patient's own intervention) will be the change of overall thought pattern
taken as a whole—it will usually not make sense to ask whether the lifting of depression is attributable to this or that individual thought as enter-
tained on some specific occasion.

5. Conclusion

I have contended in this chapter that there is no completely general argument that vindicates lower-level causal/explanatory claims at the ex-

pense of upper-level claims or vice versa. From an interventionist perspective, there are circumstances in which higher-level causal claims may be more satisfactory (roughly when they figure in answers to a wider range of "what if things had been different?" questions or perhaps just provide answers to such questions that a lower-level account does not provide) and also circumstances in which lower-level claims will be more satisfactory (roughly when they involve relationships that are more stable or variables that are more well defined for the purposes of intervention). Depending on the details of particular cases, these desiderata may trade off against one another in different ways.

ACKNOWLEDGMENT

I am grateful to Kenneth Kendler for a number of extremely helpful comments and suggestions regarding earlier drafts.

NOTES

1. Talk of "levels" in psychological and other contexts is common, but (I readily acknowledge) fraught with ambiguity and the potential for confusion. Unfortunately, sorting out the many different meanings of "level" and what is defensible in these notions is itself a project for a long paper. In what follows, I will try to exploit what I hope is a shared commonsense understanding of what "level" amounts to in the context of particular examples. I would be the first to agree, however, that this notion deserves more careful philosophical scrutiny.

2. Another logical possibility is that the correlation between *SES* and mental illness is due to some common cause or causes.

3. These relationships between the social causation and social selection hypotheses and what would happen under various hypothetical interventions are exploited in a very interesting "natural experiment" reported by Costello et al. (2003). These authors investigated the relationship between the opening of a casino on an American Indian reservation and psychopathology in children. The opening resulted in a substantial increase in the income of some poor families in the sample, while leaving others poor and non-poor families unaffected. According to the authors, this income increase was not correlated with or caused by preexisting psychological conditions in the children or by other family characteristics that could affect the children's psychological condition independently of income. In other words, the income increase had the characteristics of an intervention. Hence, the social causation hypothesis predicts that childhood psychopathology will decrease under this intervention, while the social selection theory predicts that there will be no change. In fact, what Costello et al. found was that in their sample the income increase had a major effect on some psychiatric

disorders (conduct and oppositional disorders) but not others (anxiety and depression).

4. Although not inaccurate, this claim involves a major simplification. A more general characterization of the causal claims made by path diagrams and other structural equation models would distinguish claims about total and direct causes. An arrow from one variable X directed into a second variable Y means that X is a direct cause of Y; within an interventionist framework this is cashed out in terms of the claim that Y will change under some intervention on X when all other variables in the system are fixed at some value by means of independent interventions. X is a total cause of Y when X has a non-null effect on Y when one sums over all paths connecting X and Y; this corresponds to whether Y will change under an intervention on X alone. The two notions coincide when there is an arrow from X to Y and this then only path from X to Y, as in the example under discussion.

5. See Muntaner et al. (2004). Moreover, there is reason to think that "occupation" itself fragments into several variables with distinct causal effects on health. There is a status component to occupation that varies at least somewhat independently of whether one is in a position of subordination to others. Subordination appears to have an effect on mental and physical health that is independent of status.

6. Example due to Peter Machamer.

7. *Explanans* is a philosophical term of art for whatever does the explaining in an explanation; the *explanandum* is what is explained.

8. I take this example from Murphy (2006), who uses it to make a similar point.

9. For additional discussion of the distinction between stability (or invariance) and scope, see *MTH*, pp. 268 ff. See also section below for related discussion.

10. See Caspi et al. (2003) and Lotrich and Pollock (2004) for additional discussion. This meta-analysis concludes that there is evidence for a small effect of 5-HTTLPR on monopolar and perhaps bipolar depression with an OR (odds ratio) of less than 1.2.

11. Talk of generalizations as more or less stable naturally raises the following question: what sorts of changes in background conditions matter for the assessment of stability? This is a large question and I can only gesture at an answer here, referring the reader to *MTH* and to Woodward (2006) for additional discussion. But, to an important extent, the conditions relevant to the assessment of stability will be discipline specific. For example, in psychology/psychiatry there is a prima facie expectation that fundamental explanatory principles should be stable under changes in learning history or information available to the subject. This does not mean of course that subject's behavior, etc., should not vary depending on changes in learning but rather that the generalizations governing learning should be stable under such changes, as the Rescorla-Wagner rule at least purports to be and the generalization PECK transparently is not. That is, one should be able to take the same generalization governing learning and combine it with information about different possible learning histories, showing how these lead to different outputs. Similarly, one expects that fundamental explanatory principles will be stable under changes in subject's beliefs and goals or preferences. As some readers may

recognize, these criteria are loosely reminiscent of Pylyshyn's (1984) use of "cognitive impenetrability" as a criterion for distinguishing the "functional architecture" of the mind (roughly, those properties that derive from the structure of the underlying machine) from those processes that are to be explained in terms of rules and representations: roughly, Pylyshyn requires that the "behavior" of "components" of the functional architecture be stable under changes in a subject's beliefs and goals (p. 133). But my view contrasts with Pylyshyn's in holding that we would apply this stability criterion to psychological relationships/generalizations (rather than components). For example, in connection with a generalization like "If S believes p and believes that if p, then q, then S will believe q" my suggestion is that we should ask whether this generalization would continue to hold under changes in S's other beliefs, etc. (In addition, I do not share Pylyshyn's concern with distinguishing what is explicable by reference to functional architecture from what should be explained in terms of rules and representations.)

12. Another example: the generalization (1.7.1) "If you push the key on the key board of Woodward's computer that is labeled 'Z,' a Z will show up on the computer screen" is, according to writers like Fodor, a ceteris paribus law. So also are (1.7.2) the fundamental principles of electrical engineering, transistor and circuit behavior, etc., that govern the operation of my computer's components. Needless to say, however, the latter (1.7.2) are usually though to provide a deeper and more fundamental explanation of the behavior of my computer than a list of input/output relations along the lines of 1.7.1. The interventionist account traces the greater explanatory depth of 1.7.2 in part to their greater stability. From the point of view of psychology/psychiatry, the operative question we should be asking about candidate causal generalizations is whether they look more like 1.7.1 or 1.7.2 with respect to degree of stability, not whether they qualify as ceteris paribus laws. If a candidate psychological generalization is comparable in stability to 1.7.1, this will not count as much of a vindication of its explanatory credentials.

13. In standard philosophy of science terminology, the explanandum is a sentence of proposition describing or representing the phenomenon being explained, rather than the phenomenon itself. However, it is cumbersome to write "explandandum outcome," so I will sometimes just use "explanandum" to refer to the outcome itself, trusting that the resulting conflation of use and mention will not lead to any serious confusion.

14. One set of properties, A, is said to *supervene* on another, B (the supervenience base of A), if necessarily, any change or difference in A requires a change or difference in B. Mental properties are widely believed to supervene on physical or neural properties in this sense—that is, if two organisms differ in their mental properties or states they must also differ in their physical states.

15. This conclusion is a non sequitur: there is nothing in the idea of multiple realizability per se that rules out the possibility that all of the different realizers share some common physical structure at an abstract level of description. For example, different realizations of the same intention may share some aggregate feature that is a function of firing rates exhibited by a group of neurons, just as the

same temperature may be realized by a variety of molecular configurations, all of which possess the same average kinetic energy (cf. the discussion of Andersen below). Because my interest here is just in describing the background assumptions that philosophers of mind bring to this discussion, I will ignore this complication.

16. Very roughly, the Putnam-Fodor argument was that because of multiple realizability, there will be unifying higher-level generalizations that are not "captured" by generalizations that just concern the very disparate lower-level realizers. For example, suppose that (C_1) the belief that p, (C_2) the belief that if p, then q, and (C_3) the belief that q can be realized in many different ways—in neurons, silicon, etc. Suppose in addition that explanation (3.1) it is a true causal generalization that instances of C_1 and C_2 cause instances of C_3. Then, the argument goes, information about lower-level realizers and their causal relationships will not capture or reveal the common pattern represented by explanation (3.1). To capture this common pattern, we need upper-level generalizations like explanation (3.1) formulated in terms of properties like belief and desire.

From an interventionist perspective, this argument leaves out an important consideration: to vindicate the explanatory credentials of explanation (3.1), it is not enough that there be some instances of C_1 and C_2 that cause C_3 for this is compatible with explanation (3.1) being highly unstable. In other words, if C_1, C_2, and C_3 are multiply realizable but explanation (3.1) breaks down under many or most alternative ways of realizing C_1–C_3 (because, for example, these are causally heterogeneous, in the sense described in section 4 or because explanation (3.1) holds only under very specialized background circumstances for each of its multiple realizations), this will make explanation (3.1) seem unsatisfactory from the point of view of explanation.

17. See Kim (2005) for a detailed development of this argument. My formulation is meant to make it clear how the argument depends on the assumption that a cause is just some condition that is part of a nomologically sufficient condition for its effect. If, as I have suggested, this assumption should be rejected the exclusion argument and its kindred look far less compelling.

18. I'm grateful to Richard Andersen for helpful conversations about this research.

19. In more recent research, other variables in addition to firing rate are measured and aggregated. These enable somewhat better prediction of intention than what is achieved through reliance on firing rate alone.

20. Richard Andersen, personal communication.

21. For discussion of the status of this assumption, see Dayan and Abbott (2001).

22. A paper by Briggman, Abarbanel, and Kristan (2005) provides a broadly similar illustration. These authors are interested in the neural structures that control decision-making (in particular the choice between swimming and crawling) in the medicinal leech. One extreme possibility is that such choices are controlled by a single neuron or a very small group of neurons, another is that they are controlled by the dynamics of whole populations of neurons. The authors find that recording

from populations of neurons allows for earlier prediction of choice than recording from any single neuron. While the authors acknowledge that this evidence is merely correlational, they also (in good interventionist fashion) tried manipulating (stimulating) individual neurons to see if this would bias decisions, finding only one such neuron. On this basis, they propose a "middle ground" position, according to which network dynamics (causally) determines choices but some individual neurons exert an especially important influence. To the extent that dynamical features of whole populations of neurons influence choice and these dynamical features can be realized by different combinations of states of individual neurons, it will be misleading (on the conception of explanation defended in this essay) to cite just the states individual neurons happen to assume on some particular occasion in explaining choice.

23. However, Pettit and Jackson distinguish sharply between causal relevance and what they call *causal efficacy*, where "a casually efficacious property with regard to an effect is a property in virtue of whose instantiation, at least in part, the effect occurs." According to Jackson and Petit, mental states are causally relevant to behavior but not in themselves causally efficacious in producing behavior. Instead it is the particular physical realization of the mental state on a given occasion which is causally efficacious in producing behavior. My contrary view is that this distinction between relevance and efficacy is unwarranted and (roughly) that there is nothing more to causation than causal relevance.

24. I emphasize that the example that follows is intended only as an illustration of what is meant by causal heterogeneity. For my purposes, it does not matter whether every aspect of the Blair et al. proposal turns out to be correct. In particular, Ken Kendler pointed out to me that Blair et al.'s claim that amygdala dysfunction is common in psychopaths is not generally accepted.

25. It is worth noting that just as candidate causes can be heterogeneous, so also can candidate effects. Blair et al. argue that the standard diagnostic category of antisocial behavior is like this: it really consists of two different conditions, only one of which corresponds to psychopathy, and these two conditions have very different etiologies. They claim that a more adequate explanation of both conditions thus can be found by splitting them into two more fine-grained conditions, and constructing separate explanations of each. Other examples in psychiatry come readily to mind; the splitting of depression into bipolar and unipolar variants. Some think that schizophrenia is really a heterogeneous family of diseases. So effect heterogeneity is another consideration that can lead to more fine-grained theorizing.

26. To put the point in a slightly different way, consider two extreme possibilities. According to the first, "humiliation" is with respect to other variables of psychiatric interest like "temperature" is to thermodynamic variables. There are many different ways (different molecular configurations) of realizing the same value for the temperature of a gas and all of these have the same stable effect on variables like pressure and volume. Insofar as we are interested in explaining the behavior of these latter variables, there is no motivation at all for splitting temperature into many different finer-grained variables corresponding to different microrealiza-

tions. The other extreme possibility is that even very small variations in the micro-realization of humiliation have very different effects in psychiatric variables, in which case we have at least some motivation for subdividing the humiliation variable. Now suppose that the true situation with respect to humiliation is somewhere between these two possibilities. In this case, we have some motivation both for splitting (more stable cause-effect relationships) and some motivation for not splitting (greater generality, etc.) and there may be no single best way of striking this balance.

REFERENCES

Blair, J., D. Mitchell, and K. Blair. 2005. *The Psychopath: Emotion and the Brain.* Malden, MA: Blackwell.

Briggman, K., H. Abarbanel, and W. Kristan. 2005. Optical Imaging of Neuronal Populations during Decision-Making. *Science* 307:896–901.

Caspi, A., K. Sugden, T. Moffitt, A. Taylor, I. Craig, H. Harrington, J. McClay, J. Mill, A. Braithwaite, and R. Poulton. 2003. Influence of Life Stress on Depression: Moderation by a Polymorphism in the 5-HTT Gene. *Science* 301:386–89.

Costello, E., S. Compton, G. Keeler, and A. Angold. 2003. Relationships between Poverty and Psychopathology: A Natural Experiment. *Journal of the American Medical Association* 290 (15):2023–2029.

Dawkins, R. 1982. *The Extended Phenotype.* New York: W. H. Freeman.

Dayan, P., and L. Abbott. 2001. *Theoretical Neuroscience.* Cambridge, MA: MIT Press.

Dohrenwend, B., I. Levav, P. Shrout, et al. 1992. Socioeconomic Status and Psychiatric Disorders: The Causation-Selection Issue. *Science* 255:946–952.

Earman, J., J. Roberts, and S. Smith. 2002. Ceteris Paribus Lost. *Erkenntnis* 57:281–301.

Fodor, J. 1987. *Psychosemantics.* Cambridge, MA: MIT Press.

Kendler, K. 2005. "A Gene for . . . ": The Nature of Gene Action in Psychiatric Disorders. *American Journal of Psychiatry* 162:1243–1252.

———. 2006. Toward a Comprehensive Developmental Model for Major Depression in Men. *American Journal of Psychiatry* 163:115–124.

Kim, J. 2005. *Physicalism or Something Near Enough.* Princeton, NJ: Princeton University Press.

Lotrich, F., and B. Pollock. 2004. Meta-Analysis of Serotonin Transmitter Polymorphisms and Affective Disorders. *Psychiatric Genetics* 14:121–129.

Muntaner, C., W. Eaton, R. Miech, and P. O'Campo. 2004. Socioeconomic Position and Major Mental Disorders. *Epidemiologic Reviews* 26:53–62.

Murphy, D. 2006. *Psychiatry in the Scientific Image.* Cambridge, MA: MIT Press.

Musallam, S., B. Corneil, B. Greger, H. Scherberger, and R. Andersen. 2004. Cognitive Control Signals for Neural Prosthetics. *Science* 305:258.

Pettit, P., and F. Jackson. 1990. Program Explanation: A General Perspective. *Analysis* 50:107–117.

Pylyshyn, Z. 1984. *Computation and Cognition*. Cambridge, MA: MIT Press.

Salmon, W. 1984. *Scientific Explanation and the Causal Structure of the World*. Princeton, NJ: Princeton University Press.

Scheines, R., and P. Spirtes. 2004. Causal Inference of Ambiguous Manipulations. *Philosophy of Science* 71: 833–845.

Spirtes, P., C. Glymour, and R. Scheines. 2000. *Causation, Prediction, and Search*. Cambridge, MA: MIT Press.

Woodward, J. 2003a. *Making Things Happen: A Theory of Causal Explanation*. New York: Oxford University Press.

———. 2003b. There Is No Such Thing as a Ceteris Paribus Law. *Erkenntnis* 57:308–328.

———. 2006. Sensitive and Insensitive Causation. *Philosophical Review* 115:1–50.

Yablo, S. 1992. Mental Causation. *Philosophical Review* 101:245–280.

* * *

Comment: Psychological Causation without Physical Causation
John Campbell, Ph.D.

1. Interventionist versus Mechanistic Approaches to Psychological Causation

Woodward remarks that "for X to count as a cause of Y on the interventionist account, there must be a 'stable' or regular response of Y (or the probability distribution of Y) to some interventions on X, at least in some background circumstances" (p. 147). Correlations under interventions on X between X and Y can be more or less stable or, as Woodward also puts it, invariant. As he says, "Some relationships (and the generalizations that describe them) are stable under a wider range of interventions and under a wider range of background conditions than others" (p. 147). No one has done more than Woodward to articulate this deeply intuitive conception of causation and display its philosophical significance. My first point in these comments is that this approach explains how the following situation is possible. Suppose we have a purely physical system, that is, one consisting entirely of physical particles governed by deterministic physical laws. Suppose that this system has psychological states, supervening on the physical properties of the particles constituting it. Those psychological states may be causes of the behaviors of the system, even though we can find no physical variable that causes those behaviors of the system.

In such a system, the causal exclusion problem does not arise. The causal exclusion problem is that we can't have both psychological and physical variables acting as causes of the same phenomena, for then those phenomena would be overdetermined, and they aren't overdetermined. But even in a wholly physical system we can have psychological causation without physical causation. If we have psychological causation without physical causation, the problem of causal overdetermination does not arise.

It is usually assumed that in a physical system, if we have psychological causation, we must have physical causation, too. One motive for this assumption is a mechanistic view of causation, against which Woodward sets his face. The mechanistic view of causation, first developed in the seventeenth century, says, in its prototypical form, that all causation has to be understood as ultimately the communication of motion by impulse; a number of more sophisticated and more recent formulations keep the same basic intuition (Salmon 1994; Dowe 1992). They all share the implication that psychological causation cannot be understood in isolation from physical causation. If what we are looking for, when we are looking for a causal link, is the communication of motion by impulse, we will not find that at the psychological level; similarly, if what we are looking for is the exchange of conserved quantities (Dowe 1992). We will not find conserved quantities among the psychological variables, so any causation we might claim to find among psychological variables will count as such only because of the relations between the psychological variables and physical variables. In fact, on a mechanistic approach to causation, it is natural to wonder whether what we have at the psychological level is properly thought of as causation rather than something that may at best have heuristic value in pointing us toward the true underlying physical mechanism.

The great virtue of the interventionist approach to psychological causation is that it frees us from this idea, that talk of psychological causation is a best a pointer toward underlying physical mechanisms. The interventionist approach allows us to view psychological and physical causation as phenomena that each exist in their own right. It provides a much more powerful framework for thinking about what the relations between psychological and physical causation might possibly be and exploring what those connections actually are.

In the next two sections of this chapter, I provide a frame for looking at Woodward's reaction to the causal exclusion problem. In section 2 I set out an elementary point about the relation between high-level and low-level causation in a simple physical system, with no psychological properties. The point is that, even in a deterministic physical system, there can be high-level physical outcomes that have no physical cause. In section 3 I extend the point to physical systems in which we have psychological properties that supervene on the physical properties of the system. Here, too, we can have physical outcomes that have no physical cause, but in this case the absence of a physical cause is consistent with there being a psychological cause of the outcome. In section 4 I set out Woodward's reaction to the causal exclusion problem, that is, to the case in which we have both psychological and physical causes. In section 5 I suggest some ways of pursuing his interventionist approach to this case.

2. Physical Outcomes without Physical Causes

Suppose we take a simple example of a causal relationship, such as, to borrow a case from Woodward and Hitchcock (2003), the relation between the height of a plant (Y) and the amount of water ($X1$) and fertilizer ($X2$) applied to it. Suppose that the relation is given by some such equation as:

$$(E) \; Y = a1X1 + a2X2 + U$$

where $a1$ and $a2$ are constants and U represents some source of error. Interpreted causally, this generalization says that interventions on $X1$ will make a difference to Y, as will interventions on $X2$. The demand that the generalization be invariant under a wide range of background conditions demands that it should not matter too much what temperature the plant is kept at, for example, and the demand that the generalization should be invariant over a wide range of interventions is the demand that it should not matter too much that the values of $X1$ and $X2$ are in question. Obviously, E is not a limit case of either type of invariance: it will cease to hold in some background conditions, for instance under extremes of temperature, and it will stop holding when we are considering large quantities of water or fertilizer. Nevertheless, in its limited way it is a truly causal generalization, for it does have invariance across certain limited ranges of background conditions and for a certain range of values of its variables.

Woodward emphasizes the contrastive nature of causation: when we ask about whether X causes Y, we are always at least implicitly asking whether particular changes in the value of X cause particular changes in the value of Y. Suppose the plant will die if I don't water it, and I give it some water, but not enough. Does the plant grow because I watered it? It depends what the contrast classes are. The plant grows, rather than dying, because I water it rather than not watering it at all. The plant grows less than it should because I gave it less rather than more water. When we ask these contrastive questions, we are probing the underlying general relation (E) between growth and watering (compare Hitchcock 1995).

In this kind of case, we can speak of the amount of water applied as being, in its limited way, a "control" variable for the height of the plant: we can control what height the plant reaches by manipulating the amount of water applied. It is only in a relatively limited way—in certain conditions and for certain volumes of water—that this control is possible. That is why we would speak of a "superficial" explanation here: a better causal account would make more of the background variables explicit and thus achieve a higher degree of invariance. I want now to consider a different kind of case: one in which there is no restriction on invariance, but we do not seem to have any systematic relation at all between variables.

Suppose we have a relatively frictionless billiard table. The balls, once set in motion, will roll for months, perhaps years. We are going to set them all in motion with a cue applied to a single ball. And suppose that once set in motion, the balls on the table constitute a deterministic physical system. That is, from (a) the laws governing the system and (b) the initial positions of the balls and the vector describing the force, location, and direction of the initial cue shot, one can derive, for each of the balls, just where it will be at any subsequent time. If anything is a physical system, this is.

How many possible initial configurations of the balls are there? Lots; there is no particular restriction here on where we put them all. How many possible initial cue shots are there? Lots; we can apply the cue to any ball with any force or direction. Consider an arbitrary time after the initial cue shot, say, the following Wednesday at 2:00 P.M. How many possible configurations of the balls are there for that time? Well, doing the mathematics here, the answer is lots. Depending on the initial conditions and the initial cue shot, the balls may be in any random configuration the following Wednesday at 2:00 P.M.

Among all those possible configurations, there is one in which all the balls have congregated in the top left corner of the table on the following Wednesday at 2:00 P.M. There is no special significance to this; it is simply one among many random configurations that the balls may take for that time, depending on the initial conditions and the initial cue shot.

Consider now that the balls are rolling for months. Suppose, for a given initial condition and cue shot, we look over a period of, say, 15 weeks, at where all the balls are each Wednesday at 2:00 P.M. In general, we won't find any pattern here. But suppose we find a particular initial condition and cue shot for which, each Wednesday at 2:00 P.M., all the balls congregate in the top left corner of the table. There is, again, no special significance to this. It is simply one among many random configurations we might find at that time, depending on the initial conditions and the cue shot. It is just the special case of a random configuration in which there is repetition of the configuration and the configuration is briefly describable.

Suppose I do in fact do the initial setup of the balls and the cue shot in just this way, and, to my astonishment, over the next 15 weeks I observe this pattern. "Why do they all collect in the top left corner on Wednesdays at 2:00 P.M.?" I ask. "What is the cause?" Now there is a sense in which there is a cause of the balls all collecting like this, and I know it already. It was the initial setup together with my cue shot, but that does not answer my question. What I am wondering is whether there is some cause of the balls all collecting in the top left corner rather than the bottom left corner; and is there some cause of their all collecting on Wednesdays at 2:00 P.M. rather than on Tuesdays at 2:00 P.M.? Is there some variable, or pair of variables, that stands to place and time of congregation as amount of water and fertilizer stand to height of plant? It is to this question that the answer seems negative. There may be no variable whose values are systematically correlated under interventions with the place and time of congregation of the balls. It is for this reason that we naturally say that it is merely "random" that the balls happen to congregate at that time and place. If, for example, I systematically manipulate the force of the cue shot, I do not make systematic differences to the place and time of congregation. Most changes to the force of the cue shot lead to there being no congregating of the balls at all. Notice that the point here is not about whether some generalization such as E is sufficiently invariant across background conditions or types of intervention. The problem is that there is in this case no analogue at all of the generalization E. We do not have any systematic relation between, on the one hand, the basic physical variables in terms of which the billiard balls and cue shot are characterized, and, on the other hand, the place and time of congregation.

Any philosopher reading this will reflexively suggest the possibility of "gerrymandering" a complex physical variable, a big disjunction of more specific variables characterizing the initial conditions and cue shot, that you could regard as systematically related to the place and time of congregation. For the moment, my only comment on this proposal is that we would not in fact regard the construction of such a gerrymandered variable as "discovering the cause of the pattern." Consider a real case, the documented tendency of eels to congregate in the Sargasso Sea. What's the cause? Why there rather than anywhere else? The kind of factor that is usually suggested is some use of geomagnetic patterns in navigation by all the eels. An ingenious philosopher might proceed by another route: you might give a more basic physical description of the eels and their physical environment and claim that this specifies "the cause" of the eels meeting at one place rather than another. Now in fact, although we might applaud the ingenuity, we would regard it as wasted: you have not discovered the cause of the eels meeting in one place rather than another. And suppose you did manage to face us down, so that no one could think of a good reason to complain about the gerrymandered variable. You would produce only dismay. For you would have destroyed what seems like a perfectly good and important distinction: the distinction between the congregation of the billiard balls, which is an *accident,* and the congregation of the eels, which is not an accident.

This explains the sense in which, even in a deterministic physical system, there can be a physical outcome without a physical cause. There can be patterns that appear "by accident"; there is no causal explanation of why we have this pattern rather than another, related pattern. There is no causal explanation for why the billiard balls are congregating at that particular place and time, rather than some other place and time. It is in that sense that their congregating at that place and time is "merely random," "only an accident," or "an epiphenomenon." The randomness, in this sense, is of course entirely consistent with this being a deterministic physical system. The point is emphatically not that there are nonphysical forces at work.

3. Psychological Causation without Physical Causation

Suppose now that we consider not billiard balls, but people. Let us suppose, though, that people are physical systems. In fact, let us suppose that they are deterministic physical systems, just as our billiard balls are, and, although they have psychological states, those psychological states supervene on the underlying physical reality. Once you have fixed the physical facts, you have fixed all the psychological facts.

Suppose we have a group of people, such as the members of a seminar or a committee. They agree to meet weekly for the fifteen weeks of term, at a particular place, lecture room 3, and time, say, Wednesday at 2:00 P.M.. So every week they congregate at that place and time.

Suppose you don't know that these organisms are sentient, but you do have a complete physical description of them. At the most fundamental physical level, you know all about the physical environment, and know all the relevant physical laws. Because we are dealing here with a deterministic physical system, you will be able to predict the movements of all these things, so you will be able to predict that they will congregate at that place and time. But why do they congregate at that place and time, rather than any other? Well, you say, it's random. It's just an accident. There is no particular reason why they are congregating at that place and time rather than any other. There is no physical variable whose values are systematically correlated with variations in the place and time of meeting. An ingenious philosopher might point out that "in principle" you could come up with a "gerrymandered" physical variable whose values are related to variation in place and time of meeting, but you would not allow that as a demonstration that this is not an accidental pattern. You would not in practice allow that kind of ingenuity to destroy the contrast between this case and the case of the congregation of the eels at one place rather than another, for with the eels this is really not an accident.

What about the situation of an ordinary person observing the class, who does know something the psychologies of the people involved? This observer knows that everyone in the group agreed to meet in lecture room 3 on Wednesdays at 2:00 P.M. That is why they all keep coming. This observer therefore really does know a variable that is systematically related to the time of congregation: having agreed to meet at place P and at time T. Systematic variation in the value of this variable is correlated under interventions with changes in the place and time of meeting. So there is a variable here that stands to the place and time of meeting somewhat as the volume of water and fertilizer stands to the height of the plant. Of course, in neither case is the generalization fully invariant across all background conditions or values of the variables. There are, for example, natural disasters that will disrupt the seminar, and the correlation would break down if, for instance, everyone had in the seminar had foolishly agreed to meet on a mountaintop at midnight. Nonetheless, there is enough invariance in the relationship for us to say that we have a causal connection here.

In this situation, we have a deterministic physical system, comprised of all those organisms and their environment. Although the organisms have psychological states, those states supervene on the basic physics. We have a physical outcome, that everyone is congregating at a particular place and time. There is a psychological cause for this congregation, the initial agreement, but it has no physical cause. From a physical point of view, the congregation is only an accident.

Now I think that we do feel a strong resistance to the idea that the explanatory story might end there. We tend to feel strongly that, in the case I described, we should look for some brain variable that is the cause of everyone meeting as they do. There must be, somewhere in the pattern of electrical activity across the brain, something recognizable as a diary. There must be some physical variable—perhaps a complex physical variable relating to the activity of massive assemblies of cells—whose systematic manipulation would make systematic changes to when everyone met. (By saying it may be complex, I of course don't mean that it will be "gerrymandered" in the sense I discussed earlier, but that it may be far removed from being, for example, simply the firing pattern of a single cell.) Much research on the brain is built around some such idea as this: that it should be possible to find such complex physical variables, and it is when we find those high-level physical variables that the causal exclusion problem arises, if it arises at all. I don't at all want to resist the idea that we should search for these complex brain variables, but I do want to reflect on the status of the idea that these physical variables "must" exist, and on what difference it makes to our thinking about psychology whether they exist.

Why should we think that there must be a (nongerrymandered) physical variable whose values are systematically related to the time at which everyone meets, in our example? Notice that the existence of such a variable is not a consequence of the fact that we are dealing with a deterministic physical system in which all the psychological facts supervene on physical facts. We have already seen that there seems to be no contradiction in the idea that such a deterministic system might have psychological causation without physical causation. Or is the existence of such a physical variable somehow already implicated in the very idea that we are dealing with a causal relation? As I stated at the outset, a mechanistic conception of causation does seem to imply that the only causation is physical causation, but when we leave mechanism behind and operate within an interventionist framework there is no particular reason to think that causation as such must involve physical variables. So, if we already have a psychological cause for a phenomenon, what exactly do we gain by looking for a physical cause?

4. Causal Exclusion

The causal exclusion argument says that we can't have both psychological and physical variables acting as causes of the same phenomena, for then those phenomena would be overdetermined, and they aren't overdetermined. Woodward expounds the substance of his response to the causal exclusion argument in terms of a single example, work by Andersen and colleagues on the neural coding of intention (Mussalam et al. 2004). The working hypothesis of the group here is that the aggregate firing rate of a population of neurons in the parietal reach region of the posterior parietal cortex in macaque monkeys (PPR) encodes intentions to reach for targets. Suppose now that we want to explain why a monkey exhibits reaching behavior R_1 rather than reaching behavior R_2. We might appeal to a finely detailed specification, N_{11}, of the exact behavior, along many dimensions, of each of the neurons in a particular population in the PPR. Woodward's point here is

> What we are interested in explaining (finding the cause of) is variations in reach toward different goal objects—why the monkey exhibits reaching behavior R_1 rather than different reaching behavior R_2. To explain this explanandum we need to identify states or conditions, variations in which, when produced by interventions, would be stably correlated with changes from R_1 to R_2. Ex hypothesi, merely citing N_{11} does not accomplish this, because it tells us nothing about the conditions under which alternatives to R_1 would be realized. This is because many variations on N_{11} (N_{12}, N_{13}, et cetera) are consistent with I_1 and hence will lead to R_1, rather than some alternative to R_1, and the proposed explanation which appeals just to N_{11} does not tell us which of these variations on N_{11} will lead to alternatives to R_1 and which will not. (p. 165)

And, more positively,

> By way of contrast, both appealing to the monkey's intentions *and* appealing to the abstract facts about patterns of neural firing that distinguish the en-

coding of one intention from the encoding of a distinct intention will accomplish this: it is the fact that the monkey has intention I_1 rather than intention I_2 that causes behavior R_1 rather than R_2. Similarly, it is the fact that the PRR exhibits the pattern of neural firing P_1 rather than the different pattern of firing P_2 (which encodes a distinct intention) that causes the monkey to exhibit R_1 rather than R_2. (p. 165)

This leaves us with the claim that if we ask, "What causes the monkey to exhibit reaching behavior R_1 rather than reaching behavior R_2?," there are two answers we can give:

(1) the monkey has intention I_1 rather than intention I_2, and
(2) the monkey's PRR exhibits pattern of neural firing P_1 rather than P_2.

Woodward does not explain how we should think of the relations between these two causal claims. Arguably a comprehensive discussion of the causal exclusion argument should address this question. Otherwise, it might seem that the resulting behavior is overdetermined; and it isn't overdetermined.

5. Does Psychological Causation Depend on Physical Validation?

From an interventionist perspective, what would be wrong with saying that reaching behavior, for example, is overdetermined by the two factors, intention and neural firing in the PRR? From an interventionist perspective, the mistake would be to suppose that intention and neural firing are factors that could in principle be manipulated independently of one another, to make differences to behavior. The important point, in avoiding this conclusion, is to remark that psychological and physical variables cannot in general be manipulated independently of one another, and certainly intention and firing in PRR cannot be manipulated independently on another. That point, however, is already an implication of the supervenience of the mental on the physical.

What was the point of finding this high-level variable, neural firing in PRR, in the first place? We already had a perfectly good cause for the outcome behavior, namely, possession of an appropriate intention. What insight do we gain by finding the right high-level physical variable? The principal advantage, I want to suggest, is that now a whole new range of potential interventions come into play. We now understand how there can be physiological or genetic manipulations that make a difference to reaching behavior, and we understand how an intervention on PRR might result in the paralysis of an individual. If we stayed at the folk-psychological level, we would have none of that. This point resonates throughout psychiatry. The reason we need to find high-level physical variables underpinning disorders is to bring into view, so far as we can, the multiplicity of manipulations there can be of factors that make a difference to those disorders.

This way of explaining the importance of finding high-level physical variables that affect psychological outcomes contrasts with the motivation provided by a more traditional, pre-Humean mechanism. For the pre-Humean mechanist, all causation is the transmission of motion by impulse, and any talk of "psychological causation" is a lot of hot air, to be supplanted eventually by the biological identification of the true causes of things. Methodologically, the difference between the interventionist perspective and that of the pre-Humean mechanist often does not matter much, because both can agree on the importance of the search for high-level physical causes of things. Where the interventionist and the pre-Humean mechanist part company is over the implications of a failed search.

Let me illustrate with a dramatic example. Consider cases in which a killer, K, has both a desire for revenge again the victim V, and a desire to defend himself against V. Among those cases, we distinguish cases in which the desire for revenge causes the killing from cases in which the desire for self-defense causes the killing. This is not merely a scholar's distinction: whether a court instructs that Y be executed or that Y be freed may depend on how they apply this distinction. But are we going to find a neural correlate for this distinction? Will we ever find a high-level physical variable that correlates with one motive rather than the other being the motive for which person acted? Will it ever happen that a brain scanner directed at Y during those critical few minutes of the struggle in which X died will be able to tell us whether revenge or self-defense was the motive from which Y acted? Suppose it turns out that there is no such distinction to be drawn in neural terms. What should we conclude? Should we assume that moral psychology has been discredited and that we should abandon the distinction between one type of killing and another? For the pre-Humean mechanist, moral psychology would indeed have been discredited; it would indeed have been shown that the causal distinction on which the legal system depends does not exist. For the interventionist, by contrast, there is no such priority for the physiological level. If the intervention counterfactuals hold for the psychological variables, there is no further question waiting for a neural arbitration. Woodward perhaps hints at a certain sympathy with this attitude when he says, "It will be more reasonable to construct a plurality of different models or representations of causal relationships, embodying different tradeoffs, and appropriate for different purposes" (p. 173).

ACKNOWLEDGMENTS

Thanks to Kenneth Kendler for many rounds of comment and discussion and to James Woodward for earlier discussions. An early version was presented to the Letters and Sciences Forum at Berkeley, and I am indebted to people there for a vigorous discussion.

REFERENCES

Dowe, P. 2000. *Physical Causation*. Cambridge: Cambridge University Press.
Hitchcock, C. 1995. The Mishap at Reichenbach Fall: Singular vs. General Causation. *Philosophical Studies* 78:257–291.
Musallam, S., B. Corneil, B. Greger, H Scherberger, and R. Andersen. 2004. Cognitive Control Signals for Neural Prosthetics. *Science* 305:258–262.
Salmon, W. 1984. *Scientific Explanation and the Causal Structure of the World*. Princeton, NJ: Princeton University Press.
Woodward, J., and C. Hitchcock. 2003. Explanatory Generalizations. Part 1. A Counterfactual Account. *Nous* 24:1–24.

CHAPTER 5

Causation in Psychiatry

JOHN CAMPBELL, PH.D.

In a challenging and iconoclastic chapter, John Campbell tries to deconstruct the idea, often "taken for granted," that psychiatric explanation and causation must inevitably be multilevel. (Topics covered in this chapter are related to those taken up by several other contributors to this volume, particularly Schaffner and Murphy.) Campbell takes on a deep assumption of our field, namely, that certain kinds of phenomena *have to be* explained by other particular kinds of phenomenon. He captures this assumption in the Frith quote early in his chapter that says, in essence, that a set of neurophysiologic facts (for example, changes in firing rates of dopamine neurons) *cannot* cause certain psychological experiences (for example, thought insertion). We have, Campbell asserts, unexamined a priori ideas about what constitutes a proper explanation. They might, he suggests, reflect simple prejudice rather than being an accurate reflection of the way the world works.

Let me try to bring out the essence of this problem with a little story. Imagine in 40 years, when we can know nearly everything about everything, a famous neuroscientist (Dr. N) well known as a "hard reductionist," shows convincingly that increased neuronal activity in subregion 27-z-9 of the orbital frontal cortex is a strong and consistent predictor of persecutory delusions. Longing for a Nobel Prize, he calls a press conference to announce that he has "discovered the cause of delusions." After his triumphal presentation, a young psychiatrist (Dr. X) from the audience gets up and says,

But wait a minute, Dr. N, how can you say you have solved the cause of delusions? Delusions are false beliefs. You haven't told us anything about why a person would believe that the television is talking about him or why he believes when his stomach hurts it must be the result of the gamma rays beamed at him by his next door neighbor. I'll grant you that increased neuronal activity in subregion 27-z-9 might be part of a causal chain, but you can hardly claim to have discovered *the* cause of delusions. A small part of the puzzle maybe, but no more.

I think Campbell would respond to this by saying,

On what basis does Dr. X assume that Dr. N's explanation is not complete? Maybe the way the world is designed, the *only* consistent and stable correlate of persecutory delusions is changes in subregion 27-z-9. You might wish for all kinds of psychological correlates such as tendencies to quickly interpret ambiguous stimuli with high confidence and so forth, but what if they don't exist or exist in only some delusional patients, all of whom display the changes in subregion 27-z-9? Your claim is only based on vague a priori ideas of what should explain delusions and that is a poor basis for an argument.

In his challenge, Campbell suggests he is in the good company of David Hume, who argued that causality should be taken only by observed correlations in the world and not from our preconceived ideas of what could cause what.

Campbell's argument comes up against the wall of intelligibility—the subjective sense of what it means to be given a good explanation. What can make us walk away with a smile on our face when we ask our mechanic why we have a knocking in our engine? If he says, "Oh, your fan belt is loose and knocking against your engine block. I'll just tighten it up and it will be fine," we have a sense of satisfaction. The explanation matches the phenomenon. If, however, your mechanic says, "Your gamma ray receptor is malfunctioning but I can reprogram it and the knocking noise will go away," most people would respond with a perplexed and unsatisfied look, even if the knocking does go away. In Hume's phrase, one explanation passes the intelligibility test and the other fails. Campbell argues we have to take the world as we find it and we must "resist the demand for intelligibility." A tough proposition, but Campbell does succeed at clarifying the issues involved.

Campbell then moves to a brief review of the interventionist model of causality—a perspective that is outlined in more detail in the chapter by Woodward in this volume and in even more detail in Woodward's recent book (Woodward 2003). From this, he builds up what he calls his "many sorted explanations." He uses the now familiar serotonin plus stressful life event model. His key point is—if this is what the interventionist model tells us—these are where surgical interventions will impact on risk for depression. Who are we to say this kind of model cannot be correct because the "levels don't feel right"?

In a bit of an aside, Campbell briefly contrasts the implication of an interventionist versus mechanical view of causation, arguing that the latter, unlike the former, would support a reductionist agenda for psychiatry. That is, if the only real causation involved well-defined physical mechanisms (Campbell uses a bit of philosophy-speak where he calls it "a continuous spatiotemporal process"), then this would lead inevitably to thinking that the "one true" level of causality—the place where all the action is—would be at the level of molecular biology. The interventionist model is much more inclusive or tolerant in its approach to causality. Anything that "works" in the real world would be welcome to the table, regardless of its level of abstraction.

Campbell then turns to a discussion of a "control panel," a sort of central station through which the key causal processes would operate for a particular outcome. Campbell's idea is to use interventionist models to select our control panel and not worry about any priori intelligibility issues. The final causes in the control panel might be a motley crew of heterogeneous risk factors, but so be it.

Campbell next comments on Marr's famous three explanatory levels originally designed to help explain the mammalian visual system: computation (what function is it supposed to perform?), algorithm (how does it compute the function?), and implementation (how does the wetware work?). His take on the limitations of this approach provides an interesting and different perspective to adopted by Murphy in this volume. I understand him to be describing a variant of Fodor's modular versus nonmodular construct. Although this model will work for the highly constrained visual system, trying to generalize this to what he calls "general-purpose thinking, mood and motivation" will, he suggests, run into the "nonmodularity" problem. Too many things can influence these processes. They don't have distinct levels. It won't be clear what is implementing what. We have much less of an idea about what represents malfunction. He concludes, "There is no analogue of Marr's algorithmic level for the ordinary functioning of the regulation of mood." Further empirical and philosophical work will be needed to determine whether this pessimistic conclusion is warranted.

He concludes by advocating a "many-sorted" approach to explanation in psychiatry that will not have an organized hierarchical or "level-based" form. We will have to construct our "control panels" for psychiatric disorders as we find them from our research—a likely hodge-podge of results. We have to eschew the "myth of intelligibility," lest our preconceptions about what constitutes a "good explanation" skew our conclusions. Campbell is, in the end, advocating a hard-nosed, empirical approach to causal models in psychiatry. Let the various causes be vetted by the empirical process, and we will work from what is left regardless of whether the resulting models agree with our a priori ideas of how explanation ought to work.

Kenneth S. Kendler, M.D.

REFERENCE

Woodward, J. 2003. *Making Things Happen*. New York: Oxford University Press.

＊　＊　＊

1. Intelligibility and Levels of Explanation

It is commonplace to say that causation in psychiatry is multifactorial. Many different variables, of many different types—social, economic, physiological, genetic, and so on—are said to be involved in the causation of disorders. Alternatively, it is sometimes said that causation in psychiatry has to be understood at many "different levels." This can be understood as merely a reformulation of the first remark, that variables of many different types are involved in the causation of disorders. We do have a rough intuitive understanding of when a variable is of one type or another. Income and employment are economic variables, 5-HTTLPR polymorphism is a genetic variable, and so on. On this reading, when it is said that causation in psychiatry has to be understood at many different levels, all that is meant is the empirically well-grounded remark that variables of many different types are causally implicated in the production of disorders.

A more ambitious doctrine, however, might be suggested by the idea that causation in psychiatry has to be understood at many different levels. The more ambitious doctrine is that (a) there are many different "levels of explanation" at which a disorder can be understood—sociological, psychological, biological, and so on; and (b) comprehensive understanding of a disorder will characteristically require a grasp of its explanation at a number of these levels. (You might argue that not all levels are required in all cases. Alzheimer disease can mostly be explained on a genetic or biological level; we don't need economic variables. Some phobias after severe trauma may require only an environmental explanation—perhaps no biology is needed to describe the cause.)

This idea is not usually given formal articulation. There is, as far as I know, no serious attempt in the literature on explanation in psychiatry to give explicit characterizations of the structures of explanations at each of the various presumed levels. But that there are these various levels of explanation, perhaps arranged in some kind of hierarchy, with socioeconomic or psychological models higher up and the whole thing grounding out in something like biological explanations, is a natural idea to have. For example, the neuropsychologist Christopher Frith (1992) comments on the explanation of "thought insertion"—the experience schizophrenic patients may have of alien thoughts being pushed into their minds, characteristically by some other and perhaps malign person: "[Causal explanations of the type] alien thoughts are caused by inappropriate firing of dopamine neurons [are] 'simply not admissible'" (Frith 1992, p. 26). Frith's point is not that we do not find correlations between alien thoughts and inappropriate firings of dopamine neurons. His idea is that we can see well enough in advance that "inappropriate firing of dopamine neurons" is the wrong kind of variable to be appealing to if we want to explain thought insertion. We might find the correlations between inappropriate firing of dopamine neurons and thought insertion, but that would still leave us in the dark as to why thought insertion, rather than some other phenomenon, was being produced. To get an explanation, we have to move to a "different level" of explanation, and to that end Frith produces his own cognitive model of thought insertion (Frith 1992).

I should say straight off that I select this passage for its merit rather than because I think it embodies some obvious confusion. In fact, I have for years found it helpful in introducing students to the idea of "levels of explanation," just because Frith's point seems so immediately plausible. Nonetheless, I think that the idea of a "level of explanation" that is appealed to here is problematic. It is not the same as the idea that an explanation may have to appeal to variables of many different types; in fact, it is in tension with that idea. The passage from Frith suggests that only certain variables may figure in each "level" of explanation, without being explicit about what the general structural constraints on each level of explanation are supposed to be. The appeal is to the need for some kind of understanding that is to be provided only by variables of a particular sort, so Frith's idea seems in tension with the notion of what I will call "many-sorted" explanations, in which variables of many different types are listed together as causes of a phenomenon.

Frith's remarks are also in tension with the idea that the causal relations between variables are always purely empirical and merely reflect the arbitrary correlations that we find in nature. On the role of reason in establishing the relation between cause and effect, David Hume says,

Every effect is a distinct event from its cause. It could not, therefore, be discovered in the cause, and the first invention or conception of it, a priori, must be entirely arbitrary. And even after it is suggested, the conjunction of it with the cause must appear equally arbitrary. . . . A man must be very sagacious who could discover by reasoning that crystal is the effect of heat, and ice of cold, without being previously acquainted with the operation of these qualities. (*Enquiry* [1748] 1975, IV/I)

We naturally seek a certain kind of intelligibility in nature; we naturally try to find explanations that will show the world to conform to reason, to behave as it ought. Hume's point is that there are no such intelligible connections to be found. This point has generally been accepted by philosophers thinking about causation. In fact, it is usually now taken as axiomatic that variables that are causally related should not have any logical connection between them, for, if the variables are logically related, any correlation we find between them will merely reflect that logical relation, rather than a causal connection.

Hume's comments nonetheless do leave us in an uncomfortable position, because we do tend to look for explanations that make the phenomena intelligible to reason. We are prone to relapse, to think that after all we must be able to find intelligibility in the world. This tendency survives, I suspect, in the idea of "levels of explanation." The idea is that within certain levels of explanation, we will find a particular kind of intelligibility. This lack of intelligibility is what Frith is complaining about in the idea of an arbitrary connection between improperly functioning dopamine neurons and thought insertion. Although it would be inhuman not to sympathize with the complaint, the lesson from Hume is that there is no more to causation than arbitrary connections between independent variables of cause and effect. We have to resist the demand for intelligibility.

I want now to look at the possibility of a more free-wheeling approach to causation in psychiatry than is suggested by the idea of "levels of explanation," segregated a priori by the demand for intelligibility. I want to set out the possibility of what I am calling "many-sorted" causal explanations of disorders, in which variables of any type may be used in any combination to provide an account of the genesis and maintenance of disorders. I will first explain the main idea of an interventionist approach to causation, as developed in the work of Sprites, Glymour, and Scheines (1993), Pearl (2000), Woodward (2003), and Woodward and Hitchcock

(2003). Then, in section 3, I will bring out how this approach to causation makes it possible to think in terms of many-sorted explanations. The point is that interventionism contrasts with an approach to causation that takes causation to be a matter of mechanical processes linking cause and effect. Finally, I will contrast the free-wheeling approach I am recommending to causation in psychiatry with the more rigid approach to the cognitive science of vision taken by David Marr (1982), who famously distinguished among three levels of explanation in cognitive science, a distinction that is drawn on a relatively a priori basis. Marr's explanation has a certain a priori legitimacy, I will argue, but it does not transfer from the cognitive science of vision to causation in general psychiatry.

2. Interventionism about Causation

There is a significant correlation between insomnia or hypersomnia and unipolar depression; disordered sleep is one of the *DSM-IV* symptomatic criteria for major depression. The existence of the correlation leaves open the question of causation. Is insomnia an effect of the depression? Or is insomnia one of the contributing causes of depression? Or are they both, rather, joint effects of some common cause?

These answers do not exclude one another; it is possible that all three are correct. But what difference does it make for one rather than another of these accounts to be correct? What is it for there to be some particular direction of causation? The interventionist answer is that to say insomnia is a cause of depression is to say an intervention on insomnia would make a difference to depression; perhaps it would be possible to rout depression altogether by treating a patient's insomnia. On the other hand, if insomnia is merely a symptom of depression, intervening on the insomnia will make no difference whatever to the depression. Similarly, if the insomnia is merely an effect of some common cause of both insomnia and depression, in this case, too, intervening on the insomnia will make no difference to the depression.

On this account, we explain what it is for insomnia to be a cause of depression by saying, were there to be an intervention on insomnia, there would be a difference in depression. An intervention on insomnia has to be a way of changing the subject's sleep patterns; but not just any way of changing the patient's sleep patterns should count as an "intervention."

We want to be able to conclude that, if depression were to change when we intervene on insomnia, insomnia causes depression.

An intervention on insomnia must have some effect on the subject's sleep. But, I said, not just any way of affecting the subject's sleep will do. We might, for example, find that administering tricyclic antidepressants makes a difference to a patient's insomnia and that this is correlated with a change in the subject's depression. But this would not establish that insomnia is a cause of depression. A better hypothesis is that the drug is affecting both the insomnia and the depression directly. We have to rule out this kind of thing from counting as an intervention on insomnia, so we can say that an intervention on insomnia should not be affecting the depression in any way other than by affecting the insomnia.

We also have to rule out cases in which we are changing the sleep patterns only of people who are about to recover from depression anyhow; we do not want our interventions to be correlated with the subject's level of depression. Otherwise, we would find that under our treatments of insomnia we are getting a correlation between goodness of sleep and recovery from depression, but this would not mean that insomnia was a cause of the depression. So our "interventions" on insomnia had better not themselves be correlated with the subject's level of depression.

Finally, the most difficult condition. Suppose that there is some common cause of insomnia and depression, perhaps an underlying chemical imbalance or some factor such as work-related stress. If this were the case, we might act to change the subject's sleep patterns and make some impact on them while still allowing this common cause—say, stress—also to affect both insomnia and depression. We will then still find a residual correlation between insomnia and depression. This correlation would not constitute a causal path from insomnia to depression. One solution is to demand that the intervention on insomnia should, ideally, be the sole factor affecting the subject's sleep patterns, that all other factors affecting the subject's sleep should be suspended from having their ordinary influence on it. In this ideal condition the underlying chemical imbalance or the work-related stress would have no effect on the subject's sleep. If in this condition we intervene on the subject's sleep pattern, taking complete control of it, and we still find a correlation between the subject's sleep pattern and level of depression, we can conclude this means the sleep pattern is causing depression. This is the distinctive mark of what Pearl (2000) calls a "surgical" intervention. The intention of randomized control trials is to find what would happen under such interventions. The idea is that by averaging across the randomly chosen cohort for each level of intervention, we can factor out the varying idiosyncratic causes of, for example, the insomnia on which we are intervening, and find what would happen if our intervention had taken sole control of, for example, the subject's sleep patterns.

I am expounding work by Woodward and Hitchcock (2003) and Woodward in his recent book (2003), which gives a succinct general characterization of this notion of intervention. Suppose our hypothesis is that variable X is a cause of variable Y (that insomnia is a cause of depression; that a peptide causes autism). Then an "intervention variable" I on X with respect to Y is a variable that meets the following conditions:

1. I is a cause of X.
2. I does not cause Y otherwise than by causing X.
3. I is not correlated with any Z other than X that is a cause of Y.
4. I suspends X from the influence of any other variable.

Woodward goes on to argue that for X to be a cause of Y is for X to be correlated with Y under interventions on X with respect to Y. (For further discussion of how the interventionist model applies to mental causation, see Woodward, chapter 4 in this volume.)

This is an intuitive approach to causation, and it reflects much of ordinary experimental methodology. In particular, it well reflects the methodology of randomized control trials. The whole point of the randomization is to ensure that condition 4 is met. Suppose, for example, we are conducting a randomized control trial (RCT) of the effect of some drug on recovery from an illness. The point of the randomization is to ensure that the average levels of the drug in the blood of each cohort of our study are due only to the experimental intervention, not to variation in endogenous production of the drug or spontaneous ingestion. The RCT is telling us what would happen if these idiosyncratic mechanisms were suspended from having any impact on the level of drug in the blood.

3. Many-Sorted Explanations

I now turn to how this approach to causation makes it possible to give many-sorted causal explanations of disorders, in which variables of different types are used together in any combination. An example from the literature on major depression is illustrative. I will simplify the example and push the data a little bit further than they actually go, so it gives a readily comprehensible model of the type of explanation I have in mind. Although it is simplified, the model I propose is representative of a vast range of findings in psychiatry, in which it is shown that variables of many different types—social, economic, psychological, physiological, genetic— are relevant to the causation of one or another disorder.

It has long been known that catastrophic life events such as bereavement or divorce are predictors of later depression. In a longitudinal study of 7,000 subjects, Kendler and colleagues (Kendler et al. 2003) tried to find just which catastrophic life events are the best predictors of major depression. In brief, their finding was that episodes of humiliation—in particular, humiliation with some significant social dimension—were the best predictors of later depression. Let us suppose that it is correct to give this finding a causal interpretation: that humiliation is one of the causes of major depression.

It has also long been thought that that there are genetic factors in depression and suspected that genetic deficiencies in the serotonin transporter mechanism may be at the root of the problem. It now seems likely that recent attempts to identify a specific genetic basis have been unsuccessful (Lotrich and Pollok 2004); it may be that we are looking at effects of multiple genes. For ease of exposition, though, suppose that we simplify the situation. Suppose it is indeed a genetic abnormality in some aspect of serotonin function that matters. Not everyone who is humiliated becomes depressed; let us suppose that the individual variation in serotonin transporter underpins resilience, so typically the two variables together, perhaps in combination with other factors, yield major depression. We can diagram the situation as in Figure 5.1.

Figure 5.1 is an example of what I mean by a "many-sorted" causal explanation. Variables of different levels are put together in a single causal account of the disorder. As I said, this is a simplified example, but it is representative of a vast class of more complex cases in which the causation of a disorder is found not only to be multifactorial but also to involve variables of different types.

Is there any reason why we should rule out such explanations a priori and say that they somehow involve a confounding of variables of different types? On the interventionist approach, it is difficult to see why there should be any such prohibitions. The meaning of the diagram is perfectly

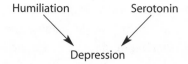

Figure 5.1. Multisorted explanation. A simple example of a "multi-sorted" explanation, in which variables of different levels play coordinate roles as causes of an outcome.

clear. Intervene on the humiliation, and there will, in some cases at any rate, be a difference in the risk for depression. Intervene on serotonin function, and there will, in some cases at any rate, be a difference in the risk for depression. Do we need any more than this to establish the legitimacy of the many-sorted explanation? Isn't it perfectly obvious that the many-sorted causal account is legitimate?

There is a significant philosophical tradition of arguing that causation has to be understood as a matter of there being mechanical processes connecting cause and effect (Fair 1979; Salmon 1984; Dowe 2000). The many-sorted explanation, interpreted in interventionist terms, makes no attempt to find mechanical processes connecting cause and effect. It allows that there may be causal relations in the absence of any such mechanical processes. The existence of such mechanical processes is not constitutive of the existence of a causal relation, on the interventionist account.

It has not proven straightforward for advocates of a mechanical approach to causation to say exactly what kind of processes they think constitute the causal relation. Still, evidently a mechanistic approach to causation does have a tendency to elevate one particular "level" of understanding—that involving the preferred mechanical level, whatever exactly it is thought to be—above any other type of causal understanding. The mechanical level, whatever it is in general, would naturally be supposed, as far as mental causation goes, to be some level of biological understanding. This kind of approach to causation does promote the idea of a hierarchy of levels of understanding, because all other variables than those relating to the mechanism are thought to be relevant to causation only by virtue of some relation they have to the underlying mechanical variables. The merit of the interventionist approach to causation is that it makes plain that we don't have to think like this: we can regard many-sorted explanations as having their own autonomy, and not as being merely programmatic steps toward some more basic level of understanding.

I want to mention one line of thought in favor of a mechanistic approach simply because it is intriguing rather than because it seems convincing. My discussion so far has concerned what is usually called "type" or "general" causation, statements such as "smoking causes cancer" rather than "singular" claims such as "John's smoking caused his cancer." It has been argued (Sober 1985) that claims of singular causation do require the existence of a continuous spatiotemporal process connecting the episodes of cause and effect. So, for example, for John's smoking to have caused his cancer, there must be processes that spatiotemporally link his smoking to his cancer; in principle, we could identify the particular pathways that lead from the inhalation of tobacco to the proliferation of cancer cells. In general, Sober argues, singular causal claims require spatiotemporal processes linking cause and effect. Applying this idea to the psychological case would mean that, if particular psychological episodes are to be viewed as causing particular further events, there must be continuous spatiotemporal processes connecting them. Because those processes would presumably be biological, this line of thought suggests a certain priority for use of biological variables in psychological explanation. Indeed, if we view general causal claims as merely generalized versions of the singular claims (Carroll 1991), this priority of the biological would apply to all causal claims in psychology.

As I said, I mention this line of thought because it seems intriguing. It would connect with another idea argued a long time ago by Martin and Deutscher (1966): an implicit materialism in folk psychology appears when we reflect on what it takes for an individual to be truly remembering a past event rather than merely being able to make a reliably correct report about it. Martin and Deutscher argued that folk psychology is informed by the notion of a "memory trace," the physical trace laid down by the past event, and that we ordinarily think of remembering as a matter of that physical trace being fired up in the current context. So it is intriguing to ask whether our ordinary conception of singular causation in the psychological case might not similarly be informed by a kind of folk materialism, so the question of the particular psychological cause of a particular event hinges on whether there is some biological path from the psychological episode to the effect; however, I can see no sign of this idea in our ordinary thinking. In courts of law, where much often turns on the question whether someone's motives were the motive for which they acted, there seems never to be an appeal to this idea (Hart and Honore 1985).

One might ask, nonetheless, whether the truth in the doctrine of "levels" of explanation is not this: there is only one level of causal explanation in psychiatry, the biological. All the rest—sociological, economic, or psychological explanations—are merely way-stations, preliminary roughings—out of the shape of what ultimately must be biological explanation. I have said that the obvious motivations for this view lack weight, but can we give any positive reason for thinking that it is right to find causation at the level of, for example, psychology? We have a complex system, the human being, that can be characterized in many different ways, using many different sets of variables. Can we find a general reason for thinking that one rather than another variable set is the one to use in describing, for example, the causes of psychological disorders?

The interventionist approach does not of itself tell us how to select a variable set; as I have explained it, the approach presupposes that we have already made our choice of variables to use, but with its suggestion that the point of an interest in causation has to do with our interest in manipulation, the interventionist approach gives us a steer toward a way of choosing a variable set. In 1965 the epidemiologist Austen Bradford Hill proposed a number of criteria for the existence of a causal relation between, principally, an environmental hazard and illness. Hill proposed that the argument for a causal relation between hazard and illness is greatly strengthened if we find that there is

(a) A dose-response relation between the two—For example, the case for a causal link between smoking and lung cancer is strengthened if we find that the greater the number of cigarettes smoked each day, the greater the probability of contracting lung cancer.

(b) A big change in the probability of the effect—If we find that smoking is correlated with a large change in the probability of contracting lung cancer, again the case for a causal relation between the two is strengthened.

(c) A correlation specifically with this outcome rather than any other— That is, if, for example, smoking is correlated specifically with the contraction of lung cancer, this correlation improves the case for saying that smoking causes cancer.

These criteria for the existence of a causal relation are evidently plausible, and their plausibility does not seem confined to the epidemiological context. At the same time, their status is not obvious. Are they somehow a priori conditions on the existence of a causal relation? Or is there some empirical argument to be given for them? I want to propose that we find the right status for these criteria if we think of them as criteria for the choice of a variable set, criteria for finding the right variable set to use in characterizing a complex system. They are perhaps not exactly stated, these criteria, but they do not have to be. We are looking for a way of finding the best candidate, the best set of variables to use in characterizing a complex system, out of a pool of competitors. On the interventionist approach, what we are looking for is a set of variables that can serve as the "control panel" for the system, and obviously we would want a control panel to have controls that meet those criteria. Suppose, for instance, that you think of the controls of a car. You want each control to have a systematic impact on its effect; the further you press the accelerator, the faster the car goes. You want the control to have a large effect on the output, and you want it to have an effect specifically on that output. That is what a good control panel looks like. In the case of a psychological disorder, we want to find a set of variables whose manipulation will give us systematic, large, and specific effects on the disorder. The best set of variables to use will be the one that best meets those criteria. There are no absolute standards to meet here; we simply want to find the best set of control variables we can.

Incidentally, I am of course not suggesting that the case for thinking that smoking is a cause of cancer could be undermined by showing that smoking is correlated with many other outcomes than cancer itself. The point is rather that smoking is one of a family of variables that jointly provide us with a control panel for cancer. We make the case for thinking that this whole family of variables, of which smoking is a nonredundant member, is the right set of variables in terms of which to think of the causes of those diseases, by showing that we can by manipulating the various variables in the set jointly have systematic, large, and specific effects on our outcomes. If we could not, by freely manipulating this whole set, have specific effects on cancer itself, this would indeed undermine the case for thinking that we had found the right family of variables in terms of which to think of the causes of the disease.

From this perspective, the argument for many-sorted explanations in psychiatry is that many-sorted explanations provide our best control panels for disorders. Intervening on a level of humiliation or on serotonin levels may each be the best ways there are of intervening on depression, given the criteria of systematicity, size, and specificity. Restricting ourselves to variables of any one type simply may not provide the best possible control panel for the disorder.

Of course, putting it in this way presupposes that we have a fixed set of disorders in whose causation we are interested, and that is not quite the situation, because the diagnostic criteria are themselves open to challenge. And one element in finding the right set of diagnostic criteria may be that we want to find ways of classifying the disorders that will allow us to find efficient sets of "control variables" for them.

4. Marr's Three Levels of Explanation

In *Vision,* Marr famously distinguishes among three levels of explanation in cognitive science, to be discriminated among when we are considering the explanation of vision in particular. The idea is that we can characterize the ordinary or healthy functioning of vision at different levels:

(a) The level of computation, at which we specify what the visual system is computing. We do not at this level say how the visual system is going about this, only what the end result is. Of course, the problem may be broken down to specify what is being computed by visual subsystems. For example, consider the problem of defining the "correspondence" that holds between successive visual perceptions of the same scene. This is a matter of formulating what has to be matched with what. Making explicit just what correspondences the visual system is managing to compute says nothing about how the visual system manages to do it.

(b) The level of the algorithm, at which we describe the information processing that the visual system uses to achieve its goals. For example, one might want to describe the process whereby vision manages to spot that it is the object that was on the left that is moving toward the right. In general, there must be a specification of the input and output representations, and the operations that are typically performed to transform inputs into outputs.

(c) The level of implementation, at which we say just how the information processing described at the level of the algorithm is realized biologically.

In Marr's approach, the study of vision proceeds through the study of various modular subsystems, processing, for example, information about shape, motion, orientation, color, and so on. For each module, we have a specification of its computational point, how that task is achieved by operations on representations, and ultimately a characterization of the biology that implements the system. We need the level of the algorithm because generalizations are available at that level that simply could not be stated in more directly biological terms. If, for example, the visual system is using a particular set of operations defined over a particular type of syntactic representation to find movement in the visual field, the generalizations we shall find about the kinds of error to which the system is prone will not depend on the details of the biology. Moreover, the algorithmic level will in one way defy comprehension in terms of the biological level, because the choice of variables to characterize the syntax of the representations will depend on what computational task we suppose is being performed. If we consider only the biological level, we will not be able to identify the relevant aspects of syntax.

As I said, these three levels relate to the ordinary or healthy functioning of the system. There are generalizations about what computational task a visual system is ordinarily or typically performing and about how it typically does that, that we would lose if we confined ourselves merely to detailed biological descriptions of the system. The idea of "levels" is that generalizations at the level of the algorithm are stated in terms of one kind of vocabulary; generalizations at the biological level are stated in terms of a distinct, disjoint vocabulary.

When we try to apply this model to the kind of general-purpose thinking, mood, and motivation that are traditionally the domain of psychiatry, a number of problems emerge. First, we do not find disjoint sets of variables in terms of which various types of generalization about the ordinary or healthy functioning of the system can be stated. Take, for example, mood regulation. In an ordinary, healthy individual, mood can be affected by variables of many different types. In the evening I settle down to try to cope with an alarming piece of news. I have just been for a swim and I am slowly ingesting a glass of whisky. Whether I've had bad news, my metabolic rate and my whisky consumption are variables of different types, but they are all equally determinants of my mood. We cannot find generalizations at one level—the "psychological" level, say—that relate to the determination of my mood and that are merely implemented by lower-level generalizations about my biology. Increased metabolic rate and whisky are, as determinants of my mood, coordinate with psychological factors such as my just having had a piece of bad news. The effect of swimming on my metabolic rate and my whisky consumption are not merely implementations of some higher-level algorithmic computation. So there is no analogue of Marr's algorithmic level for the ordinary functioning of the regulation of mood; there is no level at which we find a distinctive family of generalizations stated in a vocabulary disjoint from that of biology.

There is certainly a distinction to be drawn between a functional, "box-and-arrow" characterization of general-purpose thinking, mood, and motivation and a characterization of the whole system that describes it merely in terms of local properties. The box-and-arrow characterization depends on some identification of the point of the system, what its eventual output is taken to be, that will typically demand that we look at the context in which it is functioning. In contrast, identification of local properties, such as low-level physical properties of the system, may not depend at all on the context in which the system is operating. But, in general, the point of a system need not be a computational point. When we characterize the workings of a car, for example, it is certainly illuminating to be told about the carburetor and the pistons, and this kind of description can be contrasted with a description of the local physical properties of the thing. But the car is not fundamentally a computer, even if it has chips here and there allowing it to find the exact gas-air mixture in the tank, for instance. Similarly, it is illuminating to know that humiliation causes major depression, and there may be related computations about, for example, one's own social standing going on in the transition from humiliation to depression, but that is not to say that transition is fundamentally computational. Even though humiliation has an adaptive point, there is no reason to suppose that this must be a computational point.

Although we can distinguish between box-and-arrow characterizations and local characterizations of a system, there is in general no presumption that there is just one box-and-arrow characterization of a system to be given. Even in the case of a classical input module, there may be nested levels of box-and-arrow classification, but in the case of general-purpose thinking, mood and motivation, there may be no limit to the divergent ways in which we can give functional descriptions of the system. Does the phenomenon of humiliation have just one adaptive point? We have a complex system whose various elements developed together in a complex environment with many different demands on the organism. In the case of a domain-specific module, we can at any rate identify the kind of problem that the system is dedicated to solving. In the case of general-purpose thinking, mood, and motivation, there is no such thing as giving a concise description of the kind of problem that that the system is dedicated to solving; the system is not domain specific. The phenomenon of humiliation feeds into endlessly many processes other than merely the production of depression. There is no reason to suppose in advance that we will find just one kind of output that defines the point of the phenomenon.

Finally, in the case of vision, we have a relatively plain distinction between the ordinary or healthy functioning of the system and the way it functions in abnormal cases, or cases of partial breakdown. One approach to psychiatric cases is to suppose that we are dealing with a system whose healthy functioning can be characterized in terms of Marr's three levels but that as the result of an organic disturbance something has gone wrong with the running of the algorithm. Something like this picture underpins Frith's account of schizophrenia, on which an algorithm whose point is to assign the ownership of thoughts and actions malfunctions as a consequence of organic disturbance. The trouble with this as a general model for psychiatry is that in general we do not have a firm grasp on the contrast between the healthy and the abnormal functioning of the system. Consider again the production of major depression. If humiliation produces major depression, is that a consequence of the malfunctioning of the humiliation-depression system? What about the role of grief in producing depression? If, as the result of bereavement, you show the symptoms of depression, is there a dysfunction for which we should seek an organic basis? On the face of it, the production of the symptoms of major depression is "perfectly normal," and there is no particular reason to look for an organic disturbance that is making possible the transition from grief to the symptoms of depression. But we evidently do not have a firm grasp of the contrast between the cases in which the symptoms of grief-related depression are the result of the healthy functioning of some system and the cases in which they are the result of the abnormal functioning of a system.

Marr's approach has obviously been an illuminating approach to vision. It can also, obviously, be generalized to many other areas too. I think, though, that it is just a mistake to suppose that the right direction of generalization is to more and more psychological phenomena. I want to suggest that there will be no easy generalization of the cognitive science approach to ordinary psychological or psychiatric phenomena. Rather, the most fruitful direction of generalization will be to nonpsychological, biological phenomena: work on biological information processing. For example, it is arguable that the human immune system is best viewed as a computer whose point is to detect and respond to pathogens, a computer capable of learning and flexibility in response. That is, we should take a broadly "cognitive science" approach to the immune system, at all of Marr's three levels. This is a tribute to the power of a cognitive science approach. It also suggests, however, that the approach is unlikely to illuminate the phenomena that have traditionally been thought of as specifically psychological: the phenomena of consciousness and thinking that are central to psychiatry.

5. Explanation without a Hierarchy of Levels

My conclusion is that we should take at face value the flood of empirical work that suggests causation in psychiatry is multifactorial and that causal explanation will characteristically be "many sorted," using variables of many different types. The idea of a hierarchy of levels of explanation has no place in psychiatry, however powerful a tool it is in characterizing systems such as vision or the immune system.

The idea of a hierarchy of levels of explanation, with biology as the base level, has a number of sources. One is the appeal of a mechanistic model of causation that insists a priori that all causation must involve contact phenomena; biology is seen as the level that characterizes the contact phenomena. The point of appealing to an interventionist model of causation is that it makes it evident we do not have to think about causation in mechanistic terms. And interventionism allows for many-sorted explanations: we can find that an intervention on any type of variable will make a difference to the value of any type of variable, and the whole network of causes may turn out to have any assortment of types of variable. Our best control panel for the disorders in which we are interested may turn out to involve combinations of variables of any sorts.

Another source for the appeal of a hierarchy of levels of explanation, with biology at the base, is the success of an approach in terms of Marr's three levels in the study of vision. As I stated above, this approach does indeed seem capable of generalization to the study of biological information processing across a broad swathe of subject matters, such as the immune system. But it does not seem applicable to general psychiatry, because general-purpose thinking, mood, and motivation do not have the kind of computational point required for Marr's analysis to apply.

The deepest source of the idea of a hierarchy of levels of explanation is, I suspect, the pull of a pre-Humean demand for intelligibility in causal explanations: the idea that reason discovers for us what a level of explanation must look like so that, when we look to find what is causing what, we know in advance how nature must conform. This demand for intelligibility still lingers even in our thinking about physics, even though most philosophers would officially repudiate it. But I do not think it is too strong to say that the myth of intelligibility constitutes the idea of levels of explanation in psychiatry. I think we do have to let go of that idea. It is possible that there will turn out to be empirical conditions on what types of variable can combine with what types of variable to yield what types of outcome. In recent work on the notion of "causal grammar," Tenenbaum et al. (2007) suggested that strategies for finding out about causation will work better if we look not just for what is causing what, but for more general empirical conditions on what types of variable can combine with what. The torrent of empirical evidence for many-factorial causation in psychiatry, however, suggests that if we do find empirical evidence for any such causal grammar, the grammars will bear little resemblance to anything currently identified as a "level" of explanation.

REFERENCES

Carroll, J. 1991. Property-Level Causation? *Philosophical Studies* 63:245–270.
Dowe, P. 2000. *Physical Causation.* Cambridge: Cambridge University Press.
Fair, D. 1979. Causation and the Flow of Energy. *Erkenntnis* 14:219–250.
Frith, C. 1992. *The Cognitive Neuropsychology of Schizophrenia.* Hillsdale, NJ: Lawrence Erlbaum Associates.
Hart, H. L. A., and T. Honore. 1985. *Causation in the Law.* Oxford: Clarendon Press.
Hill, A. B. 1965. The Environment and Disease: Association or Causation? *Proceedings of the Royal Society of Medicine* 58:295–300.
Hume, D. (1748) 1975. *An Enquiry Concerning Human Understanding.* Oxford: Clarendon Press.
Kendler, K. S., J. M. Hettema, F. Butera, C. O. Gardner, and C. A. Prescott. 2003. Life Event Dimensions of Loss, Humiliation, Entrapment, and Danger in the Prediction of Onsets of Major Depression and Generalized Anxiety. *Archives of General Psychiatry* 60:789–796.
Lotrich, F. E., and B. G. Pollok. 2004. Meta-Analysis of Serotonin Transporter Polymorphisms and Affective Disorders. *Psychiatric Genetics* 14:121–129.
Marr, D. 1982. *Vision: A Computational Investigation into the Human Representation and Processing of Visual Information.* San Francisco: W. H. Freeman.

Martin, C. B., and M. Deutscher. 1966. Remembering. *Philosophical Review* 75: 161–196.

Pearl, J. 2000. *Causation*. Cambridge: Cambridge University Press.

Salmon, W. 1984. *Scientific Explanation and the Causal Structure of the World*. Princeton, NJ: Princeton University Press.

Sober, E. 1985. Two Concepts of Cause. In P. Asquith and P. Kitcher (eds.), *PSA 1984*, vol. 2 (pp. 405–424). East Lansing, MI: Philosophy of Science Association.

Spirtes, P., C. Glymour, and R. Scheines. 1993. *Causation, Prediction, and Search*. New York: Springer-Verlag.

Tenenbaum, J. B., T. L. Griffiths, and S. Niyogi. 2007. Intuitive Theories as Grammars for Causal Inference. In A. Gopnik and L. Schulz (eds.), *Causal Learning: Psychology, Philosophy, and Computation* (pp. 301–322). Oxford: Oxford University Press.

Woodward, J. 2003. *Making Things Happen: A Theory of Causal Explanation*. Oxford: Oxford University Press.

Woodward, J., and C. Hitchcock. 2003. Explanatory Generalizations. Part 1. A Counterfactual Account. *Nous* 37:1–24.

Comment: Levels of Explanation and Variable Choice
James F. Woodward, Ph.D.

Let me say at the outset that I agree with virtually all that John Campbell says in his interesting chapter—both what he has to say about the topic of levels of explanation and what he takes an interventionist account of causation to imply about this topic. So, to a substantial extent, I will elaborate and expand on ideas in his chapter here, rather than registering disagreement—a departure from the disciplinary norms of philosophy, although perhaps not those of psychiatry.

As Campbell says, the idea that explanation, not just in psychiatry but in many other disciplines, can occur at many different "levels" is a commonplace idea in methodological discussion. Properly understood, I think that it is a correct idea. It is also, however, an idea that can be interpreted in many different ways, not all of them equally plausible or defensible. In what follows, I will try to sort out and comment on some different versions of this doctrine. To summarize my conclusions, I argue that we should distinguish two different ways of thinking about levels of explanation. According to the first approach, there is some independent way of identifying a hierarchy of levels, either in nature or in our understanding, and we can then use this information to provide general constraints on the explanations we give, perhaps via the idea the factors we cite in explanations must be at the same level as the effects we wish to explain or via the idea that for each kind of effect there is some privileged level of explanation. (That is, it is claimed that facts about a subject's psychology must be explained at "the psychological level," the state of his brain must be explained just by "neurobiological factors" and so forth.) According to the second approach, it is a mistake to suppose that we can appeal in this way to general considerations about levels to tell us that certain explanations are appropriate and others inappropriate. Instead, the constraining goes in the other direction: the right level or levels to use are just those that are best from the point of view of our explanatory and modeling purposes. On this second view, there are real, nontrivial issues about the appropriate level at which we should frame explanations, but it is most perspicuous to think of these as issues about the variables we should employ in those explanations, and this in turn depends both on what we want to explain and on specific empirical considerations. On this second approach, there is thus no general, a priori reason for insisting that all legitimate explanations must involve factors at some single, privileged level— which level or levels will be most appropriate will depend on the specific details of the case at hand. In agreement with Campbell, I argue for the second approach and then, all too briefly, take up the issue of what principles should govern the choice of variables that should be included in the explanations we construct.

Let me begin, though, with the notion of a "level" itself and some of the different meanings that have been assigned to this notion. One reason for proceeding in this way is that, if we are going to discuss this notion, we should have at least some idea of the various meanings that might be assigned to it and how they are related to one another. Although talk of levels of explanation is widespread in many areas of science, we shall see that the notion itself is elusive (or at least multifaceted) and difficult to pin down. Another motivation is that once one becomes aware of all the rather different things that are sometimes meant by "level" (and the unclarity of many of these), this ought to make us suspicious of highly general or quasi a priori advice about the appropriate choice of level of explanation. Here then are some possible notions of level:[1]

1. *Levels understood in terms of relative size or in terms of spatial part/whole relationships.* It is an ubiquitous feature of the natural world that larger things contain smaller things as parts, and they in turn often have

still smaller parts; atoms are parts of molecules, which in turn are parts of subcellular structures like membranes, cells are composed of such substructures, multicellular organisms like people contain many distinct organs or systems, societies are made up of individual people, and so on. Often when investigators talk about levels, they have in mind a (partial) ordering generated by these part or whole or compositional relationships: atoms are at a "lower level" than molecules, which are in turn at a "lower level" than structures like cell membranes, and so on, because in each case, the first member of these pairs is smaller in size than and literally a proper part of the second member of the pair. The ordering generated by the part-to-whole relation is "partial" because it does not tell us how to compare levels for factors that do not stand in this relation (for example, an environmental variable such as "low social status" is not a part of a subject's neural state [or vice versa], so the part-to-whole ordering does not tell us whether these variables are at a "higher" or "lower" or the "same" level with respect to each other).

2. *Levels understood in terms of relative abstractness versus concreteness.* Here the idea is that the same process or feature of a system can be described either in a relatively specific, detailed, or fine-grained way or, alternatively, in a less-specific (more coarse-grained) way that abstracts away from at least some of this detail. The more abstract description reveals what the process has in common with other processes that may differ from it at a fine-grained level. The more abstract description/representation is regarded as at a different and "higher" level than the more concrete description. This seems to be the most natural way of understanding David Marr's famous discussion of levels of explanation in visual processing. When some aspect of visual processing is described at the algorithmic level and then at the computational level, it seems most plausible to think of this as a matter of the same process being described at different levels of specificity or abstractness. (That is, it is not as though the computational characterization describes some process that is over and above or distinct from whatever is described by the algorithmic characterization—it is the same process, differently described.) What characterizes the computational level is the function being computed. Different algorithms may be employed to compute the same function, and, in any given case and insofar as visual processing is computational, one specific algorithm rather than another will be employed on any given occasion. When we describe the processing at the computational level, we simply abstract

away from details having to do with the specific algorithm employed. Presumably, a similar relationship holds between the algorithmic and implementational level. The latter might involve a description of some neural network or circuit, and how the firing rates of various components are influenced by their inputs and the connectivity of the entire system. The algorithmic level involves a description of this processing in a way that abstracts from this detail and just tells us about the algorithm being implemented.

Notice that this is different from the part-to-whole notion of level described above. The algorithm (or whatever is described by the algorithmic characterization) is *not* a spatial part of the computation (or whatever is characterized by the computational level of description).[2] Although the abstract/specific contrast is a matter of different descriptions of a single process, the whole/part relation (or the description of a whole versus a description of one of its proper parts) is not a matter of the same thing being described in different ways, at different levels of abstraction. It is true that it often turns out that if we wish to provide a tractable explanation of the behavior of a whole, we will need to find a way of characterizing it that abstracts away from various details of the behavior of its parts (see below for examples) so that, in this sense, the part/whole distinction and the specific/abstract distinction are correlated. Nonetheless, what makes a whole be at a higher level than its parts in sense 1 is the part/whole relationship in which it stands rather than how abstract/specific its description is. Whereas the relationship between part and whole is "out there" in nature, the abstract/specific contrast is a contrast in different ways that *we* may choose to describe nature—that is, it is a feature of our descriptive practices, albeit a feature that is influenced in various ways by relationships that exist in nature.

3. *Levels understood in terms of theories, disciplines, or characteristic concepts.* Another common line of thought associates the notion of level with a general kind of theory or research tradition or perhaps with an entire scientific discipline or concepts or vocabulary employed in that discipline. Arguably, it is in this sense that one finds commentators talking about "the psychological level," "the biochemical level," sometimes even "the physical level," and so on. (This may of course be accompanied by the thought that each discipline or kind of theory is concerned with objects of some characteristic size or which are represented at some distinctive level of abstraction—that is, level in the sense of 3 can be combined

with ideas about levels along the lines of 1 and 2.) When the notion of level is understood in this discipline or theory-specific way, however, it is difficult to see how it can have any fundamental methodological significance. For example, if "the psychological level" merely means something like employing vocabulary, concepts, descriptions, theories, and so forth that currently figure in the discipline of psychology as currently practiced (or referring to processes and so on that are characterized in terms of this vocabulary), this would appear to be a notion with vague boundaries that shift over time and that reflect facts about the interests and practices of psychologists, rather than any fundamental features of nature. On this characterization, for example, as psychologists employ neural imaging techniques and begin to talk about specific brain regions that are involved in the processes they study, these become part of "the psychological level." It is difficult to see how considerations having to do with levels in this sense could serve as a constraint on the content of our theories—rather it is our theorizing that is dictating what we think of as belonging to the same or different levels.

In light of these different notions of level, what follows for how we should think about the notion(s) of levels of explanation? Let me begin with some ideas that (in agreement with Campbell) I see as misguided. It is sometimes suggested that explanations should always involve causes or effects (or characterizations of these) that are all at the same single level— that is, that multilevel (or what Campbell calls "multisorted") explanations should be disallowed as a matter of general principle. The underlying thought is perhaps something like the following: nature segregates naturally into distinct levels (or alternatively the theorist or scientific disciplines must assume such a segregation), we identify the level L to which the effect we want to explain belongs, and then the explanation must be entirely in terms of factors that are also at the same level L. Obviously, this idea might be spelled out in a number of different ways depending on the notion of level that is employed—thinking of nature as segregated by size/part/whole relationships or by perhaps by disciplinary subject matter are two of the most common choices. The common thread running through this approach is that the appropriate level at which an explanation is to be constructed is identified independently of and before the construction of the detailed explanation itself: the choice of level tells us what sorts of factors are appropriately cited in the explanation. On this conception, we end up with claims like the following: psychological phenomena must be explained in terms of factors that are themselves at the psychological level rather than in terms of "lower-level" factors such as levels of neurotransmitters, the behavior of groups must be explained in terms of group level or social factors rather than in terms of facts about individual psychology, biochemical effects should be explained exclusively in terms of biochemical causes, and so on.

Put in this bald way, I think that there is almost nothing to be said for this idea, no matter how the notion of level is to be interpreted. To begin with, even if we accept one or more of the ideas about levels canvassed above, they do not, for the reasons I have already noted, give us a general way of determining whether factors or phenomena are at the same level or not: at best they yield a partial ordering. That is, even if we can say that some factors, states, or processes are at a higher level than some others (according to some appropriate conception of level), this doesn't give us a general recipe for determining whether various factors that we are considering, including in an explanation are or are not at the same level as others. (For example, according to the part/whole conception brains are at a higher level than neurons, but, as we have seen, this doesn't tell us whether, say, [a] the experience of humiliation is at a higher or lower or the same level as [b] the state of a subject's brain or some part of his brain, because [b] does not stand in a part/whole relationship to [a].) In other words, it looks as though, for most of the conceptions of level described above, the notion of sameness of level is just too vague and indeterminate to give us much guidance in trying to implement the proposal, even if it were otherwise defensible. In practice, I suspect that the proposal may amount to little more than the advice that explanations should appeal only to factors that are currently studied within single disciplines: explain the sorts of phenomena that psychologists or psychiatrists study in terms of other factors they currently study or theorize about. Needless to say, there is no serious methodological justification for this advice.

A similar conclusion follows if we try to motivate the idea that explanations should appeal to factors at the same level by appealing to a size-based conception of level. Some writers[3] seem to be tempted by the following line of thought: objects of the same general size tend to interact more often or more strongly with one another than with objects of different sizes—atoms with atoms, molecules with molecules, and so on. If something like this size principle were true, we might have a rationale for thinking that it is likely that the most satisfactory explanations will relate factors at the same level, when level is understood in terms of size. The size principle, however, seems dubious, at least in the biological and psychological sciences. For example (compare Bechtel and Hamilton 2007; Craver 2007), structures such as membranes can mediate the transport and interactions of ions and molecules despite being a much larger size than the latter, levels of neurotransmitters in particular neural structures can affect the behavior of entire organisms, the social environment can affect levels of neurotransmitters and gene expression and so on.

Suppose, however, that we put aside the fact that it is difficult to specify what the notion of level amounts to and rely instead on whatever intuitive understanding we may have of this notion—that is, we take it that we are able to identify sameness or difference of levels in specific cases, even if we have no good general theory of what a level is. I believe that it is still true, for the reasons Campbell elaborates, that there is no reason to think that explanations that appeal to factors that are at a single level are in general superior to explanations that appeal to factors at number of different levels. First, as a number of commentators have observed, multilevel explanations are extremely common (and are accepted as legitimate) in the biomedical sciences, including psychiatry; arguably, they are the rule rather than the exception in these disciplines. Whatever one thinks of the empirical credentials of the claim that genetic variations in the serotonin transporter mechanism influence whether subjects respond to stressful or humiliating life experiences by becoming depressed, there does not seem to be anything objectionable about the abstract structure of this claim, which involves the idea that an environmental or social event, like humiliation, can interact with features of a subject's genotype to influence gene expression and this in turn can influence the level of certain neurotransmitters (serotonin) or other biochemical substances that in turn can influence both neural architecture, cognition, mood, and behavior. Other examples of explanatory claims having this sort of structure include claims about the influence of position in a social hierarchy on serotonin levels and immunological functioning, claims about the influence of stress and social isolation on immunological functioning, and claims about the influence of maternal nurturing on gene expression within the brain and resulting changes in neural structure. (For further discussion of many of these examples, see Cacioppo et al. [2000].) According to any intuitive notion of level, such explanations certainly counts as multilevel if anything does. They appeal to factors that run the gamut from macroenvironmental events (humiliation, position in a hierarchy), to genetic and biochemical factors, to psychological level factors such as depression or confidence, and to factors having to do with overt behavior. Second, as Campbell notes, from the point of view of an interventionist account of causation and explanation, there is absolutely nothing wrong methodologically with such explanations. From an interventionist perspective, finding factors that figure in the explanation of some outcome is (roughly speaking) simply a matter of finding factors such that manipulation of those factors is stably and systematically related to changes in the outcome one wants to explain. (For more detail about what this means, see my accompanying chapter in this volume and also below.) Which factors satisfy this requirement is always an empirical matter, and in principle they can be found at any level; there is no a priori reason for thinking that they must all be found at a single level. Thus, as long as it is true that under interventions that alter whether subjects experience humiliation H, variations in such experiences are stably associated (perhaps just for a subset of subjects with a certain genotype) with variations in neurotransmitter level S and they in turn with variations in mood and behavior M, then H counts as a legitimate cause of S, which in turn counts as a legitimate cause of M, despite the fact that these three variables are, at least intuitively, at different levels.

Parallel observations apply to another idea, also discussed by Campbell, which is also associated with the idea of levels of explanation. This is the idea that certain levels of explanation can be seen as a priori more intelligible or preferable than others, at least for certain phenomena. Historically, one of the most popular versions of this idea has been that explanations that are "mechanical" in some appropriate sense are more intelligible or illuminating than other kinds of explanation, at least for many phenomena. This was a widely espoused idea in the early modern period, with many major scientists and philosophers (Galileo, Boyle, Descartes, among others) insisting that theories that involve contact action, or geometrical modes of reasoning and understanding, or which model natural phenomena in terms of simple, well-understood machines (levers, springs, and so on) provide a kind of intelligibility that is not provided by theories that are not at this "level." As Campbell says, echoes of this idea persist in the causal process accounts of causation developed by philosophers like Wesley Salmon (1984) and Phil Dowe (2000), with their idea that the causal explanation consists in tracing or exhibiting spatiotemporally continuous processes of a sort that transmit energy and momentum and that lead to the phenomenon we want to explain.

If we take this conception of explanation literally, it would mean that an account that appealed to the role of episodes of humiliation in producing depression, without tracing in detail the neural and biochemical processes that connect the exposure to humiliation to this outcome, would count as unexplanatory because there is no tracing of intervening causal processes in the same sense as Salmon and Dowe. Again, the view taken by the interventionist model is that this is a mistaken assessment. Exhibition of a stable pattern of dependence according to which interventions on whether a subject is humiliated are associated with changes in the incidence of depression is enough for explanation, even in the absence of information about intervening causal processes. This is *not* to say that there is no motivation within the interventionist framework for providing this additional information about connecting processes, but how much information should be provided will depend on what it is we are trying to explain and other empirical considerations.[4] There is no automatic, universal preference for the mechanical level, however this is understood.

A similar point holds for another candidate for a privileged level of intelligibility that is often invoked in psychological or psychiatric contexts. This is the idea that explanation of psychological level facts (for example, that a subject holds a certain belief or is motivated to act in a certain way) should be in terms of common sense or folk psychological categories (or at least should appeal to factors that are interpretable in terms of these)— categories such as belief, desire, and so on that rationalize the belief or behavior in question. Thus, one gets the idea that, say, monothematic delusions must be explained in terms of rational processes of belief formation in response to unusual sensory or emotional experiences and that addicts simply have unusual preferences, and act rationally, given these. Once again, the interventionist account does not imply that such explanations are necessarily mistaken, but it does insist that there can be no automatic preference for them. Suppose it turns out that there is a stable relationship between interventions on the level of some physiological factor P and whether a subject exhibits a delusional belief—indeed, that this relationship is more stable than any explanation that is framed purely in terms of other beliefs B' and desires D' that the subject possess and the relationship possesses other characteristics that make it explanatorily powerful. Then appeal to P will provide a good explanation for B, even though P is, intuitively, at a different (nonpsychological) "level" from *B*. In other words, nothing within the interventionist guarantees a priori that a subject's beliefs and desires are best explained by appealing to facts about other beliefs, desires, or psychological level facts about the subject, rather than in some other way.

So far I have been expressing skepticism (in agreement with Campbell) about the idea that appeal to levels can be used to provide a source of independent constraint on the kinds of explanation that are appropriate in psychiatry or in any other discipline. This does *not* imply, however, that the idea that there are levels of explanation is mistaken or confused, or that there are not important issues about the choice of an appropriate level of explanation that we face when we investigate empirical phenomena. Instead, the moral we should draw is that the choice of appropriate level of explanation is dictated by more specific and local considerations (just what it is we are trying to explain, where, as an empirical matter, the stable relationships are to be found, which details can be safely neglected as irrelevant, given what it is we want to explain and so on). As Campbell suggests, I think that to a large extent, issues about the choice of level of explanation are most naturally viewed as issues about which variables to use in framing our explanation. In what follows, I want to develop this idea.

I begin with an illustration of "levels" talk that seems to be entirely unproblematic. In a recent paper in *Science* (entitled "Modeling Single-Neuron Dynamics and Computations: A Balance of Detail and Abstraction"), Herz et al. (2006) discuss what they describe as five "levels" at which the behavior of a single neuron may be modeled. At the most detailed or fine-grained level (level *I*), they consider what they call "detailed compartmental models," which aim to be "morphologically realistic" and to capture how the detailed anatomy of the neuron and its spatial structure "contributes to its dynamics and function." Such models are highly dimensional but can help us understand how "spatial aspects of synaptic integration in dendrites support specific computations" carried out by single neurons such as logical or mathematical operations like conjunction and multiplication.

At level II, there are "reduced compartmental models." Commenting on these, the authors write,

Although detailed compartmental models can approximate the dynamics of single neurons quite well, they suffer from several drawbacks. Their high dimensionality and intricate structure rule out any mathematical understanding of their emergent properties. Detailed models are also computationally expensive and are thus not well suited for large-scale network simulations. Reduced models with only one or few dendritic compartments overcome these problems and are often sufficient to understand somatodendritic interactions that govern spiking or bursting. (2006, p. 81)

Continuing through the intermediate III–IV levels (single compartment models, cascade models), we reach level V, or "black box" models. They are constructed to "understand and quantify the signal-processing capabilities of a single neuron without considering its biophysical machinery" (p. 83). Here the neuron is "best regarded as a black box that receives a set of time-dependent inputs—sensory stimuli or spike trains from other neurons—and responds with an output spike train." This input-output relationship is represented by an overall conditional probability distribution $\Pr(R/S)$, where S is the stimulus and R the response. The authors comment that "although models on levels I–IV make specific assumptions about neural processes and hence about the functional form of $P(R/S)$ such assumptions can be overly restrictive at level V. Here it is often advantageous to work with non-parametric estimates of $P(R/S)$," taken directly from measurements.

These remarks illustrate several general points about the considerations that influence choice of levels in modeling and explanation. Note first that the appropriate level at which to construct a model is purpose-relative and that it will be strongly influenced by (among other considerations) just what it is that we want to explain or understand—what the *explanandum* is, in philosophical terminology. If we want to understand how detailed anatomical features of a single neuron influence the computations that it is able to perform, level I may be the most appropriate. If, instead, we want a "quantitative understanding" of phenomena such as spike train generation or to understand how "neurons alter their response when input statistics are modified," a higher-level model (levels III and IV, respectively) will be more appropriate. When models or explanation at different levels of abstraction are directed at different explananda, we should not think of them as necessarily competing with or excluding one another. Both may be good explanations of the different explananda at which they are directed. This observation alone undercuts the idea that there must be a single privileged level at which all explanations should be framed.

A second, closely related point is that which factors should be included in a model or what level of detail should be employed depends on whether such factors or detail are *relevant* to what it is we are trying to explain, where relevance is understood along the interventionist lines described in my chapter in this volume: roughly, a factor F is relevant to some phenomenon E that we are trying to explain, if changes in F (when produced by interventions) are associated with changes in E. F is irrelevant when this is not the case. It is, of course, an empirical question, not to be decided on the basis of a priori considerations, whether a particular F is relevant or irrelevant to E in this sense. (More generally, one may think of relevance as coming in degrees—perhaps changes in F will make some difference to E, but this is only a "small" or "unimportant" difference in comparison with the difference made by other factors—see below for more on what this might mean.) Whether F is a relevant factor to include in a model will thus depend on the E we are trying to explain: certain anatomical details may be relevant to the specific computations that a neuron is able to perform but may matter less if we just want to understand how general features of the output spike train such as firing rates are influenced by general feature of the neuron's input or how the neuron works together with other neurons to perform calculations that involve interactions between many neurons. In other words, one reason why we have "levels" of explanation is simply that there are different features of the behavior of the same system that we may wish to explain and details that are relevant to some of these features may not be relevant to others.[5]

Another general consideration influences choice of level of explanation and choice of variables in science: *tractability.* Even if some set of factors may be relevant (or we may suspect that they are relevant) in the sense just described, it may be that if we attempt to include all of them in our model, it will be intractable. I take the general idea of tractability to be this: when we attempt to explain an outcome we attempt to exhibit patterns of dependency that show how in the outcome depends on changes in various explanatory factors. These patterns of dependency should be tractable in the sense of being graspable, surveyable, or comprehensible by us. Whether a model is tractable depends on a number of different considerations. If the model is mathematically complex, representing the phenomenon of interest by means of a large number of complicated equations, we may want those equations to have exact analytical solutions which we are actually able to find. Or, failing that, we may at least want to insist that we be able to achieve some understanding of general features of the mathematical behavior of the model, perhaps by using simulation techniques of various kinds. In the absence of this, we may think that the model fails to provide any real understanding. (Recall Herz et al.'s remark that, despite the usefulness of level I models for some purposes, their "high dimensionality and intricate structure rule out any mathematical understanding of their emergent properties.") Even if the model is not mathematical, if there is too much detail (even relevant detail) this may make it impossible for us to grasp the patterns of dependency that are implicit in the model. In such cases, it may make sense to omit some relevant detail (abstract away from it) for the sake of improving tractability— in effect, one trades off realism for improved understanding. Herz et al. have this sort of tradeoff in mind when they talk of modeling neuron behavior at various levels as "require[ing] a delicate balance between incorporating sufficient detail to account for complex single-cell dynamics and reducing this complexity to the essential characteristics to make the model tractable" (2006, p. 80). They go on to add, echoing my remarks about purpose relativity above, that "the appropriate level of description depends on the particular goal of the model. Indeed finding the best abstraction level is often the key to success" (2006, p. 80). Note that "level" is used here in the second of the various senses distinguished above—as a matter of degree of abstraction.

So far I have been arguing that the choice of level or of which variables to employ in an explanation is influenced by considerations of relevance and tractability. Can we say anything more about the considerations that should influence variable choice? Let me conclude with some additional comments on this issue, again connecting with Campbell's remarks. As he says, in standard presentations of intervention-oriented treatments of causation and explanation (including my own)[6] there has been a tendency to take the set of possible variables (or the appropriate level of analysis) as given and then to simply apply interventionist ideas to these. However, although this aspect of the interventionist position is relatively underdeveloped, I think (again in agreement with Campbell) that the core interventionist idea that causal relationships are those relationships are exploitable for purpose of manipulation and control can also provide some guidance in the choice of variable set or appropriate level. Some of the respects in which this is true are at least implicit in my accompanying chapter in this volume. In brief, I suggest there that, other things being equal, we should choose variables for which there is a well-defined notion of manipulation rather than those for which this is not true. We also should choose variables that are related in a uniform, stable way to other variables of interest, rather than variables that have inconsistent or heterogeneous effects depending on how they are realized (as my total cholesterol example illustrates), and we should choose variables that figure in relationships that are stable or invariant in the sense that these continue to hold across changes in other conditions. In addition, we should choose causal variables that are "proportional to" their effects in Yablo's (1992) sense.[7]

In his comments, Campbell draws attention to additional considerations, including finding variables that exhibit stable dose-response relationships and involve "large" effects, which are discussed in the epidemiological literature under the somewhat misleading characterization of "criteria for causation"[8] and which can guide the choice of variables. I want to conclude by commenting in a bit more detail on one of these considerations that I find particularly interesting (and which has tended to be neglected in philosophical discussion): the notion of "specificity" of association, which I see as related to the inclusion in one's explanation of what Campbell calls "control variables."

To illustrate (what I take to be) the basic idea, consider an ordinary radio with (a) an off/on switch and (b) a rotary dial, the position of which controls the volume. The state of the off/on switch is causally relevant to the state of the volume in the sense that if this switch is off, the radio will produce no sound at all, and, if it is on, the radio can produce some sound or other. On the other hand, there is an obvious sense in which the position of the volume dial gives one (provided the radio is on) a kind of specific, fine-grained control over the level of volume that is not provided by the on/off switch. This notion of control can be usefully related to the philosopher David Lewis's (2000) notion of "influence." Lewis does not employ an interventionist framework for thinking about causation, but we may (roughly) capture his basic idea in the following way: suppose that C and E are variables and that there are lots of different possible states or values of C and lots of possible different states of E. Moreover, different states of C are associated with different states of E and most of the different states of E are associated with some state of C. Furthermore, these associations are relationships of dependency involving relatively stable, interventionist counterfactuals. When a condition like this is met, we may think of C not only as having a lot of "influence" on E (both in Lewis's sense and as a matter of ordinary speech) but also as a good control variable for E in Campbell's sense and also of the state of C as having a causally specific impact on E. The relationship between the position of the volume dial and the volume of the radio satisfies these conditions: there are many possible positions of this dial, many possible levels of volume, and something close to a stable one-to-one relationship between the two, provided the switch is on. We accordingly think of the state of the dial as having a substantial influence on and a causally specific impact on the level of the volume, as well as allowing for fine-grained control over the volume. By contrast, the off/on switch has just two possible states (it is, after all, a switch). One of these (the off position) is associated with a specific level of volume (= no sound), but the other is not. We accordingly think of the position of the off/on switch as having less influence on the volume, less specific impact, and as affording one less control over the volume—one can't modulate or fine-tune the volume by varying the state of the off/on switch.

A similar contrast between variables that have substantial amount of influence over other variables and provide for the possibility of fine-grained control over those variables and those that are not is important in many biological and psychological contexts. For example, Eric Davidson (2001, pp. 1–2) argues that there is an asymmetry between, on the one hand, what he calls the "control circuitry embodied in the DNA" and, on the other hand, "other cellular machinery" (that is also involved in protein synthesis) in answering the question of where do the "causal differences responsible for morphological diversity reside and how exactly do they function?" The state of the former has rather specific influence in something like Lewis's sense and exerts a fairly fine grained control over which proteins are synthesized, whereas the role of the other cellular machinery is arguably more generic and switchlike—if it is absent or disrupted there may be no protein synthesis at all, but one can't change which proteins are synthesized by modulating the operation of this machinery in a fine-grained way. One might of course argue about whether this asymmetry is as sharp as Davidson makes it out to be (at least in eukaryotes), but let us assume that his claim is broadly correct. Davidson argues that this justifies focusing on the control structures embodied in the DNA as particularly important variables in explaining development and generating diversity. In effect, what he is arguing is that DNA serves as a good control variable in Campbell's sense and that this warrants focusing on it in modeling efforts and paying less attention to other causally relevant variables, particularly in cases in which the systems with which we are dealing are too complex to model everything. The latter may be relegated to the status of "background conditions."[9]

As another illustration of the same idea, consider performance on a test measuring memory retrieval. Whether a subject experiences massive damage to his heart while taking the test will certainly be causally relevant to his performance, but in realistic cases the impact of any such changes is likely to be fairly coarse grained or switchlike—nonspecific rather than specific. Such damage may kill the subject or render him unconscious or make him highly confused or distracted, thus dramatically affecting test performance, but it is unlikely that it will be possible to control test performance in a fine-grained way by introducing various specific changes in the state of his heart. To the extent this is so, the state of the subject's heart is a nonspecific cause of (and not a good control variable for) test performance. Examples of good control variables for test performance are arguably harder to find, but one might imagine, for example, that the length of a list of items to be memorized or the amount of time allowed for memorization might influence test performance in a more specific and fine-grained way than measures that interfere with general health. To the extent this is so, there may be an argument for assigning a more central role to such variables in explaining test performance and relegating variables like state of the subject's heart to the status of a mere background condition. (Notice that, in this case, the better control variable may be found at the "psychological" level.)

As a final illustration, return to Campbell's example of thought insertion. As we have seen, there is no in principle barrier to explaining whether thought insertion occurs in terms of the state of the subject's dopamine system—it all depends on whether there is a stable, intervention-supporting relationship between these two variables. It is, however, considerably more difficult to believe (although it is not a priori impossible) that the state of a subject's dopamine system could be a control variable for exactly which thoughts (among the many possible candidates) are inserted. If this latter possibility was correct, one could influence or modulate in a fine-grained way which thoughts are inserted by manipulating the state of a subject's dopamine system, and this seems unlikely. It may be instead that to the extent there is *any* control variable for which thought is inserted (when there is some suitable derangement of the dopamine system), this is more likely to have to do with variables that look more psychological in

character—the subject's attributional style, the presence of various reasoning biases, or features of his or her personal history.

Why attach any particular explanatory significance to control variables, as opposed to other, noncontrol variables that are relevant to what
we want to explain? Like Campbell, I take our inclination to focus on such
variables (when it exists) to be connected to what, on the interventionist
account, is the underlying motivation for engaging in causal thinking in
the first place: our concern with finding relationships in nature that are
exploitable for purposes of manipulation and control. Control variables,
and particularly control variables that are connected to their effects via
relatively stable or invariant relationships, give us the possibility of detailed, fine-grained control over particular outcomes that is not available
with other, less causally specific variables. We don't always care about
achieving such fine-grained control, but often, particularly in biomedical
(including psychiatric) contexts, we do. Often, we want to be able to tweak
our bodies and minds in small, specific, targeted ways, rather than affecting them in coarse, switchlike ways—to lower blood pressure to something close to 120/80 rather than just making it a lot less, to kill cancer
cells differentially rather than such cells and all surrounding tissue, to re-
lieve or moderate depression while not at the same time altering other features of affect and cognition in undesirable ways. The search for variables
having these features is thus yet another feature influencing the choice of
level of explanation.

NOTES

1. Obviously, this list is far from exhaustive. The discussion of different notions
of level that follows is substantially influenced by Craver (2007), which contains
by far the best discussion of the notion of levels in neurobiology that I am aware of.

2. As observed in Craver (2007).

3. Wimsatt (1976) is one of the more prominent defenders of this position.

4. See below and my accompanying chapter in this volume (chapter 4, this volume) for additional discussion. One advantage of providing information about
connecting processes and intervening causal links is that this often furnishes more
detailed, fine-grained information that is relevant to manipulation and control—
additional points at which intervention may occur, better control variables (in the
sense described below) and so on. From an interventionist perspective such information is highly relevant to increased understanding. Thus, if we have a detailed
account of the connecting processes by which humiliation produces depression
(via changes in gene expression, levels of neurotransmitters, changes in neural

structures like the amygdala, and so forth) this will yield much more information relevant to intervention. In addition, for reasons described in chapter 4 of this volume, the causal links spelled out in connecting processes will often be individually more stable or invariant than the overall humiliation-depression connection. The general point, though, is that, although there will often be good reasons within an interventionist framework for seeking information about connecting processes, it will also be true that (a) relationships between variables can be explanatory even in the absence of information about connecting processes and (b) how much such information should be provided will depend on what we are trying to explain and local empirical issues about the relevance of such information and how well it furthers our explanatory goals such as our interest in finding stable relationships.

5. This is a feature of explanation and modeling in general and is not in any way confined to biological or psychiatric contexts. Suppose I hold a large rock four feet directly above a wine glass and then drop it, shattering the glass. If I merely wish to explain why the glass shattered (rather than not), it will probably be sufficient to mention that the rock transfers energy and momentum above a certain threshold to the glass and perhaps some general features of the glass—as long as these features hold, the details of exactly how the rock strikes the glass and with exactly what energy/momentum won't matter. By contrast, suppose that I want to explain the exact details of the shattering—why the shards have just the shape they do and end up in one particular position rather than another. Now many more details, including the exact momentum of the rock, facts about the microconstitution of the glass, and so on, will probably be relevant and will need to be included in the explanation. Again, the moral is that what we want to explain (the contrast we want to account for) plays an important role in dictating the appropriate level of abstraction in our explanation.

6. I should add, though, that although there is no systematic discussion of variable choice in my recent book (Woodward 2003), a number of suggestions are scattered throughout the book (for example, that we should include in our models only variables that represent serious possibilities, that mechanisms that are independently disruptable should be represented by different variables, rather than by different values of a single variable, and that we should avoid variables that are logically or conceptually connected to one another).

7. Yablo's idea is discussed in section 3 of chapter 4 in this volume. Basically, the constraint is that causes should neither be too detailed and specific, nor too general, but should involve just enough detail for their effects. As an illustration, recall Yablo's example of a pigeon that is trained to peck at targets of any shade of red and only at targets of this color. Yablo argues that, if a target of a specific shade of red (such as scarlet) is presented and the pigeon pecks, it is misleading to cite the scarlet color of the target as the cause of the pigeon's pecking. Instead, one should cite the red color of the target as the cause of the pigeon's pecking. Citing the scarlet color of the target is to describe the cause of the pecking in an overly specific way that includes irrelevant detail (because any shade of red would have

caused pecking). By contrast, when we cite the redness of the target we are citing a cause that is appropriately "proportional" to its effect.

To spell out the idea of proportionality a bit more explicitly in interventionist terms: a cause is proportional to its effect to the extent that there is a pattern of systematic counterfactual dependence (the dependence being understood along interventionst lines) between different possible states of the cause and the different possible states of the effect, where this pattern of dependence at least approximates to the following ideal: the dependence (and the associated characterization of the cause) should be such that (a) it explicitly or implicitly conveys accurate information about the conditions under which alternative states of the effect will be realized *and* (b) it conveys *only* such information—that is, the cause is not characterized in such a way that alternative states of it *fail* to be associated with changes in the effect. (Recall that it is this condition that identifies the red rather than the scarlet color of the target as the appropriate level of description in the pigeon example.)

8. This characterization is misleading because the "criteria" in question are neither necessary nor sufficient in general for a relationship to be causal. Rather than being conditions that distinguish causal from noncausal relationships, it seems more appropriate to view them as marking distinctions *among* causal relationships—as describing features that causal relationships may or may not possess but that, when possessed, are important or noteworthy. Thus, in agreement with Campbell, I see these criteria as more plausibly viewed as considerations or guidelines for the conduct of inquiry and the construction of explanations; look for causal relations having certain features (stable dose-response relationships, specificity, and so forth) and choose variables and levels of explanation that represent or capture causal relationships having these features.

9. Another biological example is provided by Kenneth Kendler. Consider the difference between two major classes of base pair–changing mutations in genes. The first has a major disabling effect on gene function either by terminating protein translation (by a stop codon) or producing a nonsynonymous base pair change thereby changing a critical amino acid, and rendering the protein product nonfunctional. The effect of such mutations on phenotypic traits is typically nonspecific-variations in these mutations don't exert a fine-grained influence on the character of phenotypic traits. The second class includes subtle changes in up-stream control sequences that affect the specific timing or amount or cell type in which the protein is expressed. Here the protein is unchanged but the amount or place or time of its expression is altered. In these cases, the change in the control sequence will often have a much more subtle, fine-grained influence on phenotypic traits.

REFERENCES

Bechtel, W., and A. Hamilton. 2007. Reduction, Integration and the Unity of the Sciences. In T. Kuipers (ed.), *Philosophy of Science: Focal Issues* (pp. 377–430). Vol. 1 of *Handbook of the Philosophy of Science*. New York: Elsevier.
Cacioppo, J., G. Bernston, J. Sheridan, and M. McClintock. 2000. Multilevel Inte-

grative Analyses of Human Behavior: Social Neuroscience and the Complementing Nature of Social and Biological Approaches. *Psychological Bulletin* 126:829–843.

Craver, C. 2007. *Explaining the Brain: Mechanisms and the Mosaic Unity of Neuroscience.* Oxford: Oxford University Press.

Davidson, E. 2001. *Genomic Regulatory Systems: Development and Evolution.* San Diego: Academic Press.

Dowe, P. 2000. *Physical Causation.* Cambridge: Cambridge University Press.

Herz, A., T. Gollisch, C. Machens, and D. Jaeger. 2006. Modeling Single-Neuron Dynamics and Computations: A Balance of Detail and Abstraction. *Science* 314:80–85.

Lewis, D. 2000. Causation as Influence. *Journal of Philosophy* 97:182–197.

Salmon, W. 1984. *Scientific Explanation and the Causal Structure of the World.* Princeton, NJ: Princeton University Press.

Wimsatt, W. C. 1976. Reductionism, Levels of Organization, and the Mind-Body Problem. In I. Savodnik (ed.), *Consciousness and the Brain: A Scientific and Philosophical Inquiry* (pp. 202–267). New York: Plenum Press.

Woodward, J. 2003. *Making Things Happen: A Theory of Causal Explanation.* Oxford: Oxford University Press.

Yablo, S. 1992. Mental Causation. *Philosophical Review* 101:245–280.

PART II

PHENOMENOLOGY

Varieties of "Phenomenology"

On Description, Understanding, and Explanation in Psychiatry

JOSEF PARNAS, M.D., DR.MED.SCI.,
AND LOUIS A. SASS, PH.D.

Chapter 6 is important to include in this volume because it represents the meeting point of philosophy and psychiatry as seen from the perspective of the *Continental* philosophical tradition in general and the philosophical movement of phenomenology more specifically. This philosophical perspective, deeply influenced by the works of Husserl and Heidegger, can be contrasted with the *Analytic* philosophical tradition (sometimes called *Anglophonic*), which has provided the philosophical framework of the preceding chapters in this volume. This is not the place to describe in detail these two major branches of twentieth-century philosophy. For those who are interested, I suggest consulting a brief but clear article on this topic in Wikipedia (http://en.wikipedia.org/wiki/Schism_between_Analytic_and_Continental_Philosophy). Suffice it to say that each major tradition has something of value to bring to those interested in the deeper problems of psychiatry.

This chapter begins with the central question of what should be the nature of description in psychiatry. Parnas and Sass (P&S) remind us of the critical importance of this task. After all, what symptoms and syndromes psychiatry decides to attend to, in their words, "dictates the targets of scientific activity and influences the treatments that are developed and offered to patients." P&S proceed to argue forcefully that the *DSM* enterprise has, as an end product if not by design, largely shut off discussion about the nature of description in our field. Why have we arrived at the particular categories we have in our *DSM* and *ICD* manuals and not others? We, as a field, have pretended that these deep descriptive issues have been "solved." We become embarrassed if we are reminded that there remain fundamental issues about

the nature of our assessments. We shuffle our feet nervously if someone asks the specific justification for why we have chosen this particular set of symptoms and syndromes to include in our manuals and not
others. Are we sure we got the right ones?

I might editorialize for a moment to suggest that we need to be
humbler and realize the arbitrary (or "historically contingent") nature
of the particular diagnostic categories and criteria that we have. Many
of them were decided sitting around a conference table first in Washington University, St. Louis, during the creation of the Feighner criteria (Feighner et al. 1972) and later in various hotel rooms during the
DSM-III deliberations and sometimes even on the back porch of Robert
Spitzer's home in Westchester County, New York! (For some further
discussion of these issues, see Kendler and Zachar [chap. 9] in this
volume.)

P&S proceed to provide a helpful historical and philosophical
background to the concept of operationalized criteria that have become so influential in psychiatry but little understood or examined.
They briefly take up the central concept of delusion to illustrate the
substantial limitations of the standard "operational" approach to psychiatric assessment. Their main point here is to "raise consciousness"
about the limitations of the "fundamentalist" or non-self-critical operationalism that has dominated much DSM discourse.

P&S then turn to examine a central figure who sits at the crossroads
of psychiatry, philosophy, and phenomenology, Karl Jaspers. They
summarize what they see as the key points of Jaspers's magnum opus,
General Psychopathology (Jaspers 1963). No easy reading, this book is
unfortunately little known, especially in modern American psychiatry. They note that Jaspers might be credited with some prophetic ability to see potential limitations of the post-DSM world of psychiatry
with our "compendiums" of symptoms and signs. P&S emphasize the
key role that Jaspers ascribed to recreating "the patient's anomalous
experience" through a process of empathic "imaginative actualising"
and the critical attention to both the content and the form of psycho-
pathologic experience.

Next, P&S review the work of what they term "Continental phenomenology," here referring largely to the work of Husserl and
Heidegger, which they see as an extension and elaboration of the
Jasperian approach to psychopathology. This section of the chapter is
likely to be challenging to readers whose prior experience in philosophy has predominately been with the Anglo-American analytic tradition. It is also difficult to summarize and so my comments here are
especially sketchy. The problems confronted by Continental phenomenology are in some sense more global and deeper that those tackled by
analytic philosophy, striking at the heart of what assess and measure

when we think about the nature of psychiatric symptoms, signs, and syndromes. However, it also can be hard to get a detailed grip on concepts like the "embedded nature of human subjectivity" or "Lifeworld." My advice to a reader new to this kind of material is to strive at first reading only for a "gestalt" understanding and to avoid getting frustrated if the concepts seem obscure. The goal should be one of a general familiarity with the approaches of these thinkers rather than a detailed grasp of the specifics.

P&S examine four major issues as articulated in the Continental phenomenological tradition. The first of these, "ontological issues: lived world, lived body." As P&S emphasize, concepts of the multiple layers of the "lived world" map onto ideas of integrative pluralism or patchy reductionism commented on by authors in earlier parts of this book. This link provides a potentially important connection between the analytic and continental traditions as they apply to problems of causation and understanding in psychiatric illness.

If this wasn't hard enough, next they try to summarize the phenomenological approach to the central issue of "consciousness." They emphasize the unique and central place of consciousness in the phenomenological perspective—the process that relates itself *comprehendingly to both self and world.*" Critically, phenomenology approaches consciousness both from a first- and from a third-person perspective—as both object and subject—and thereby stands in opposition to hard reductive approaches that would marginalize inquiries into consciousness.

From there, the chapter moves to the major topic of the phenomenology of mental disorders. They emphasize that phenomenology approaches psychopathology from a perspective of both content and context, context here meaning how the disordered experiences fits into or disrupts the other contents and structures of consciousness. They outline three key aspects of the phenomenological approach: (a) typification, (b) search for invariances, and (c) the exploration of subjective structures. The first two issues reflect the problems of developing a vocabulary of pathologic phenomenon that reflects both the richness of individual experience and the key commonalities. The third issue reflects the need to articulate the modes of experience that frame anomalous experiences.

P&S then turn to the central issue that cuts deeply across the face of both the clinical and scientific work in psychiatry—the distinction between understanding (through our innate human empathic ability) and explanation (third-person causal/scientific reasoning), particularly outlining the approaches of Jaspers and Husserl to these issues. (For a good discussion of this issue that should be relatively accessible to those without a strong philosophy background, see Fulford, Thornton, and Graham 2006, chap. 10.) The former involves the key concepts of meaning and intention which are absent for the "bloodless" scientific view of the world. Appropriately, P&S relate these two classes of approaches to psychopathology back to the broad issue— taken up by several authors in this volume—of pluralism.

Finally, in the closing section of their chapter, P&S turn to schizophrenia to provide a good "taste" of what a modern-day informed phenomenological analysis would look like. They summarize their previously published work suggesting that the diverse symptoms of schizophrenia can be understood as the result of a fundamental disturbance of consciousness, specifically in the sense of self. They propose the term *ipseity,* which they define as the fundamental configuration of self-awareness. They argue that a small number of defects in ipseity underlie the observed diverse characteristic symptoms of schizophrenia.

Their work in this area, while informed by prior descriptive and phenomenological analyses, was driven by clinical experience, by a concerted effort to try to understand the fundamental aspects of the schizophrenic experience. Of importance, P&S did not stop at the level of theory. Rather, they developed rating scales and now exciting prospective studies of symptoms whose structure has been understood from a phenomenological perspective. This is an important step that attempts to marry the observational approaches of the phenomenologists with the more scientific methods with which the analytic philosophical tradition is more at home. Their work represents an important synthetic step that could enrich both disciplines. Two implications of this approach are noteworthy. First, from a clinical perspective, P&S argue that their phenomenological analyses can allow clinicians to expand their sense of understanding—to see that the superficially bizarre symptoms of schizophrenia such as delusions of influence can be seen as arising in an understandable sense from the deeper disorders of ipseity. Second, this theory is not "merely descriptive" but can be of explanatory relevance and suggest specific etiologic models for understanding the development of the schizophrenic syndrome.

In summary, I see this chapter as a passionate call for deeper efforts to understand at a phenomenal level the experiences of our patients. Their goal is not only to make us better clinicians, which it surely would. This approach also holds promise to enrich our impoverished psychopathological conceptual vocabulary and generate etiologic hypotheses that can feed into our empirical research.

Kenneth S. Kendler, M.D.

REFERENCES

Feighner, J. P., E. Robins, S. B. Guze, R. A. Woodruff, Jr., et al. 1972. Diagnostic Criteria for Use in Psychiatric Research. *Archives of General Psychiatry* 26:57–63.

Fulford, B., T. Thornton, and G. Graham. 2006. *Oxford Textbook of Philosophy of Psychiatry: International Perspectives in Philosophy and Psychiatry.* New York: Oxford University Press.

Jaspers, K. 1963. *General Psychopathology.* Chicago: University of Chicago Press.

* * *

1. The Problem of Description in Psychiatry

Descriptions of abnormal or disordered experience and expression—comprising sensory, cognitive, volitional, affective-emotional, and behavioral phenomena—are the basis of psychiatry as a scientific field and a pragmatic-therapeutic discipline. We often refer to this descriptive level as *phenotypic* (pertaining to a level of directly visible or observable phenomena, in contrast to the "invisible" genotypic or endophenotypic level) or as *phenomenal* (pertaining to what is manifest or given in a conscious experience). At this level, we delineate "signs" and "symptoms," and we aggregate these phenotypes into classes or dimensions relevant to diagnostic categories. Through its power to declare which symptoms exist or are important enough to be the focus of attention, psychiatric description dictates the targets of scientific activity and influences the treatments that are developed and offered to patients.

Despite its obvious importance, description as such is rarely discussed in the contemporary psychiatric literature. Bluntly put, it is as if psychiatry, after its conversion to operationalized diagnostic criteria some 35 years ago, decided to silence any debate about the nature of description or descriptive concepts, perhaps even viewing such topics as embarrassing or shameful vestiges of a preoperational era that was readily equated with *prescientific* psychiatry.

The search for adequate methods and forms of description in psychiatry seems to be caught in a *rationalist-empiricist* dilemma—a version of the classic "sophistic paradox" or "paradox of knowledge" described in Plato's *Meno* (Plato 1961, p. 363).[1] Either we know in advance *what* (and *how*) to describe (in other words, we have some a priori knowledge, however dim, of the entities to be described) or, assuming a rigorously atheoretical stance (programmatically stated in *DSM-III, DSM-III-R, DSM-IV,* and *DSM-IV-TR* and *ICD-10* [APA 1980, 1987, 1994, 2000; World Health Organization 1992]), we do not know what to look for and are therefore doomed to an endless process of accumulating unrelated atomistic empirical observations, with little prospect of synthesis into larger meaningful wholes. This second option has dominated the field of psychiatric diagnosis and research for many years, but not without obvious problems. As Manfred Spitzer pointed out, "The impossibility of pure description brings with it a corollary that might be even more important: If everything that we have so far regarded as 'pure' data is a result of certain steps of interpretation, these steps should be the subject of thorough reasoning. So any attempt to get better descriptions and a better understanding of (disturbed) perception, thought, and the experiencing I can only consist in reflections on the theories we have and use, i.e.: in philosophical reasoning" (Spitzer 1988, p. 15).

This chapter offers a synoptic overview of some of the philosophical issues pertaining to description that have been unduly neglected in psychopathology. The relevant questions are disparate and extremely complex. They are, however, also clearly interrelated and must be considered together, even at the risk of some inevitable oversimplifications. We shall begin with a critical analysis of contemporary operational "phenomenology" before turning to the phenomenology of Karl Jaspers. (Whereas *phenomenology* refers simply, in mainstream psychiatry, to the level of observable signs and symptoms, in Jaspers and the continental approach, it refers more specifically to the description and understanding of the patient's subjectivity or "lived experience.") We present our own preferred perspective: the continental-phenomenological approach. We conclude discussion of the latter approach by considering, in the context of schizophrenia, whether phenomenology (in this latter sense) can be relevant to the critical project in psychiatry of explanation—including causal explanation—as well as of description.

2. Operational "Phenomenology"

From its beginning in 1838 (the publication year of what is widely considered to be the first psychiatric textbook, *Des maladies mentales,* by

Esquirol) until the end of the 1960s, modern psychiatry was theoretically eclectic and diversified along national and linguistic boundaries, with locally dominating "schools of thought." At the end of the 1960s, the World Health Organization launched a series of international collaborative studies. One of these, the U.S.-U.K. diagnostic project, had a dramatic impact on the entire domain of description (Cooper et al. 1972). This project demonstrated an alarming lack of diagnostic agreement between American and British clinicians. It was clear that a *science* of psychiatry was not compatible with such variations in diagnostic habits. Adding to the sense of crisis was the emergence of biological treatments that seemed to emphasize the crucial importance of differential diagnosis (for example, lithium salts for bipolar disorders). It was also an era of rapid expansion of biological research, pushing into the forefront the issues of nosology. The solution to this crisis was to embrace a positivist-behaviorist epistemology, usually called "operationalism"—a term relevant to multiple aspects of psychiatric description.

Operationalism stems from the ideals of logical empiricism or logical positivism, a philosophical position inaugurated in Austria and Germany in the end of the nineteenth and the beginning of the twentieth centuries and imported to academic psychiatry in the United States, partly due to the strong influence of positivist philosophers Rudolph Carnap and Carl Hempel. Logical positivism claims that sensory experience, along with the rules of logic, is the only valid source of knowledge about reality. Although in its original, *antimetaphysical program,* it refrained from claims about the *essence* of reality, it gradually slipped into a position currently designated as *objectivism* and *physicalism.* Reality is *as* it is, independently of any human perspective on it: objectivism. Also, the nature of reality is wholly physical: physicalism. Supposedly, whatever exists is ultimately reducible to subatomic particles and forces and their interactions governed by physical laws.

Physicalism underlies various programs of strong biological reductionism. The physical reality (roughly as we know it today) is considered to be the only *truly existing reality* and presumably gives rise, through ascending effects, to naturally occurring *biological* categories such as lions and humans and to more esoteric entities such as perceptual processes, concepts, and patterns of social behavior. Physicalism—as it is ordinarily understood[2]—pictures reality as stable and graspable in a certain substantive mechanical sense, akin to the vicissitudes of movements.of objects in

Newtonian mechanics. Physicalism has important consequences for psychiatric description because of the tremendous and widespread impact of its views on the *nature of consciousness:*

1. Consciousness and experience are considered to be on a par with other spatial-temporal, *substantive* objects of the natural world (that is, things) and, therefore, to be describable in the same manner (namely, in third-person perspective, through the thing's defining features).

2. The ontology (that is, *nature of the being*) of consciousness is typically seen as *epi*phenomenal (in other words, as being, in itself, causally *impotent,* and *devoid* of any causally relevant *meaning structures*). Consciousness can supposedly be reduced to causally efficient neurobiological processes; indeed, it is *nothing other than these processes.* Successful reduction in psychiatry was first envisaged as a local match between a given phenotype and a given specific brain dysfunction. The nature and extent of the putative dysfunctions have progressively expanded, however, in response to accumulating failures of the strictly focal or monofactorial research approach (with a talk of networks replacing that of modules).[3]

Logical positivism was strongly preoccupied with the issue of how theories and concepts, stated in language, might correspond to extralinguistic reality. This preoccupation came to mark decisively the descriptive psychiatric approach. In the early years of logical empiricism in the philosophy of science, it was hoped that "reality" might be faithfully described by means of simple, atomistic, theory-free "observational" statements or "record" statements (respectively, called *Beobachtungssätze* or *Protokollsätze*). A criticism of the original positivist program made it clear, however, that language is never theory-free (see Putnam 1987). In his famous essay "Two Dogmas of Empiricism," William Quine (1951) offered what many have considered as a knock-down refutation of "reductionism" (that is, of "the belief that each meaningful statement is equivalent to some logical construct upon terms which refer to immediate experience"). An important response to some of the early criticisms of logical positivism was the development, originally in physics, of the notion of *operational definition,* supposed to assure an objective link between a concept and its referent or counterpart in nature (Bridgman 1927). This notion was presented in a famous and influential address that Carl Hempel delivered to the American Psychiatric Association: "An operational definition of a term is conceived as a rule to the effect that the term is to apply to a particular case if the performance of *a specified operation in that case yields a certain characteristic result*" (1965, p. 123; italics added).

For example, the term *ice* can be operationally defined as a volume of water that *changes into a solid state if* brought to a specified measurable temperature under a specified measurable barometric pressure. Such a definition specifies a process or tells us *how to act* (to operate) to make an empirical check on the concept of ice. This way of defining does not, however, seem either theoretically appropriate or practically applicable for the vast majority of psychiatric terms. No *operation,* for example, can be envisaged to check up on a patient's first-person avowal that "I feel as if there are electric migrations in my spine." Hempel himself considered operational definitions to be *provisional* tools only. He believed that *mental terms* would *eventually* be replaced by an appropriate vocabulary of physical science and their reality established via lawfully predictable regularities. A contemporary version of this view is known as *eliminativism,* a position that claims that mental terms (for example, hoping, desiring, remembering) are merely illusions, with no referent in nature, and should be ultimately eliminated and replaced by neuroscientific terms about brain events (Churchland 1986).

If viewed in critical perspective, what operationalism finally amounted to in psychiatry was the idea that descriptions of mental or subjective phenomena should be cast at the *"lowest possible level of inference"*—that is, ideally in *external behavioral* description, or else in *simple lay language* (for example, "affect is to mood as weather is to climate"). It was hoped that clinicians would consistently use low-order, ordinary language to frame nonjudgmental, acontextual, and atheoretical definitions and thereby improve the reliability of their descriptions. These operational hopes, however, invariably seem to confront the fact that what words signify is always framed by their local context, which (by its very nature) cannot be specified in advance. In other words, there are no acontextual definitions. There is now a nontrivial literature on the pitfalls of psychiatric operationalism, which is beyond our scope (but see, for example, Sadler et al. 1994; Parnas and Bovet 1995; Heinimaa 2002; Howsepian, 2007). Here, we will briefly touch on the issue of "defining delusion," to illustrate the operationalist epistemological and practical dilemmas in addressing this

core domain of psychopathology. Classic key features of nearly all definitions of delusion—(1) falsity of content, (2) strong conviction, and (3) incorrigibility[4]—are also incorporated in the operational systems such as
DSM-IV and *ICD-10*. However, neither Karl Jaspers nor Kurt Schneider (to
both of whom this defining triad is frequently ascribed), nor their contem-
poraries, considered these three features to be defining *what a delusion
was*, but rather as its "external indicators" (*aussere Merkmale*); that is, to
suggest or indicate the presence of delusion rather than to *define its essential nature*. The search for the essence of delusion, for "what it is," always
implies a broadening of the context to include the level of a *person* (for example, the subject's history, her experiences, her "mental frame" of other
beliefs and her more overarching attitudes and orientations). Such context
precludes the possibility of an unequivocal definition, as the one proposed in the *DSM-IIR:* "A false personal belief based on incorrect inference about external reality and firmly sustained in spite of what almost
everyone else believes and in spite of what constitutes incontrovertible
proof or evidence to the contrary." In fact, delusion needs not be (and
sometimes is not) empirically *false* (for example, delusions of jealousy
may be empirically true); it may not be *personal* but involve other people;
it is not always about *external reality*, for it may involve body or mind as
themes; it needs not to be, and frequently is not, based on *inferential reasoning;* nor does it need to be believed with full "conviction" to be clinically significant.[5]

A somewhat similar illustration is provided by the attempts to improve
interrater reliability of the concept of "bizarre delusions" (low interrater
reliability continues to be a problem here [Bell et al. 2006]), which are
defined as delusions that are *"clearly implausible and not understandable."* This definition seems rather incoherent given that the very notion
of "clear implausibility" would seem to imply a clarity of understanding
(the imagining of plausibility and implausibility under certain circumstances) that would indicate that the statement is not, in fact, truly incomprehensible (Heinimaa 2002). It has been suggested that "bizarreness"
could perhaps best be specified as referring to delusional content that is
physically or empirically impossible (for example, the patient claims that
he is able to influence the weather patterns by his thinking [Flaum et al.
1991; Spitzer et al. 1993]). It turns out, however, that the content-based
definitions do not, in fact, accurately identify the relevant class of delusions (Parnas 2004). The reason for this is that there is no discussion of

what may *give rise* to the observer's sentiment that something appears bizarre.[6] For example, the bizarreness aspect of any mental content or behavior may often rely on an implicit perception of profound *changes in the subjective orientation or framework* of the patient, changes that transpire or are revealed *through the content or action,* rather than based on the content "as such" or "in itself" (for example, when the patient's experience apparently violates normal frameworks of time, space, or intersubjectivity). In our view, what characterizes *schizophrenia-typical* delusions is the alteration of the structural (formal) aspects of experience, which the formation of a "bizarre" delusion seems to presuppose (for example, a solipsistic sense of omnipotence, immediate, direct resonance between the subject and the world, or failing sense of privacy of consciousness [Bovet and Parnas 1993; Parnas 2004]).[7]

Unfortunately, neither the *DSM* system (for example, Webb et al. 1981) nor the *ICD* nor any major contemporary psychiatric textbook offers a *descriptive or conceptual* account of the nature of consciousness, experience, and expression, and associated epistemological issues. This conceptual void makes it difficult, if not impossible, to conceptualize the qualities and vicissitudes of subjective life or to envision links and relations (including causal relations) between various mental states and contents.

The point of this critique is *not* to say that we should abandon striving for clear definitions and for reliability of "technical terms." What we should abandon, rather, is the illusory, deceptive, and ultimately counterproductive simplicity of operationalism to strive, instead, for a more adequate, even though more complex and demanding, conceptual framework for the science of psychopathology.[8]

3. Karl Jaspers on Descriptive Phenomenology

Karl Jaspers—a psychiatrist who later became a famous philosopher in the phenomenological tradition—is an emblematic figure in psychiatric theory. His *General Psychopathology* was first published in 1913, then substantially rewritten and expanded in 1923 and 1946, and published in the English translation in 1963. This remarkable book provided the first systematic description and discussion of anomalous mental phenomena. Typically, Jaspers's expositions of anomalous phenomena are preceded by discussions of the relevant *normal* modes of experience, as when he analyzes the normal sense of reality before turning to the topic of delusion.

Jaspers's core assumption was that psychiatry was interdisciplinary. This interdisciplinarity was not an *option*, a possible path out of many, but psychiatry's very condition and raison d'être. As Jaspers notes, mental disorders are at the intersection of subjective experience, psychological mechanisms, nonconscious biological processes, and the sociocultural frameworks. Jaspers therefore believed that familiarity with the methods and viewpoints of philosophy and other human sciences was indispensable for psychiatry. Philosophy in particular was necessary for fostering a curious and sophisticated attitude of mind, an attitude allergic to "platitudinous speculation, dogmatic theorizing, and absolutism in every form" (Jaspers 1963, p. 46). Jaspers believed that, if psychiatrists lacked a sufficient level of general intellectual sophistication—if, for example, they knew only "compendiums" of symptoms and the like—their supposed expertise would in fact be "superficial pseudo-knowledge . . . more subversive for practice than total ignorance" (pp. x–xi).[9]

As we have seen, in mainstream psychiatric usage, the term *phenomenology* refers to a description of psychiatric signs and symptoms of mental disorders that relies on a behavioristic or commonsense view of how things seem to appear. Jaspers proposed a more restrictive use of the term *phenomenology,* closely bound to its meaning in philosophy, *phenomenology* as a descriptive study of *experience:*[10] "We should picture only *what is really present in the patient's consciousness*" (1968, p. 1316; emphasis added). He notes that mental phenomena are given as a flow of experiences and do not possess a thinglike character or a reality status akin to *medical* signs and symptoms: "the *psyche* itself does *not* become *an object.*" Mental phenomena cannot be accessed through a disengaged ("behaviorist," in today's parlance) epistemic operation. The primary task of the psychiatrist, in Jaspers's view, is to *seize in detail and to recreate* the patient's anomalous experience through a process of empathic "imaginative actualizing." The patient's spontaneous statements and written self-descriptions are particularly valuable sources, Jaspers believed, because they picture the patient's inner life in a maximally faithful way, undistorted by questioning. A phenomenological investigation emphasizes the *form* of experiencing rather than its *content* only. Thus, for example, it is not sufficient to note that a patient is excessively preoccupied with jealousy as a theme (content) dominating his mind. What is crucial for the psychopathologist is to recognize the particular *mode* of his jealous experience (for example, whether it presents as an obsession, an overvalued idea, a delusion, or a hallucination), and each of these modes would need to be grasped in terms of the distinctive subjective attitude that it involves.

Jaspers's *General Psychopathology* achieved a limited dissemination and influence in the Anglophone world. The epistemological project of operational psychiatry, however, never distanced itself explicitly from Jaspers's views on the nature of psychopathology.

Jaspers must be credited with a profound insight that the study of anomalous subjective experience has no analogue in somatic medicine, and therefore requires a suitable method, *a phenomenology,* a point to which we will return below. Despite its foundational importance, *General Psychopathology* suffers from certain theoretical and philosophical inadequacies. Most important, Jaspers *never really solved the problem of description* or the rationalist-empiricist dilemma associated with the "sophistic paradox" (mentioned above). He recognizes that to describe and classify the processes of experience we need a conceptual framework and a vocabulary suitable for description. The phenomena to be investigated need to be isolated, characterized, and *conceptually determined,* for, as Jaspers notes, "knowledge only consists in psychological determinations." Jaspers realizes that *we cannot get the concepts from descriptions because the former are the tools for performing the latter;* and for this reason, he writes of a "phenomenological analysis" that would provide the conceptual tools for description. But Jaspers does not actually provide any detailed discussion of this phenomenological mode of analysis; nor does he direct us toward any specific phenomenological alternative. As Manfred Spitzer pointed out, "Jaspers refers to single cases when he speaks of his method in general and refers to his general method when he discusses single cases. What is left is his emphasis on detailed descriptions of single cases and on the necessity to clarify concepts. How this should be done— in other words, what the science of psychopathology consists in—*he does not say"* (Spitzer 1988, p. 9; emphasis added).

4. Continental Phenomenology

Here we refer to an approach (or set of approaches) to psychiatric phenomenology that differs both from the operational approach and from Jaspers's restrictive concept. We refer to a tradition, specifically aiming at grasping the essential structures of human *experience* and *existence* that was inspired by phenomenological philosophy—especially by the work of Husserl and Heidegger, but also by Merleau-Ponty, Sartre, Scheler, and the protophenomenologist Henri Bergson. The themes of phenomenological reflection as understood in this tradition exceed Jaspers's narrow definition (namely, study of experience). They include not only perceptual, cognitive, and emotional *experiences,* but also *actions,* bodily *expressions,* and even *cultural* practices and institutions, including language.

During the articulation of the main domains of psychiatric research in the early twentieth century, phenomenology provided one possible approach for in-depth case studies (for example, in the work of Binswanger [1956] and Minkowski [1927]), and they, in turn, often permitted general insights into the nature of particular psychiatric disorders, not unlike the qualitative case studies that founded modern neuropsychology. Like all philosophy, phenomenology offers conceptual analyses, but in this case the analyses are always anchored in concrete human experience. Edmund Husserl, the founder of philosophical phenomenology, used a slogan of returning "to the things themselves," implying the foundational priority of experience.

Phenomenology should account for its abstractive steps when it moves from the level of experience to the level of concepts. For example, a reflection on the nature of an ordinary perceptual experience of a three-dimensional object may help us to elucidate and anchor the highly abstract concepts of objectivity and reality. In the act of perception we always see the things from a limited perspective. The object never presents itself to me in its totality, with all its features lying bare, as if from a godlike point of view. This nonactual, yet potential, surplus of further appearances is accessible through *other perspectives* or a *further exploration.* These potentials are not just purely abstract possibilities but are, so to say, defining features, *co-present* in the actual perceptual act. Such basic structure of ordinary perception is the experiential prerequisite or condition of the ability to consider the things as demarcated or *individuated entities,* existing *independently of the mind* and as being public, *accessible to others.* In other words, the perspectival, partial or incomplete appearance is a constitutive dimension of the experience of objectivity and reality (for an excellent introduction, see Sokolowski 2000). Thus, the experience of objectivity is viewed by phenomenology, in a continuity with the Kantian approach, as a function or *achievement* of the human subject, one that is *made possible by various organizing structures or principles that the subject brings to the process of cognition* (Hanna 2006). In looking at a saucer—whether from on top, or the side, whether in shade and in bright light—all the time it looks like a saucer, despite the radically different image that each time falls on our retina (Zahavi 2001).

We will list some of the distinctive features of phenomenology in a schematic way.

Ontological Issues: Lived World, Lived Body

According to a widespread misconception, phenomenology is a form of speculative, subjectivistic, Cartesian introspectionism, or even a kind of latter-day idealism. In reality, contemporary phenomenology represents a radical critique of both the subject-object and the mind-body dualisms of Cartesianism and emphasizes the *embodied* and *embedded* nature of human subjectivity—the crucial relevance both of the lived body and of one's immersion in the world.

The mind is not a camera-like "interior space" or "theater"; nor is perceptual experience an inner movie screen that confronts us with mental *representations* projected on it. Instead, perceptual experience should be understood in transactional terms, as (in successful cases) *an acquaintance with the genuine properties of external objects,* unmediated by any "intramental images." Rather than saying that we experience *representations,* we might say that our experiences are *presentational* and that they *present* the world as having certain features. The subject does not (of course) *create* the world but contributes actively to its articulation and significance. The organism is world directed, and consciousness is intentional (consciousness *of something*); the world itself—the lived world—we might say, offers its own best presentation: "The world is inseparable from the subject, but from a subject which is nothing but a project of the world, and the subject is inseparable from the world, but from a world which the subject itself projects. The subject is a being-in-the-world and the world remains 'subjective' *since its texture and articulations are traced out by the subject's movement of transcendence* [that is, movement towards the world]" (Merleau-Ponty 1962, pp. 491–92; emphasis added).

Subjectivity (that is, a term, roughly corresponding to consciousness) is embodied in a way that makes it, in a certain sense, continuous with the world of objects. Distance and weight, for example, are experienced not as neutral or abstract dimensions of physics, but, rather, *in implicit relation* to one's experience of reaching or lifting (for example, that something is *too far away* for me to reach or *too heavy* for me to lift). At the most basic experiential level, my body is not just a material object of focal perceptual awareness (like when I visually inspect my hands). Rather, it is lived "from within" as a subject, namely, as an implicit and coordinated articulation of *my* inclinations and capacities directed toward the world.

An important point to recognize is the *public dimension of experience* that is perhaps too readily seen in Cartesian mind-world dualistic terms— that is, as wholly "inner" or private in nature. Although phenomenology is certainly keen to emphasize and articulate the experiential *asymmetry* between the first- and the third-person perspective, it also points to the public or intersubjective dimensions of experience, perhaps most clearly manifest in emotion. "We must reject the prejudice which makes 'inner realties' out of love, hate, or anger, leaving them accessible to one single witness: the person who feels them" (Merleau-Ponty 1964, p. 52).

In the case of emotions, the lived or subjective aspects cannot be separated from either the situational context in which they occur or from the associated bodily states, tendencies, and forms of expression with which they are associated. These forms of embeddedness and embodiment actually have a *constitutive* significance, which is to say that they *define the nature and identity of the emotion that occurs.* Anger, for example, would not *be* anger in the absence of an appropriate target and of certain actions and states of bodily tension: "I could not imagine the malice and cruelty which I discern in my opponent's looks separated from his gestures, speech and body. None of this takes place in some otherworldly realm, in some shrine located beyond the body of the angry man . . . anger inhabits him and blossoms on the surface of his pale or purple cheeks, his bloodshot eyes and wheezing voice" (Merleau-Ponty 2004, pp. 83–84). Subjectivity, we might say, is, in a certain sense, continuous with what is public, visible, and physical.[11] In this sense, experience bleeds into expression, and expression into experience.

The subject is being-*in*-the-world, but this "being-in" is radically different from the way that, say, a bunch of matches can be said to be *in* the box. *To be* is a radically different matter for a thing and a human being. The matches and the box are independent entities. They coexist in a contingent spatial juxtaposition: the matches may now be in the box, but they may also be piled up elsewhere. The subject, on the other hand, is *"always already" engaged* in moulding (*constituting*) his world by contextualizing his being through the essential purposiveness of his concerns, ways of experiencing, language, habits, and actions. All that makes his world both meaningful and inseparable from himself and possessing a multifaceted and open sense. Some aspects of this sense or meaningfulness are handed down to us by culture and tradition, including science.[12]

Such a human world (the *lived*-world) is not *a collection of things* or physical objects and their connective relations—a sort of a grand *container* universe. Rather, it is a tacit, omnipresent, unifying *frame of reference,* a background fabric, trusted in its *familiarity* and *everydayness* (for a detailed analysis, see Bégout [2005]). It is a background or a horizon coalescing disparate domains of meaning into a comprehensive whole. The forms and contents of a particular Lifeworld—a concept corresponding to Wittgenstein's notion of "form of life"—are, of course, codetermined by historical, geographic, and sociocultural contexts as exemplified by geohistorical differences in beliefs, customs, and social institutions. Yet we find invariances or commonalities as well, such as certain typical manifestations and their correlated subjective structures. An important example is the "everyday" and "familiar" character of all Lifeworlds—their repetitive, intimate and obvious, taken-for-granted, character. This typicality of the Lifeworld is correlated with the basic structures of human subjectivity, for example, the automaticity of habit and tacit, but all-pervading, awareness of living in a *shared* (intersubjective) world. *The Lifeworld*—grounded in the realities of practical activity and intersubjective life—*is our most immediate and basic reality.* We depart from it into abstractions, generalizations, and reductions of particular sciences, but these endeavors never cease to be grounded in, kept together, and practically motivated by, the Lifeworld.

The concept of the Lifeworld is sufficiently undogmatic and inclusive that it can serve as a common philosophical ground for integrative pluralism. The different domains of human reality—such as the physical, psychological, and sociological—are *neither* totally independent realms existing in isolation from one another *nor* sharply defined ontological "layers" characterized by different *densities of reality,* some "more real" than others, and inviting the ultimate translation "down" to the most real.[13] For example, we would not consider it meaningful to explain the political victory of the Social-Democratic Party at recent municipal elections in Copenhagen in terms of quantum mechanics. Rather, "levels of reality" should be best considered as *different domains of signification or sense*—different "ways of mattering" for the pragmatically engaged society of subjects, unified by their shared horizon of the Lifeworld. These domains are therefore partly or provisionally autonomous in their respective realities, yet their relations and dependencies may be philosophically analyzed and empirically investigated.

Consciousness

Perhaps the main question posed by phenomenology is how to describe consciousness. Is consciousness, in essence, just another object in the universe, like weather patterns, biochemical reactions, or subatomic forces, or does it have a unique status, one that our choice of methodology must reflect? Phenomenology begins with the assumption that consciousness is *not* like just any other object or just an object among many. Consciousness reveals a certain peculiarity: it not only is given as an empirical part of the world but also, simultaneously, *is the condition of this world's appearing.* Consciousness differs from everything else by being that which is in possession of comprehension, by being *that which relates itself comprehendingly to both self and world.*

This view has obvious but profound implications. Any investigation (including investigation in the physical or biological sciences) necessarily presupposes the epistemic and cognitive contribution of consciousness, for any investigation *whatsoever* has consciousness as its pivot and condition.

The term *phenomenology* literally means an account of a phenomenon. *Phenomenon* is that which manifests itself, an appearance. Consciousness *enables* or is *a condition of such manifestation* or appearing (*phenomenality*), for one cannot talk about an appearance or a manifestation *of* something unless there is a consciousness *for* which this something manifests itself. Consciousness, then, is the *constitutive* dimension that allows for identification and manifestation, the "place" "in" which the world can reveal and articulate itself. Phenomenology emphasizes that it is possible to investigate consciousness in several ways. It is possible to consider it not only as *an empirical object* endowed with functional properties, as a causally determined *object in the world,* but also as the subject of intentional directedness to the world (that is, as the *subject for the world* [Husserl 1970, p. 178] or, to paraphrase Wittgenstein [1922], as "the limit of the world"). Needless to say, such a view precludes reductive materialism, eliminativism, and epiphenomenalism from the range of adequate philosophical positions, because they all deny, or explain away, the pivotal role of consciousness.

Phenomenology of Mental Disorder

Phenomenology does not consider consciousness as a spatial object but instead emphasizes its intrinsically *non*spatial nature. As many philosophers have noted, consciousness is a temporal flowing, a flux, or a "stream" of intertwined experiences. Consciousness does not consist of sharply separable, *substantial* components, exerting mutual mechanical effects. "Rather, it [is] . . . a . . . network of interdependent *moments* (i.e., nonindependent parts) . . . founded on intentional *intertwining, motivation* and mutual *implication,* in a way that has no analogue in the physical" (Husserl 1977, sect. 37). These views on the holism of consciousness have many implications for psychopathology. This was the reason behind Jaspers's denial of any analogy between phenomenological description and description in somatic medicine.

Thus, most important, what defines a given psychiatric symptom as *a certain kind or type of phenomenon* (say, a phenomenon of "audible thoughts," at the prepsychotic phases of anomalous experience) is not the thinglike qualities or characteristics of the phenomenon such as it would be in the case when identifying a physical object in the third-person perspective (for example, "*this* tall tree, in front of you!") or, in the case of "audible thoughts," a presumed acoustic intensity or pitch. The anomalous experience or a symptom, severed from its inherence in the stream of consciousness, is *individuated or defined* not only through its sheer content (its intrinsic characteristics) but *also* through its position in the implicative web of dependencies on *other contents* and associated *forms* of consciousness. Thus, the presence of "audible thoughts" may be *suspected* in the case of a dissociation of inner speech into its components of meaning *and* expression (for example, when the patient seems to *attend to his "spoken" thoughts* to grasp *what* he is thinking). Phrased differently, psychopathology does not identify its symptoms independently of the context and flow of consciousness in which these symptoms emerge and articulate themselves. Rather, *the symptoms' defining phenomenological characteristics articulate themselves through the implicative relations to other experiences and structures of consciousness.* This is a crucial epistemological issue in the psychiatric interviewing.

Jaspers notes that reports from a few patients, who are able to describe their experiences in great detail, may in fact be more informative regarding the nature of a given disorder than are large-sample studies that are necessarily performed in a simplified manner. We shall describe three interrelated aspects of investigation in phenomenological psychopathology: (a) typification, (b) search for invariances, and (c) exploring subjective structures implicated in experience.

Typification

The process of typification is based on "seeing as" (Hanson 1965), namely, the fact that we *always* perceive the world aspectually—in a certain way, from a certain perceptual and conceptual perspective. We see objects, situations, and events as being certain *types* of objects, situations, or events. The notion of typicality and of a *prototype* is crucial in this context[14] and plays an important role in cognitive research. *Prototypes* are central exemplars of a category in question (for example, a sparrow is more typical of the category "birds" than is a penguin, which can not fly and does not seem to have wings) (Cantor, Smith, and French 1980; Rosch 1988). Typification is mainly an automatic process that occurs outside explicit thinking. In a diagnostic encounter, for example, the psychiatrist quickly senses a patient as being in *a certain way* (for example, withdrawn, hostile, sympathetic, guarded, eccentric, and so on). Such quick global typifications depend on our knowledge and experience and become modified by further interactions with the patient (Schwartz and Wiggins 1987). But, as suggested by Jaspers, we can also engage in more focused, reflective attitudes to make such typifications more explicit, and to subject them to criticism and revision. Through the *eidetic* and *phenomenological reductions* (described below), we may arrive at the essential features or configurations of the examined gestalt. In this process, we move between a holistic grasp of the gestalt and an inquiry into its component aspects or parts, better to comprehend the sense of the whole—a procedure known as the "hermeneutic circle."

The prototypes acquired through clinical experience are not simply a matter of averaging, over time, of a series of *mutually independent* sensory experiences. The prototypes emerging from experience are codetermined by a quest for *meaningful* interrelations between the observed phenomenal features, as when one looks for an "ideal type" (Schwartz and Wiggins 1987).[15] Processes of describing and understanding cannot be sharply separated; description itself is an act of complex pattern recognition that requires comprehending the essence or the whole. One goal of psychiatric typification is to analyze the character of the Lifeworld in major mental disorders—how it manifests itself and also how it can come to be formed, a point illustrated at the end of this chapter with reference to the schizophrenia spectrum disorder.

Search for Invariances

The search for invariances in anomalous experience is the attempt to disclose essential structures by means of imaginative variation. This imaginative variation is a conceptual operation whereby one attempts to imagine a phenomenon as being different from how it currently is to discover which features or aspects are essential—namely, which features cannot be varied without preventing the phenomenon from being the *kind* of phenomenon that it is. Imaginative (eidetic) variation is a form of conceptual analysis that may be shared among investigators and is therefore open to refutation and rejection. By no means does phenomenology promote the notion that infallible insights into the essence of any object (or any subjective world) could be obtained by means of a passive contemplative gaze—whether conceived as an infallible introspective look or as some kind of immediate empathic or mystic intuition.

As an ordinary example, we can mention identifying "thought pressure," a particular prepsychotic symptom that should be distinguished from a variety of phenomena—including ruminations, reflections, and obsessive thoughts—with which it may be confused. Only mental episodes characterized by involuntary, parallel-simultaneous, or quickly alternating thoughts—*sometimes* with a certain experiential alienation (not felt as fully one's own), *frequently* experienced in a spatialized manner (for example, with a specific location or other quasispatial qualities), and *always* with a loss of meaning or lack of common theme and confusion—would be considered as the phenomenon of thought pressure *prototypically described* in the phenomenological literature (for example, in the BSABS scale [Gross et al. 1987] and in the EASE scale [Parnas et al. 2005]). These qualities are, under the optimal circumstances, progressively elucidated over the course of a diagnostic interview that is not based on a series of preformed questions but on a mutual, naturally unfolding, patient-doctor reflective dialogue, supported by concrete examples.

Exploring Subjective Structures

Jaspers emphasized the formal aspect of description, namely, interest in the *form* rather than only the *content* of experience: not in what the experience is *about* as much as in *how* it articulates itself in consciousness. Phenomenology offers here a method called *phenomenological reduction,* a kind of reflection that enables our access to the structures of subjectivity. In general, the term *reduction* refers in phenomenology to an analytic process, which tries to purify the investigated theme of experience by getting rid of the obscuring influences exerted by habits, conceptual distortions and prejudices. This reduction is meant to let the investigated phenomenon unfold itself more fully and clearly.

Phenomenological psychopathology is obviously concerned with comprehending the patient's subjectivity and, in particular, the experiential dimension of his abnormality or disorder. As indicated above, *subjectivity,* in the tradition of continental phenomenology, also encompasses action, volition, and the subject's relations to the world and other humans.

Phenomenological analysis focuses not just on characteristics of what is manifest as the *object* or *field* of awareness (that is, the manifest experience); it also concerns experiential *structures* or *modes* of consciousness with which these appearances are correlated (the act aspects). Insofar as we are confronted with the appearance of an object as perceived, judged, evaluated, and so on, we are led to the experiential *structures,* to the modes of consciousness with which these appearances are correlated. We are led to the *acts* of perception, judgment, and valuation and thereby to the *subjectivity* in relation to which the object as appearing must necessarily be understood. In other words, we do not simply focus on the phenomenon exactly as it is given but also on the subjective side of consciousness and thereby gain access to *the structures of subjectivity that are at play in order for the phenomenon to appear as it does.*

These formal configurations of experience include the modes and structures of *intentionality* (its object-directedness), *spatial* and *temporal* aspects of experience, *embodiment,* modes of *self-awareness* or sociality (*intersubjectivity*), and so forth. To explore these formal or structural aspects of anomalous experience, the clinician must be familiar with the basic organization of consciousness or phenomenal awareness. Otherwise, he will have at his disposal only a superficial, commonsensical grasp of the nature of experience. The absence of such familiarity has typically resulted in a tendency to focus only on the *content* of experience while neglecting formal or structural aspects.

5. Continental Phenomenology: Description, Understanding, Explanation, and Mental Causation

Like many thinkers in his time, Jaspers accepted the sharp distinction between understanding and explanation. For him, explanation was synonymous with physical/biological accounts referring to deterministic and efficient forms of causality and applicable to organic brain disorders. Understanding, by contrast, involved the recognition of *meaningful* connections through *empathic comprehension* of human experience, expression, and action—as when an historian shows the reasons that motivated a politician or when a psychologist traces the development of an inferiority complex to childhood experiences of defeat.

For Jaspers, a crucial criterion of the understandability of a mental content (for example, of a belief or a mood) was that it is essentially *normal,* either differing *quantitatively* from normal states (for example, lowered mood) or involving some *combination* of normal experiences (for example, "secondary delusions" of morbid jealousy, grounded in more primary feelings of inferiority and shame). Understanding thus requires that the experience to be understood be accessible to an empathic act of a normal layperson, as, for example, when one readily grasps that a depressive attitude is triggered by the death of someone's spouse. What Jaspers termed *psychogenesis* had, in this view, to conform to this commonsense perspective and be imaginable within such a framework. If a mental disorder violated such standards of comprehension, said Jaspers, it could be subjected only to a causal-organic explanation. Moreover, the emphasis in this type of understanding seems to fall largely on the supposed interaction of mental *contents,* especially beliefs and emotional states (for example, as allegedly involved in the genesis of the so-called mood-congruent delusions, in which depressed mood is assumed to cause delusions of guilt) but *leaving much of the structure of subjectivity outside the causal consideration.*

Similar assumptions about mental explanation continue to be widely held in current philosophy of mind in the analytic tradition as well as in derivative work in the philosophy of psychiatry, though now the emphasis is typically placed on issues of logical coherence rather than empathic access (Bolton and Hill 1996; Bermúdez 2005). The philosopher Donald Davidson, in particular, argued that mental causation and explanation required that the subject's mental state could be described in terms of sentence-like propositions organized in terms of the practical syllogism (for example, "I took an umbrella *because* I believed it was going to rain" [Davidson 1980]). When this could not be done, the only possible form of explanation would be in terms of physical causation.

This line of argument was quickly adopted by biological reductionism, which views certain key psychiatric symptoms and syndromes (especially in schizophrenia) as devoid of meaning and therefore beyond empathic understanding (for example, bizarre delusions). Such symptoms or syndromes were instead only considered as indicators of the underlying neural—predominantly localized—pathology, a research paradigm vigorously pursued with ever new technologies over the past 40 years (but with modest results).

Neither of the distinctions introduced or implied by Jaspers—understanding versus explanation; description versus *both* understanding and explanation—was, however, ever fully accepted within phenomenological philosophy. We have already emphasized that elements of understanding are necessarily involved in the descriptive processes (for example, in typifications and eidetic-imaginative variations), because these cognitive operations are always influenced by the search for meanings—a point emphasized by various writers in the tradition of continental phenomenology and hermeneutics (Sass 1998). Also worth noting is the fact that both distinctions (understanding versus explanation; description versus understanding *and* explanation) have a rather ambiguous status in contemporary philosophy.

The authoritative *Cambridge Dictionary of Philosophy*, for example, defines "explanation" in rather general terms (and—*nota bene*—by employing the term "understandable"): as "an act of making something intelligible or understandable, as when we explain an event by showing how or why it occurred" (Audi 1999, p. 298). A paradigm case of explanation is, indeed, *causal* explanation; and the paradigm cases of *causal explanation* do typically refer to *efficient* causality in the *physical* world. There are, however, also concepts of both "mental" and "motivational" causation, formulated in the terms of analytic and continental philosophy, respectively (Husserl 1989; Heil and Mele 1993). Indeed, "causal relevance" can be defined broadly—as requiring only that a given attribute or factor (the cause) "makes a difference" to the probability of the occurrence of a given property (the effect) (Grünbaum 1993, p. 163; Woodward 2003; Woodward, chap. 4 in this volume).

Also significant is the fact that *the possible forms of explanation need not be restricted to causation alone:* they can also involve *other* forms of relationship that may reveal the underlying unity or interdependence of a group of phenomena, including forms of logical as well as phenomenological *implication* (see below). Indeed, explanatory factors can be said to cover "*all* those things to which any event or process can be ascribed, *anything* in the light of which it can be said to make sense" (Lawson-Tancred 1995, pp. 418–419; emphasis added). Explanation is perhaps best defined, therefore, in general terms—simply as "an apparently successful attempt to increase the understanding of [a given] phenomenon" (Wilson and Keil 2000, p. 89). This broad view of explanation appears, in our opinion, well-suited for psychopathology, given the variety of factors, patterns, and experiential qualities that can be relevant to issues in mental health. We think that phenomenology provides psychopathology with a variety of concepts, tools, and investigative guidelines—closely linked to phenomenology's methods of description—that are necessary elements of an integrative or pluralistic approach to explanation in psychiatry.

In the early phase of his work, Edmund Husserl (1859–1938) presented phenomenology as a purely descriptive approach that excluded all concern with both genesis and causation (Bernet, Kern, and Marbach 1993, p. 195). Later, however, he adopted a broader and more ambitious view, advocating the need to supplement what he called "static" or "descriptive phenomenology" with phenomenology of a "genetic" or "constructive" type. Indeed, Husserl himself came to speak of "*explanatory*" phenomenology—a "phenomenology of regulated genesis" (1999, p. 318). Genetic phenomenology, for Husserl, included the study *of how complex objects and modes of experience come to be constituted,* over time, via the synthesis of simpler or more basic processes or "lived experiences" (1999, p. 319). Thus, Husserl (1989, p. 402) eventually moved away from the sharp opposition between description (as the goal of the human sciences) and explanation (as the goal of the natural sciences).

A key concept for Husserl (1989) was that of "*motivation,*" which in his view provides the *"fundamental lawfulness of spiritual life"* and implies a kind of "motivational *causality*". Unlike blind physical causality, this motivational causality involved the subject's attitude or orientation, his or her viewpoint on, or interpretation of, the world (1989, pp. 231, 241f). Husserl's concept of motivation transcends the narrow frame of Jaspers's view of understanding and is broader than the everyday-language concept of motive, disposition, or ground for action. In a quote already cited, Husserl says that "consciousness consist(s) of . . . a network founded on intentional *intertwining, motivation* and mutual *implication,* in a way that has no analogue in the physical" (1977, sect. 37). Motivation can operate through associative and other links (including logical ones) among the *contents* of awareness. Presumably, these would include the kinds of links emphasized by analytic philosophers who speak of "mental causation" or the "practical syllogism." But motivation (in Husserl's sense) can also operate through *formal* or *structural* aspects of the *act* of consciousness itself—as, for example, when inner time consciousness serves as a necessary condition for the unity of the flux of experiences, or when an anomalous mode of self-experience is expressed in specific kinds of delusional beliefs (Husserl 1989, p. 238). Motivation thus covers many forms of what might be termed *interdependence* between mental acts and experiences that contribute to the coherence and unity of consciousness, both in its synchronic (simultaneous) and diachronic (successive) aspects (1989, pp. 223–293).

To have a phenomenological grasp of the mind of another person is to *grasp the motivational relationships that lend coherence and continuity to that person's consciousness.* This requires that one move beyond descriptions focusing on isolated aspects of subjective life and beyond mere static understanding of particular mental states toward an understanding of both the overall unity of that person's subjectivity and its development over time. This inclusive approach is, as indicated above, already at play in assessing the single symptoms. A phenomenological understanding of a disturbed overall mode of consciousness or lived-world may allow one to make sense out of seemingly bizarre actions or beliefs that might otherwise seem completely incomprehensible. One may, for example, come to see how the person's actions or beliefs can be understood in the light of general features of the person's experience of time, space, causality, or selfhood or how they are, in some respects, *inspired* or *justified* by the kinds of experiences the person is having and has had.

6. Forms of Explanation in Phenomenological Psychopathology: The Case of Schizophrenia

As far as we know, the current literature contains no comprehensive and clear discussion of the variety of forms of *explanation* that phenomenological psychopathology can offer. We ourselves recently attempted (Sass and Parnas 2007) to provide just such a scheme, one that details how a phenomenological account, rather than being purely descriptive, can be seen to have *explanatory* or even *causal* relevance. We will try to illustrate these explanatory issues by turning our attention to schizophrenia. We have proposed a phenomenological theory (Parnas 2003; Sass 2003; Sass and Parnas 2003) asserting that schizophrenia involves a particular kind of disturbance of consciousness, more specifically, of the sense of self or ipseity that is normally implicit or prereflectively *given* in each act of awareness. Ipseity derives from *ipse,* Latin for "self" or "itself." *Ipseity refers to a fundamental configuration of self-awareness* (that is, *of all experiencing in first-person perspective).* It is a crucial sense of *subjectivity of experience,* as it were, of *coinciding* with oneself at any given moment of experience (Henry 1973; Ricoeur 1992; Zahavi 2005). Ipseity is not something willed or mobilized through a reflective effort. Rather, it is a given, automatic, passive, and immediate (that is, direct) mode of the articulation of consciousness (Zahavi and Parnas 1998; Zahavi 1999).

The self-disorder or *ipseity disturbance* characteristic of schizophrenia has two complementary aspects: *diminished self-affection*—a decline in the (passively or automatically) experienced sense of existing as a living, unified, and self-coinciding subject of awareness—and *hyperreflexivity*— a transformation of the field of awareness into a form of ongoing, exaggerated self-consciousness, a sort of objectifying focal attention that is directed toward processes and phenomena that would normally be "inhabited" or experienced only implicitly as part of oneself. In other words, the primary problem lies in *the structure of self-awareness* and *not* in one's self-image, self-esteem, or self-representation, although these self-representational problems will often follow and accompany the primary experiential disorder.

This hypothesis has important precursors in many classic texts on schizophrenia, most clearly and comprehensively formulated by Joseph Berze and Hans Gruhle (Berze 1914; Berze and Gruhle 1929), in more recent phenomenological literature (Minkowski 1927, 1997a; Binswanger 1956; Blankenburg 1971) and in the discussions on the nature of schizotypy (for review, see Parnas et al. 2005). Our own approach—while aware of the historical resources—was strongly inspired by daily clinical work with young, first-contact schizophrenia spectrum patients in Denmark and Norway (Parnas et al. 1998; Møller and Husby 2000). Extensive, in-depth interviews with such patients revealed certain typical complaints (often considered by the patients as the most disturbing aspects of the illness): a diminishment of a basic and normally automatic—immediate sense of identity or of self-coinciding, a sentiment of a pervasive inner void or lack,[16] an increasing anonymity ("depersonalization") of the field of awareness, characteristically associated with a hyperreflexive self-conscious stance. Such a stance involves certain cognitive and perceptual disturbances in which elements of the stream of consciousness become autonomous, almost like focally demarcated, spatialized entities or objects that are experienced as possessing their own life and existing at a distance from the self. The patients report feeling isolated and detached, a stance from which they are unable to grasp the "natural," everyday significations or meanings in the world and in relations to others. In summary, the disorder of ipseity (that is, a diminished self-affection and hyper-reflexivity) may be considered as an enduring, trait-like "altered state of consciousness."

In subsequent empirical studies, systematic evaluations of experiential anomalies were performed with semistructured interviews conducted by senior clinicians, using a phenomenological-prototypical scale ([BSABS] Gross et al. 1987), supplemented by a few additional items derived from our clinical experience and literature. The interrater reliabilities of the scale's measures of subjective experience were good or excellent (Vollmer-Larsen et al. 2007). These studies demonstrated that, among first-contact, nonorganic patients (Copenhagen Prodromal Study, $n = 151$), self-disorders aggregate in *ICD-10* schizophrenia *and* schizotypy ($n = 101$) but *not* in other, "nonspectrum," psychiatric diagnoses ($n = 50$) (that is, *self-disorders occur selectively in the schizophrenia spectrum disorders)* (Handest and Parnas 2005; Parnas et al. 2005). A study showing no aggregation of self-disorders in psychotic bipolar illness buttressed the observed affinity of self-disorders to the *schizophrenia spectrum* (a comparison of patients with residual schizophrenia with remitted bipolar *psychotic* patients [Parnas et al. 2003]). In a recently completed, prospective 5-year follow-up study of the Copenhagen Prodromal Study, the development of schizo-phrenia or schizotypy (n = 14) in the group of nonschizophrenia spectrum patients (n = 38) was predicted by the initial presence of self-disorders (OR = 12, p = 0.003) (Vollmer-Larsen 2008).

We consider self-disorders as the fundamental subjective trait features of the schizophrenia spectrum disorders, as markers of vulnerability, a "generative disorder" with causal implications. The concept of generative disorder refers to basic phenomenal (experienced) configurations of con-sciousness that are detectable already in the early stages of the evolution of schizophrenia and that, in conjunction with certain expressive or be-havioral features (for example, disorders of affectivity and language), con-fers on schizophrenia its distinctive phenomenological typicality and, in our view, grounds its conceptual validity. In describing the potential causal relevance of this key *ipseity* disturbance, we distinguish two gen-eral perspectives according to whether the focus is on features of the dis-order that are primarily *synchronic* (simultaneous) or *diachronic* (occur-ring in succession).

Here we will discuss only one particular example of the synchronic re-lationship: the *expressive* type. Expressive relationships involve situa-tions in which a mental *content* (for example, a delusion) seems to repre-sent, express, or emblematize, in a specific way, what appear to be *general formal or structural* characteristics of consciousness or mental life. This is akin to the philosopher Merleau-Ponty's notion of "emblems of being" (Merleau-Ponty 1968, p. 270; Dreyfus and Wakefield 1988, p. 280).[17] It should be noted that the relation between a *form* and its expressive, man-ifest *content* is intimate: one never grasps a pure structure or a formless content but always a content that is structured in a certain way. To grasp the expressive relationships is a matter of delineating, not *causal* relations but relationships of mutual phenomenological *implication*. The manifest symptoms or contents always embody the larger wholes or structures, which condition the formation of these contents. The symptoms, so to say, always carry the traces of the underlying formal alterations of subjectiv-ity. Phenomenological investigation is here a matter of *unfolding* these different facets of conscious life to arrive at a richer grasp of its *lived tex-ture and internal structure*. To articulate such expressive relationships provides an integrative vision, an understanding not of patterns of causal interaction but "of style, of logical implication, of meaning and value" (Geertz 1973, p. 145), and this *does* serve an *explanatory* function.[18] The individual factors or aspects are understood as mutually implicative *aspects* or *expressions* of mental activity as a whole (Marbach 1993, p. 35; Minkowski 1997a).[19]

Consider, for instance, the famous influencing-machine delusion of the patient Natalija (Tausk [1919] 1933; Sass 1992b)—a delusion that implies that Natalija experiences herself as, at the same time, *godlike* (at the center of the world, with all other entities existing only for her) but also a mere passive entity within the world (a machine manipulated by others). The apparently contradictory situation where the self can be experienced *both* as a passive mechanism at the mercy of the world *and* as a kind of omnipotent solipsistic deity—sometimes at the same moment—can be understood if one recognizes that *both* these forms of self-experience are *implicit* in a hyperreflexive transformation of the functioning of one's own mind and its role in the constitution of the experiential world (Bovet and Parnas 1993; Sass 1998a, 1992b; Parnas 2004).

Many characteristic schizophrenic delusions (for example, delusions about dissolving, being controlled by an influencing machine,[20] or being constantly recorded by video cameras) are not, in fact, psychologically incomprehensible, as Jaspers claimed. The phenomenological approach affords us with additional resources to understand such mental contents as *arising from* and, in a sense, *expressing* the profoundly altered *forms* of experiencing that are characteristic of schizophrenia and that constitute its generative disorder (especially, the disorder of ipseity). We have described elsewhere how the ipseity disorder provides an underlying, and hence unifying, aspect of the "three syndromes" of schizophrenia: the negative, positive, and disorganized dimensions of psychopathology (Sass and Parnas 2003).

The diachronic dimension of phenomenological psychopathology concerns the development of symptoms over time and the relative *causal* primacy of various kinds of processes.[21] A grasp of this dimension requires understanding certain familiar relationships that are commonly used in psychopathology—in particular, those between more *primary* or foundational disturbances and those having a more *secondary* status, whether as *consequences* ("natural sequelae") or as *compensatory* or defensive mechanisms. In our model, self-disorders (trait-altered states of consciousness) are markers of vulnerability and considered as basic, primary phenotypes of schizophrenia.[22] A *phenomenological* approach (in the diachronic dimension) would articulate how such self-disorders, rather than possessing a merely epiphenomenal status, might actually play a causal role in the development of other symptoms. It is the *phenotypic dimension* of vulnerability (for example, a constant feeling of void, self-detachment, and low-grade perplexity) that, in interaction with other factors, leads to symptomatological consequences (for example, changes in the worldview, isolation, or "inappropriate" behavior). Thus, the altered states of consciousness *prefigure* the range of symptoms that may emerge. For example, the anomalies of self-awareness involving diminished self-affection and hyper-reflexivity, may attract further reflexive attention, thereby eliciting processes of scrutiny and self-exacerbating alienation that occur as byproducts of the primary disturbance. A patient may pay exaggerated attention to strange kinesthetic sensations or may scrutinize odd visual appearances in a way that only increases their oddness. Diminished sense of privacy of consciousness (sense of demarcation or of "ego boundaries") will be conductive to a formation of mental contents, which we designate as delusions of influence and omnipotence. The primary self-disorders do not, however, merely *elicit* fairly automatic consequences; they also *inspire* defensive or *compensatory* responses. Patients may attempt, for example, to reassert control and reestablish a sense of self by means of introspective scrutinizing or pseudo-obsessive intellectual ruminations. Defensive or compensatory processes often have counterproductive effects, however. Hyperreflexivity may, for example, become a source of *further* alienations or diminishments of self-affection and perceptual meaning. Attention may become devoted to detail, with consequent destruction of the gestalt field of experience. The inner life may become tortured and painfully self-conscious, ultimately fragmenting itself from within. There may occur a veritable "centrifuging" of the self—a process whereby phenomena that would normally be "inner" or tacit are progressively spun outward and away (Sass 1992, pp. 337–338).

Such an analysis is consistent with the results from studies of symptom progression in schizophrenia (Conrad 1958; Klosterkötter 1988; Klosterkötter et al. 1997, 2001). In a study of 118 cases of first onset schizophrenia, Conrad considered characteristic patterns of psychosis as the products of reorganizations of the field of awareness, which followed certain phenomenological regularities. Similarly, Klosterkötter (1988), in a study of 121 patients with schizophrenia, suggested that the developments of psychotic symptoms followed phenomenologically *typical sequences and patterns* of transition ("prägnanztypische Übergangsreichen"), from the stages of anomalous "*initial* experiences" (Ausgangserfahrungen) to the "end-phenomena" (Endphänomene) (namely, full-blown psychotic first-rank syndromes). In both studies, these transitions involved increasing objectification and externalization of experiential phenomena (such as proprioceptive sensations or the stream of thoughts or inner speech) that would normally be "*inhabited*" (that is, experienced in a tacit rather than explicit or focal manner).

In this way, subjective *experience* can play an important causal role in the progressive experiential transformations of a developing schizophrenic illness. The described forms of symptomatic progression can be neither understood nor explained without making reference to the subjective or phenomenological dimension. This is not to deny the key role of neurobiological abnormalities. It is not, however, neural events per se but, rather, the *experience* of, for example, certain kinesthetic sensations as focal objects that elicit ever more intense forms of hyper-reflective concentration, which, in turn, can exacerbate the experiential fragmentation. *Certain irreducible features of subjective life thus provide both the motivation and the field of possibility for the progressive symptomatic developments.*

Here we might speak of a certain "autonomy of the phenomenological." As McClamrock (1995) points out in a book on causal explanation in cognitive science, causal analysis sometimes requires that one specify a set of objects and goals that are a function of the way in which the world is *experienced* by the patient. In this sense, "irreducibly subjective" properties are sometimes able to account for a person's behavior in a way that referring to the state of the nervous system alone could not possibly do; they will sometimes constitute the "preferred level of explanation" (p. 42, also pp. 4, 45–53, 178, 187; Searle 1983, pp. 112–140; Husserl 1989, pp. 227, 241).

To clarify the diachronic dimension of motivational causality is (among other things) to specify the person's (or patient's) way of seeing things and grasp how the (perceived) environment solicits or elicits further forms of action and perception. These forms, of course, have their own consequences, thereby leading to comprehensible and predictable—but not wholly determined—progressions of behavior and experiential modes. It is not enough to say, then, that the experiential phenomenology of abnormal experiences merely *constrains* explanations on the cognitive or neurobiological levels: it can actually provide a key element of the explanations themselves.

7. Conclusion

In this chapter, we presented several approaches to the problem of description in psychopathology. Excessive and, in our view, epistemologically naïve focus on the issues of reliability created serious problems concerning the more fundamental level of validity. In the main body of the chapter, we introduced the approach of *continental phenomenology*. We presented some contributions of this set of approaches to epistemological and ontological issues in psychopathology: for example, how to establish generalizations about subjective states that are both valid and reasonably reliable and questions about the nature of subjective worlds and their psychopathological variations. In our view, continental phenomenology makes an indispensable contribution to psychopathology—relevant not only to description and understanding but also to various forms of explanation (including causal explanation).

NOTES

1. Menos's argument—that "a man cannot try to discover either what he knows or what he does not know"—is summarized by Socrates as follows: "He would not seek what he knows, for because he knows it there is no need of the inquiry, nor what he does not know, for in that case he does not even know what he is to look for" (p. 363)

2. This is a deeply enthroned habit of psychiatric thinking to consider the causal relations in a *mechanical* way, which is not necessarily consistent with the contemporary physical theories of, for example, general and special relativity or the quantic processes. See John Woodward, chapter 4 in this volume.

3. These are the latest vicissitudes. A similar alternation between modular and holistic views of the brain functions already happened some 100 years ago (Lantéri-Laura 1998).

4. In fact, only two features, because "conviction" and "incorrigibility" are two aspects of the same phenomenon.

5. Clinically, this is a difficult feature to assess, because patients often do not reveal their innermost convictions and may conceal their delusional ideation.

6. To discuss it within the operational perspective is almost contradiction in terms: we are confronted here head-on with the issue of subjectivity, whose very existence and clinical importance operational psychopathology tries to deny or explain away.

7. These problems in defining delusions have of course serious consequences on the issues of conceptual validity and reliability of the concept of *psychosis,* and

of more marginal, yet diagnostically important, classes of other *operational terms* related to psychoticism (for example, overvalued idea, paranoid ideation, self-reference, pseudo-obsessive ruminations, and magical thinking).

8. Operationalism, no doubt, stimulated explosion of empirical studies, yet it is difficult to say—from a global point of view—whether operationalism entailed a progress, led to stagnation, or even halted potential developments in psychiatric knowledge. It certainly entailed reification of diagnostic criteria into real kind categories and to an extinction of interest in (and familiarity with) the domains of psychopathology that were not listed as the diagnostic criteria. There are many voices drawing attention to a rather alarming decline in psychopathology (for example, Maj 1998; Tucker 1998; Andreasen 1998).

9. Karl Jaspers himself wrote, "The opinion has been expressed in medical quarters that this book [Jaspers's own *General Psychopathology*] is too hard for students, because it attempts to tackle extremely difficult and ultimate problems. As far as that is concerned, I am convinced that either one grasps a science entirely, that means in its central problems, or not at all. I consider it fatal simply to adjust at a low level. One should be guided by the better students who are interested in the subject for its own sake, even though they may be in a minority. Those who teach should compel their students to rise to a scientific level. But this is made impossible if 'compendia' are used, which give students fragmentary, superficial pseudo-knowledge 'for practical purposes,' and which sometimes is more subversive for practice than total ignorance. One should not show a facade of science" (*General Psychopathology*, pp. x–xi).

10. Descriptions of expression and behavior are the respective tasks of the psychology of expression (*Ausdruckspsychologie*) and the psychology of performance (*Leistungspsychologie*).

11. In fact, a claim may be made with respect to thoughts, concepts, and other so-called inner phenomena—as always being individuated through their relations of intersubjective references (Bennett and Hacker 2003).

12. For example, when people—laypeople and psychiatrists—talk today about neurotransmitters when they mean a phenomenal depression.

13. Such a view would eventually entail a physicalistic metaphysics, which is precisely incompatible with our claim of the ontological primacy of the Lifeworld.

14. Wittgenstein's notion of "family resemblance" (1958) is a similar concept. The degree of proximity of the concrete exemplar to the prototype determines classification of the former. Prototypes may organize the categories of a classification scheme while allowing for the simultaneous dimensional considerations.

15. An ideal-type analysis brings out the *ideal and necessary* connections between features of a phenomenon. The ideal type transcends what is given in experience: for example, all my possible drawings of a straight line will be somehow deficient (for instance, if examined through a microscope) compared to the very (ideal) concept of a straight line.

16. See the patient of Blankenburg (1971): "What is it that I really lack? Some-

thing so small, so comic, but so unique and important, that you cannot live without it" (pp. 42–43).

17. This distinction corresponds, in Heidegger's system, to the difference between "ontic" facts and "ontological" dimensions of existence; see Sass (1992a).

18. The logical relationships analyzed are not, however, those constituting a practical syllogism, as in contemporary analytic philosophy of mind. For discussion of this somewhat technical issue, see Sass and Parnas (in press).

19. This is what Merleau-Ponty (1962) was pointing to when he spoke of "internal links" between aspects of experience that "display one typical structure . . . standing in a relationship to each other of reciprocal expression" (p. 157).

20. Note that, in a similar vein, Schneider considered some of the so-called first-rank symptoms as conditioned on self-disorders.

21. In a certain sense, diachronic understanding is always partly involved in grasping the synchronic relation: we always need some grasp of the temporal constitution of the clinical picture to comprehend its synchronic coherence.

22. From this perspective, they may serve important function as dependent variables (explananda) for a neurobiological approach.

REFERENCES

American Psychiatric Association. 1980. *Diagnostic and Statistical Manual of Mental Disorders,* 3rd ed. (*DSM-III*). Washington, DC: American Psychiatric Association.

———. 1987. *Diagnostic and Statistical Manual of Mental Disorders,* 3rd ed, revised (*DSM-III-R*). Washington, DC: American Psychiatric Association.

———. 1994. *Diagnostic and Statistical Manual of Mental Disorders,* 4th ed. (*DSM-IV*). Washington, DC: American Psychiatric Association.

———. 2000. *Diagnostic and Statistical Manual of Mental Disorders,* 4th ed., text revised (*DSM-IV-TR*). Washington, DC: American Psychiatric Association.

Andreasen, N. 1998. Understanding Schizophrenia: A Silent Spring (Editorial). *American Journal of Psychiatry* 155:1657–1659.

Audi, R. (ed.). 1999. *The Cambridge Dictionary of Philosophy,* 2nd ed. Cambridge: Cambridge University Press.

Bégout, B. 2005. *La decouverte du quotidien.* Paris: Éditions Allia.

Bell, V., P. W. Halligan, and H. D. Ellis. 2006. Diagnosing Delusions: A Review of Inter-Rater Reliability. *Schizophrenia Research* 86:76–79.

Bennett, M. R., and P. M. S. Hacker. 2003. *Philosophical Foundations of Neuroscience.* Oxford: Blackwell.

Bermúdez, J. L. 2005. *Philosophy of Psychology. A Contemporary Introduction.* London; New York: Routledge.

Bernet, R., I. Kern, and E. Marbach. 1993. *An Introduction to Husserlian Phenomenology.* Evanston, IL: Northwestern University Press.

Berze, J. 1914. *Die primäre Insuffizienz der psychischen Aktivität. Ihr Wesen, ihre*

Erscheinungen und ihre Bedeutung als Grundstörungen der Dementia Praecox und der hypophrenen überhaupt. Leipzig: Frank Deuticke.

Berze, J., and H. W. Gruhle. 1929. *Psychologie der Schizophrenie.* Berlin: Springer.

Binswanger, L. 1956. *Drei Formen Misglückten Daseins. Verstiegenheit, Verschrobenheit, Manierertheit.* Tübingen: Niemeyer.

———. 1960. *Melancholie und Manie. Phänomenologische Studien.* Pfullingen: Verlag Günther Neske. French translation by J.-M. Azorin and Y. Totoyan. *Mélancolie et manie. Etudes phénoménologiques.* Paris: Presses Universitaires de France, 1987.

Blankenburg, W. 1971. *Der Verlust der Naturlichen Selbstverstandlichkeit: Ein Beitrag zur Psychopathologie Symptomarmer Schizophrenien.* Stuttgart: Ferdinand Enke Verlag. French translation by J.-M. Azorin and Y. Totoyan. *La perte de l'evidence naturelle: Une contribution a la psychopathologie des schizophrénies pauci-symptomatiques.* Paris: Presses Universitaires de France, 1991.

Bolton, D., and J. Hill. 1996. *Mind, Meaning and Mental Disorder: The Nature of Explanation in Psychology and Psychiatry.* Oxford: Oxford University Press.

Bovet, P., and J. Parnas. 1993. Schizophrenic Delusions: A Phenomenological Approach. *Schizophrenia Bulletin* 19:579–597.

Bridgman, P. 1927. *The Logic of Modern Physics.* New York: MacMillan.

Cantor, N., E. E. Smith, and R. French. 1980. Psychiatric Diagnosis as Prototype Categorization. *Journal of Abnormal Psychology* 89:181–193.

Churchland, P. S. 1986. *Neurophilosophy: Toward a Unified Science of the Mind/ Brain.* Cambridge, MA: MIT Press.

Cooper, J. E., R. E. Kendell, B. J. Gurland, L. Sharpe, J. R. M. Coppeland, and R. Simon. 1972. *Psychiatric Diagnosis in New York and London.* Maudsley Monograph 20. London: Oxford University Press.

Davidson, D. 1980. *Essays on Actions and Events.* Oxford: Clarendon Press.

Dreyfus, H., and J. Wakefield. 1988. From Depth Psychology to Breadth Psychology: A Phenomenological Approach to Psychopathology. In S. Messer, L. Sass, and R. Woolfolk (eds.), *Hermeneutics and Psychological Theory.* New Brunswick, NJ: Rutgers University Press, pp. 272–288.

Esquirol, J.-E.-D. 1838. *Des maladies mentales considérées sous les rapports médical, hygiénique et médico-légal.* Paris: J-B Bailliére.

Flaum, M., S. Arndt, and N. C. Andreasen. 1991. The Reliability of "Bizarre" Delusions. *Comprehensive Psychiatry* 32:59–65.

Geertz, C. 1973. *The Interpretation of Cultures.* New York: Basic Books.

Gross, G., G. Huber, J. Klosterkötter, and M. Linz. 1987. *Bonner Skala für Beurteilung von Basissymptomen (BSABS)* [Bonn Scale for the Assessment of Basic Symptoms]. Berlin: Springer Verlag. Danish translation by P. Handest and M. Handest. Copenhagen: Synthélabo Scandinavia A/S, 1995.

Grünbaum, A. 1993. *Validation in the Clinical Theory of Psychoanalysis.* Madison, CT: International Universities Press.

Handest, P., and J. Parnas. 2005. Clinical Characteristics of First-Admitted Patients with ICD-10 Schizotypal Disorder. *British Journal of Psychiatry* 187 (48):49–54.

Hanna, R. 2006. *Kant, Science, and Human Nature.* Oxford: Oxford University Press.

Hanson, N. R. 1965. *The Patterns of Discovery: An Inquiry into the Conceptual Foundations of Science.* Cambridge: Cambridge University Press.

Heidegger, M. 1962. *Being and Time.* Trans. J. MacQuarrie and E. Robinson. New York: Harper & Row.

Heil, J., and A. Mele (eds.). 1993. *Mental Causation.* Oxford: Clarendon Press.

Heinima, M. 2002. Incomprehensibility: The Role of the Concept in DSM-IV Definition of Schizophrenic Delusions. *Medicine, Health Care and Philosophy* 5:291–295.

Hempel, C. G. 1965. *Aspects of Scientific Explanation and Other Essays in the Philosophy of Science.* New York: Free Press.

Henry, M. 1973. *The Essence of Manifestation.* Trans. G. Etzkorn. The Hague: Martinus Nijhoff. French original: *L'Essence de la Manifestation.* Paris: PUF, 1963.

Howsepian, A. A. 2007. The DSM-IV-R "Glossary of Technical Terms": A Reappraisal. *Psychopathology* 40:28–34.

Husserl, E. 1977. *Phenomenological Psychology* (lectures, summer semester, 1925). Trans. J. Scanlon. The Hague: Martinus Nijhoff.

———. 1983. *Ideas Pertaining to a Pure Phenomenology and to a Phenomenological Philosophy: First Book.* Trans. F. Kersten. Dordrecht, Holland: Kluwer.

———. 1989. *Ideas Pertaining to a Pure Phenomenology and to a Phenomenological Philosophy: Second Book: Studies in the Phenomenology of Constitution.* Trans. R. Rojcewicz and A. Schuwer. Dordrecht, Holland: Kluwer.

———. 1999. *The Essential Husserl.* Ed. D. Welton. Bloomington: Indiana University Press.

Jaspers, K. 1963. *General Psychopathology.* Trans. J. Hoenig and M. W. Hamilton. Chicago: University of Chicago Press.

———. 1968. The Phenomenological Approach in Psychopathology. *British Journal of Psychiatry* 114:1313–1323.

Lantéri-Laura, G. 1998. *Essai sur les paradigmes de psychiatrie moderne.* Paris: Editions du Temps.

Lawson-Tancred, H. 1995. Ancient Greek Philosophy II: Aristotle. In A. C. Grayling (ed.), *Philosophy: A Guide through the Subject* (pp. 398–439). Oxford: Oxford University Press.

Maj, M. 1998. Critique of the DSM-IV Operational Diagnostic Criteria for Schizophrenia. *British Journal of Psychiatry* 172:458–460.

Marbach, E. 1993. *Mental Representation and Consciousness: Towards a Phenomenological Theory of Representation and Reference.* Dordrecht: Kluwer Academic.

McClamrock, R. 1995. *Existential Cognition: Computational Minds in the World.* Chicago: University of Chicago Press.

Merleau-Ponty, M. 1968. *The Visible and the Invisible.* Trans. A. Lingis. Evanston, IL: Northwestern University Press.

———. 1945. *Phénoménologie de la perception.* Paris: Gallimard. Phenomenology of Perception. London: Routledge, 1962.

————. 1964. *Sense and Nonsense.* Trans. H. L. Dreyfus and P. A. Dreyfus. Evanston, IL: Northwestern University Press.

————. 2004. *The World of Perception.* London: Routledge. Trans. O. Davis. *Causeries 1948,* Paris: Éditions Seuil, 2002.

Minkowski, E. 1927. *La schizophrènie: Psychopathologie des schizoides et des schizophrènes.* Paris: Payot.

————. 1997a. Du symptome au trouble gènèrateur. (Originally published in *Archives suisses de neurologie et de psychiatrie,* 1928; 22). In *Au-delà du rationalisme morbide.* Paris: Éditions L'Harmattan.

————. 1997b. *Traité de Psychopathologie.* Paris: Institut Synthelabo.

Møller, P., and R. Husby. 2000. The Initial Prodrome in Schizophrenia: Searching for Naturalistic Core Dimensions of Experience and Behavior. *Schizophrenia Bulletin* 26:217–232.

Parnas, J. 2000. The Self and Intentionality in the Pre-Psychotic Stages of Schizophrenia: A Phenomenological Study. In D. Zahavi (ed.), *Exploring the Self: Philosophical and Psychopathological Perspectives on Self-experience* (pp. 115–147). Philadelphia: John Benjamins Publishing.

————. 2003. Self and Schizophrenia: A Phenomenological Perspective. In T. Kircher and A. David (eds.), *The Self in Neuroscience and Psychiatry* (pp. 217–241). Cambridge: Cambridge University Press.

————. 2004. Belief and Pathology of Self-Awareness: A Phenomenological Contribution to the Classification of Delusions. *Journal of Consciousness Studies* 10–11:148–461.

Parnas, J., and P. Bovet. 1991. Autism in Schizophrenia Revisited. *Comprehensive Psychiatry* 32:7–21.

————. 1995. Research in Psychopathology: Epistemologic Issues. *Comprehensive Psychiatry* 36:167–181.

Parnas, J., P. Bovet, and D. Zahavi. 2002. Schizophrenic Autism: Clinical Phenomenology and Pathogenetic Implications. *World Psychiatry* 1/3:131–136.

Parnas, J., and P. Handest. 2003. Phenomenology of Anomalous Self-Experience in Early Schizophrenia. *Comprehensive Psychiatry* 44:121–134.

Parnas, J., P. Handest, L. Jansson, and D. Sæbye. 2005a. Anomalous Subjective Experience among First Admitted Schizophrenia Spectrum Patients: Empirical Investigation. *Psychopathology* 38(5):259–267.

Parnas, J., P. Handest, D. Sæbye, and L. Jansson. 2003. Anomalies of Subjective Experience in Schizophrenia and Psychotic Bipolar Illness. *Acta Psychiatrica Scandinavica* 108:126–133.

Parnas, J., L. Jansson, L. A. Sass, and P. Handest. 1998. Self-Experience in the Prodromal Phases of Schizophrenia. *Neurology, Psychiatry, and Brain Research* 6:97–106.

Parnas, J., P. Moeller, T. Kircher, J. Thalbitzer, et al. 2005. EASE: Examination of Anomalous Self-Experience. *Psychopathology* 38(5):236–258.

Plato. 1961. *Meno.* Trans. W. K. C. Guthrie. In E. Hamilton and H. Cairns (eds.), *The*

Collected Dialogues of Plato, Including the Letters (pp. 353–384). Princeton, NJ: Princeton University Press.

Putnam, H. 1987. *The Many Faces of Realism.* LaSalle, IL: Open Court.

Quine, W. V. O. 1951. Two Dogmas of Empiricism. *Philosophical Review* 60:20–43.

Ricoeur, P. 1990. *Soi-même comme un autre.* Paris: Les Editions Seuil.

Rosch, E. 1988. Principles of Categorization. In A. M. Collins and E. E. Smith (eds.), *Readings in Cognitive Science: A Perspective from Psychology and Artificial Intelligence* (pp. 312–322). San Mateo, CA: Morgan Kaufmann.

Sadler, J. Z., O. P. Wiggins, and M. A. Schwartz. 1994. *Philosophical Perspectives on Psychiatric Diagnostic Classification.* Baltimore: Johns Hopkins University Press.

Sass, L. 1992a. Heidegger, Schizophrenia, and the Ontological Difference. *Philosophical Psychology* 5:109–132.

———. 1992b. *Madness and Modernism: Insanity in the light of Modern Art, Literature, and Thought.* New York: Basic Books.

———. 1994. *The Paradoxes of Delusion: Wittgenstein, Schreber, and the Schizophrenic Mind.* Ithaca, NY: Cornell University Press.

———. 1998. Ambiguity Is of the Essence: The Relevance of Hermeneutics for Psychoanalysis. In P. Marcus and A. Rosenberg (eds.), *Psychoanalytic Versions of the Human Condition and Clinical Practice* (pp. 257–305). New York: New York University Press.

———. 2003. Schizophrenia and the Self: Hyper-Reflexivity and Diminished Self-Affection. In A. David and T. Kirchner (eds.), *The Self in Schizophrenia: Neuropsychological Perspectives* (pp. 242–271). Cambridge: Cambridge University Press.

Sass, L., and J. Parnas. 2003. Self, Consciousness, and Schizophrenia. *Schizophrenia Bulletin* 29(3):427–444.

———. 2007. Explaining Schizophrenia: The Relevance of Phenomenology. In M. Chung, W. Fulford, and G. Graham (eds.), *Reconceiving Schizophrenia* (pp. 63–96). Oxford: Oxford University Press.

Schwartz, M. A., and O. P. Wiggins. 1987. Diagnosis and Ideal Types: A Contribution to Psychiatric Classification. *Comprehensive Psychiatry* 28:277–291.

Sokolowski, R. 2000. *Introduction to Phenomenology.* Cambridge: Cambridge University Press.

Spitzer, M. 1988. Psychiatry, Philosophy, and the Problem of Description. In M. Spitzer, F. A. Uehlein, and G. Oepen (eds.), *Psychopathology and Philosophy* (pp. 3–18). Berlin: Springer-Verlag.

Spitzer, R. L., M. B. First, K. S. Kendler, and D. J. Stein. 1993. The Reliability of Three Definitions of Bizarre Delusions. *American Journal of Psychiatry* 150: 880–884.

Tausk, V. (1919) 1933. On the Origin of the "Influencing Machine" in Schizophrenia. *Psychoanalytic Quarterly* 2:529–530.

Tucker, G. J. 1998. Putting DSM-IV in Perspective (Editorial). *American Journal of Psychiatry* 155:159–161.

Vollmer-Larsen, A. 2008. *Copenhagen Prodromal Study: Five Years Follow-Up.* Copenhagen: University of Copenhagen, Faculty of Health Sciences.

Vollmer-Larsen, A., P. Handest, D. Sæbye, and J. Parnas. 2007. Reliability of Measuring Anomalous Experience: The Bonn Scale for the Assessment of Basic Symptoms (BSABS). *Psychopathology* 40(5):345–348.

Webb, L., C. DiClemente, E. Johnstone, J. Sanders, and R. Perley. 1981. *DSM-III Training Guide for Use with the American Psychiatric Association's Diagnostic and Statistical Manual of Mental Disorders,* 3rd ed. New York: Brunner/Mazel.

Wilson, R. A., and F. C. Keil. 2000. The Shadows and Shallows of Explanation. In F. C. Keil and R. A. Wilson (eds.), *Explanation and Cognition* (pp. 87–114). Cambridge, MA: MIT Press.

Wittgenstein, L. 1922. *Tractatus Logico-Philosophicus.* Trans. C. K. Ogden. London: Routledge and Kegan Paul.

———. 1953. *Philosophical Investigations.* Eds. G. E. M. Anscombe and R. Rhees. Oxford: Blackwell.

Woodward, J. 2003. *Making Things Happen: A Theory of Causal Explanation.* Oxford: Oxford University Press.

World Health Organization. 1992. *The ICD-10 International Statistical Classification of Diseases and Related Health Problems.* Geneva: WHO.

Zahavi, D. 1999. *Self-Awareness and Alterity: A Phenomenological Investigation.* Evanston, IL: Northwestern University Press.

———. 2001. *Husserl and Transcendental Intersubjectivity.* Athens: Ohio University Press.

———. 2003. *Husserl's Phenomenology.* Stanford, CA: Stanford University Press.

———. 2005. *Subjectivity and Selfhood: Investigating the First-Person Perspective.* Cambridge, MA: MIT Press.

Zahavi, D., and J. Parnas. 1998. Phenomenal Consciousness and Self-Awareness: A Phenomenological Critique of Representational Theory. *Journal of Consciousness Studies* 5(5–6):687–705.

Comment: Beyond Descriptive Phenomenology
Thomas Fuchs, M.D., Ph.D.

In *General Psychopathology* ([1913] 1968), Karl Jaspers tried to develop a conceptual framework for psychopathology of mental states by integrating the phenomenological methodology with hermeneutic distinction between understanding and explanation. The resulting descriptive phenomenology served as the basis for psychopathology until today, in particular, for Kurt Schneider's nosology and its offshoots in present operational diagnostic systems. In Jaspers's view, however, *phenomenology was only a subdiscipline within psychopathology.* Its primary task consisted in providing a basic taxonomy of psychopathological phenomena, thus performing a preparatory work for other subdisciplines of psychopathology and psychiatry. Jaspers was all the more anxious to keep his approach free from all explanatory claims, which he thought would contaminate the purity of description by premature inferences, theories, and speculations: "We should picture only what is really present in the patient's consciousness" (Jaspers [1913] 1968, p. 1316).

According to Jaspers, only empathic understanding is the appropriate understanding of mental life. There are, however, limits to understanding, namely, with respect to the delusional experiences of schizophrenic patients. Delusional beliefs, as well as delusional perceptions, resist any attempt to understand them by empathic or psychological methods. Even the more subtle and gradual changes of personality, apparent in the early stages of schizophrenia, are due to an incomprehensible (that is, biological) "process." Such "schizophrenic process" is to be contrasted with the understandable "developments" of the normal or neurotic personality.[1] Jaspers's doctrine of incomprehensibility not only had an authoritative influence on German and international psychopathology but also paved the way for treating schizophrenia merely as an epiphenomenon of some underlying brain dysfunction.

Further problems arise from Jaspers's tendency to draw firm distinctions between domains such as explanation and understanding, or mind and body. Thus, he reduced the notion of explanation to a causal reduction of mental phenomena to their biological underpinnings. Such an automatic, even a priori, reduction of explanation to biology leaves phenomenological analyses without any explanatory value for the psychiatrist. Moreover, by strictly limiting his descriptive psychopathology to conscious experience, he discarded any approach to unconscious or presconscious as well as to embodied, prereflective dimensions of subjectivity. This restriction, primarily intending to ward off the encroaching psychoanalysis, lead to a rigid self-limitation and, consequently, a growing crisis of psychopathology in the second half of the last century. In 1960, Schneider believed that with the forthcoming completion of the description and ordering of symptoms "the mine of psychopathology was depleted" and there would be no use in engaging in psychopathological research any more. Thus, gradually reduced to an ancillary role for syndromic diagnosis, psychopathological research and expertise in clinical psychiatry suffered an alarming decline (Andreasen 1998, 2007; Hojaij 2000).

On the level of research, however, this situation has changed over the last decade. Present phenomenological psychopathology has gained new ground by emphasizing the roots of mental illness in the patients' *prereflective or prethematic experience*. Based on the advances of phenomenological research in general, phenomenological psychopathology has its investigative focus not only on explicit mental contents (for example, delusion that . . . or hallucinations of . . .) but also—as described here by Parnas and Sass—on the basic, constitutive structures of consciousness such as self-awareness, embodiment, spatiality, temporality, and intersubjectivity. These structures are not unconscious, but they are not thematically given as objects of experience; rather they are tacit and prereflective conditions for the emergence of mental contents. Phenomenology, through its "reductions" (see Parnas and Sass), uncovers and articulates the constitutive processes effective in building up subjective experience, such as formation of perceptual meaning, temporal continuity, or implicit bodily action. Phenomenology, for example, tries to detect the critical points where this constitution is vulnerable and open to deviations that characterize the psychotic way of being-in-the-world. By gaining access to this prereflective dimension of subjectivity, the psychiatrist extends his scope of understanding to include phenomena which would otherwise be dismissed as incomprehensible products of brain dysfunctions.

This concept of understanding, however, does not mean psychological or empathic understanding. Rather, it is an understanding enriched by additional resources, namely, informed by an *explication* of the implicit constitutive structures of conscious experience. Phenomenology in this sense seeks to find the "logos" of the phenomena in themselves, not in underlying subpersonal mechanisms—even in the case of psychopathological phenomena. Understanding, description, and explanation may then no more be strictly separated, as Jaspers believed was possible, for here the explanation is based on the inherent structure of the phenomenon to be explained. By analyzing the basic constitution and explicating the implicit structure of experience, phenomenology offers another way of developmental understanding: It allows for a comprehension of the prereflective dimension of experience that is affected in psychotic disorders, and from which their manifest symptoms arise. In these disorders, as Parnas and Sass have pointed out, consciousness loses its ground in the lived body as the ensemble of taken-for-granted habitualities. It also loses its anchoring in temporal continuity and its rooting in intersubjective common sense (Stanghellini 2004; Fuchs 2007). On the other hand, even in the erosion of the basic constitutional processes, the patients still strive for a coherent worldview, though this may only be possible in the form of delusion. Phenomenology also explores the modes through which the patients try to make sense of the basic disturbances and to reestablish some form of coherence. Following these tracks leads far beyond Jaspers's claim for a strict incomprehensibility of delusional experience.

In addition to the analyses of schizophrenic experience put forward by Parnas and Sass, I would like to give one more example of such explanatory structure. It concerns the well-known alienation of the perceived environment in the initial stages of schizophrenia, usually referred to as "delusional mood." In these states, the surroundings obtain a strange, artificial, and puzzling character. They seem arranged like a stage setting and things give the impression of being only backdrops or imitations put up for an undeterminable purpose. In the midst of this alienation, however, single objects may gain a new, mysterious and frightening expression or meaning. The sight of a limping man may give the impression of the devil hunting the patient. The stroke of a bell may announce his imminent death. The term "delusional perception," coined by Schneider (1959), refers to these idiosyncratic and self-referential significances given to apparently indifferent things or situations.

Edmund Husserl's phenomenological analyses of perception may shed light on these experiences (Husserl 1950, 1952; compare Fuchs 2005). It would seem that in perceiving an object we can each time only grasp a part, an aspect or image of it. Nevertheless, the perceived object is obviously given to us in its entirety, as the real object. Normal perception is thus characterized by reaching the object as such through its appearances. It overcomes its own limited perspective by *intending* the object through its nonseen aspects. The perceived object is not just passively received into consciousness as a picture in a camera but is also actively constituted by the act of conscious perception. In each perceptive act multiple intentive processes are combined together, in a way that Husserl calls "passive synthesis." For example, as I look at a table, only its visible sides are directly given to me. On the basis of this aspect, however, other aspects of the object (for example, its invisible sides) are synthetically cointended. A second, temporal form of synthesis is the *identification* of the object as one and the same through its successive perceptions. The present aspect thus includes and reflects the totality of possible aspects making up the unity of the full object. How is this copresence possible? Husserl concluded that our perception of an object presumes reference to other subjects that could perceive and recognize this object from other sides. Thus, the Other is always already copresent in my habitual way of perceiving objects. In other words, intersubjectivity is an integral part of my subjectivity, or of my relation to the world. The perspective of the Other that is implicit in my own perspective enables me to perceive the objects as real, and not just as mere semblances or backdrops.

Moreover, it is also the synthetic intentionality of perception that bestows *meaning* to the perceived and constitutes the object as a meaningful unity. According to Husserl, perception contains an ideal component, its "sense." The general concept or the "idea" of the table is not just added to the seen object but is also itself perceived. We do not see something colored in such and such configuration which we then interpret as a table set for the meal. On the contrary, the meaningful unity of the object "table" and the situation "meal" is the primary given, and only afterward may we isolate single sensory moments out of it. In perceiving we are simultaneously aware of the meaning of the perceived, and this meaning is always embedded in the familiar and intersubjective context of the life world: the table is to sit at, the meal is prepared for me, I come in time for supper, and so forth. Intentional perception constitutes meaningful unities in a world that we share with each other as a meaningful whole.

On this basis, we can explain the fundamental alteration of schizophrenic perception by a weakening and destruction of the synthetic intentionality effective in normal perception (Wiggins, Schwartz, and Northoff 1990; Fuchs 2005). The synthetic processes, which constitute unified and identical objects, are seriously disturbed in beginning schizophrenia. Although perception normally intends the object itself through its different aspects, it is now capable only of presenting an aspect of it, an "image" or a "surface." Instead of actively grasping the objects, the patient experiences an unreal scenery or backdrop. Following Parnas and Sass, this alteration may be derived from a loss of ipseity or self-affection inherent in each act of awareness. The schizophrenic patient, as it were, watches his own perceptions rather than living in them; he "experiences his experiencing" (Parnas 2000, p. 125). Thus, he does not recognize in the active sense but instead is surrounded by puzzling images, which, like the dream images for the dreamer, all seem to aim at him. He literally becomes the visitor of a theater performance or a film projection put on by his senses without knowing what kind of play is going on.

Moreover, with the disintegration of intentional perception, the patient loses the *familiar meaning* of the perceived situations: He does not know any more "what's it all about," why the things he encounters are here at all, or what to do with them. To be sure, the patient is still able to identify and name the things, but we have to be aware here of the basic sense of the word *meaning* as opposed to *significance*. Significances are intersubjectively and historically generated, encoded in language and concepts, and acquired by socialization. They are part of the "common sense" (*sensus communis*). Meanings realize these common significances here and now: Things matter for me. This pencil is not only a pencil as such, but something *I* can write with; this chair is something *I* can sit on, and so forth. Normally, these are "matters of course." For the schizophrenic person, however, things often lose this familiarity. Their conceptual significance may be known to him as before, but they have ceased to *mean or matter* anything to him. The constitution of the everyday world is thus fundamentally disturbed.

With this diminished intentionality, the second major change in schizophrenic perception arises: the objects in the perceptual field, having lost their "objectivity" and meaning, may gain an overwhelming wealth of physiognomic expressions, and new, peculiar meanings may arise. Single aspects or details of the perceptual field, now no longer framed and kept in distance by active intention, may become prominent, leap at the perceiving subject, catch him or penetrate into him. Especially the gaze of others, the quintessence of expression, obtains a captivating and piercing power. The breakdown of the intentional, active perception thus releases an archaic communication of the lived body with its environment. Instead of the common and intersubjective significance of things or situations (for example, "this is a table set for the meal"), there arise idiosyncratic fragments of meaning, always alluding to the patient and his body. The smell of the soup on the table may suddenly appear poisonous; the white color of the tureen may evoke purity and innocence. But then the table could also be prepared to celebrate a ritual in which he shall be sacrificed; the screwed legs of the table indicate that he shall be tortured. The intersubjective constitution of reality is replaced by the idiosyncratic experience of the lived body. It creates meanings that seem incomprehensible because they are far from the commonsense significances of everyday life. The delusions arising from delusional mood carry this basic experience further by systematizing the new meanings and identifying the hidden, anonymous other, thus creating a new coherence of experience.

Although these altered structures of perception could be outlined here in only a rather sketchy way, we can already see that there is an understanding of psychotic experience beyond mere empathy, namely, an understanding informed by an explication of the implicit structures of perception. Similarly, other dimensions of conscious experience can be explored in their constitution and, hence, in their possible destruction in mental illness. In this way, phenomenology leads us beyond description and offers a method of explanation that bridges the "explanatory gap" between mere symptomatology and the underlying neural structures of experience.

NOTE

1. The older distinction between process and reactive schizophrenia has its roots in this notion of the morbid process.

REFERENCES

Andreasen, N. 1998. Understanding Schizophrenia: A Silent Spring? *American Journal of Psychiatry* 155(12):1657–1659.

———. 2007. DSM and the Death of Phenomenology in America: An Example of Unintended Consequences. *Schizophrenia Bulletin* 33:108–112.

Fuchs, T. 2005. Delusional Mood and Delusional Perception: A Phenomenological Analysis. *Psychopathology* 38:133–139.

———. 2007. The Temporal Structure of Intentionality and Its Disturbance in Schizophrenia. *Psychopathology* 40:229–235.

Jaspers, K. (1913) 1968. *General Psychopathology.* Trans. J. Hoenig and M. W. Hamilton. Chicago: University of Chicago Press.

Hojaij, C. R. 2000. Reappraisal of Dementia Praecox: Focus on Clinical Psychopathology. *World Journal of Biological Psychiatry* 1:43–54.

Husserl, E. 1950. *Ideen zu einer reinen Phaenomenologie und phaenomenologischen Psychologie.* Vol.1, *Allgemeine Einführung in die reine Phaenomenologie.* Husserliana III. The Hague: Nijhoff.

———. 1952. *Ideen zu einer reinen Phaenomenologie und phaenomenologischen Psychologie.* Vol. 2, *Phaenomenologische Untersuchungen zur Konstitution.* Husserliana IV. The Hague: Nijhoff.

Parnas, J. 2000. The Self and Intentionality in the Prepsychotic Stages of Schizophrenia: A Phenomenological Study. In Zahavi, D. (ed.), *Exploring the Self:*

Philosophical and Psychopathological Perspectives on Self-experience (pp. 115–148). Philadelphia: John Benjamins.

Schneider, K. 1959. *Clinical Psychopathology.* Trans. M. W. Hamilton. New York: Grune & Stratton.

———. 1960. *Psychiatrie heute.* Stuttgart: Thieme.

Stanghellini, G. 2003. *Disembodied Spirits and Deanimated Bodies: The Psychopathology of Common Sense.* Oxford: Oxford University Press.

Ulhaas, P. J., and A. L. Mishara. 2007. Perceptual Anomalies in Schizophrenia: Integrating Phenomenology and Cognitive Neuroscience. *Schizophrenia Bulletin* 33:142–156.

Wiggins, O. P., M. A. Schwartz, and G. Northoff. 1990. Toward a Husserlian Phenomenology of the Initial Stages of Schizophrenia. In M. Spitzer and B. A. Maher (eds.), *Philosophy and Psychopathology* (pp. 21–34). New York: Springer-Verlag.

CHAPTER 7

Self-agency and Mental Causality

SHAUN GALLAGHER, PH.D.

Shaun Gallagher, with a professional background in phenomenologi-cal philosophy, has been, for many years, an active figure in cognitive sciences. Gallagher's overarching idea is that cognitive science and phenomenology need each other. The way we experience and the workings of the nervous system cannot be examined or comprehended in isolation from one other. Cognitive science must take subjective ex-perience seriously if its claims are to be plausible. Conversely, if phenomenology (as a philosophy of subjectivity) is to step outside a purely theoretical or exegetical stance, it needs to incorporate insights emerging from cognitive sciences and neurosciences. For Gallagher, *phenomenology of the body*—how we experience the body and how the body shapes our experience—is the preferred candidate for a dia-logue with cognitive science.

The relation between phenomenology and cognitive science can be envisaged with different degrees of interdependence. Possible inter-dependences are of *mutual constraint* or of *mutual enlightenment.* The former demands that the two terms of the equation constrain each other (for example, a given particular nature of experience constrains the range of its plausible cognitive instantiations). Thus, a phenome-nological description may exert a selective influence on the range of the potential adequate cognitive models. By contrast, it would be preferable that, for example, a phenomenological account of percep-tion does not collide with the availably neuroscientific data. Mutual enlightenment is a more lax relation. It refers to a situation where any insight in one domain may act as a catalyst for comprehending the corresponding other domain.

This chapter offers good examples of collaboration between phe-nomenology and cognitive sciences. The reader should be attentive to certain terminological aspects. First, the term *bodily schematic:* it owes its meaning to a distinction between the concepts of *body schema,* which is an unconscious totality of sensorimotor correlations involved in automatic bodily skills and bodily dispositions, and *body image,* partly unconscious and partly conscious, *representation* (that is, sort of inner replica or model) of our body. A graceful dance would be an example of a performance dependent on bodily schematic abilities, whereas a phantom limb syndrome or a body-dysmorphic syndrome would point to potential problems in the body image.

Gallagher addresses the issue of mental causation, which is a central topic in philosophy of mind and highly relevant for psychopathology (see Parnas and Sass, this volume). Mental causation is a familiar, frequent, everyday experience, in which our thoughts and desires (mental occurrences) lead to certain behaviors or actions in the physical world. My desire to have Italian food tonight (a "mental event") may be realized by consuming minestrone, carpaccio and spaghetti Bolognese in a nearby Italian restaurant ("physical event" or action in the physical world). My desire, given appropriate context, *causes* me to have an Italian supper at a restaurant, but such a causal account is considered as illusory by epiphenomenalism, a philosophical position claiming that mental phenomena are devoid of any true causal powers; they are illusory and superfluous constructions, exhaustively reducible to the neural level. There is no free will, only blind physiological processes. Gallagher argues against the epiphenomenalist position, insisting on the account of human action as being something *more* than just an instantaneous muscular movement. Action is *embedded, situated, and extended in time.* It is *embedded* because it is directed to goals in the world, meaningful, and codetermined by social significations. It is *situated,* which means that it is dependent on a particular subjective perspective, taking place in a particular situation or context. Being embedded and situated are not some contingent, inessential features but additional facets of action and cognition. Actually, these dimensions *define* (individuate) certain behaviors *as actions* and as actions of a certain kind.

The concept of free will is naturally associated with the notions of self, subject, or person. This concept of self-hood is complex, vast, and hotly debatable. Fortunately, Gallagher spares his reader from the abyss of this debate. Instead, he introduces two basic dimensions *of the ways in which we are self-aware:* as *agents* or authors of actions (self-agency) and as *owners* of our experiences (self-ownership). These two ways of being self-aware are normally intimately fused, but may, under certain circumstances, become dissociated. Gallagher shows how the concept of self-agency may be helpful in the research aiming to naturalize (bring closer to biology) the complex psychological phenomena.

Josef Parnas, M.D., Dr. Med. Sci.

* * *

In this chapter, I explore one small corner of the concept of mental causality and how it relates to questions about free will and agency. It's the corner where discussions about mind-body interactions and epiphenomenalism take place. My basic contention is that these discussions are framed in the wrong terms because they are infected by a certain conception of action that defines the question of mental causality in a classic or standard way. The standard way of asking the question is this: How does a mental event cause my body to do what it does? Setting the question in this way has consequences for ongoing interdisciplinary (psychological, neuroscientific, and philosophical) discussions of mental causation, as well as for the concepts of free will and agency. These concepts, in turn, have much to do with our understanding of what goes wrong in certain instances of psychopathology. Let me begin by setting the historical scene of what I am calling this standard way of understanding the problem of mental causality.

1. The Standard Approach to Mental Causation

The epiphenomenalist position explicated by Shadworth Holloway Hodgson in 1870 states that the presence of consciousness does not matter in regard to action because it plays no causal role; neural events form an autonomous causal chain that is independent of any accompanying conscious mental states.[1] Hodgson thus denies mental causation. William James calls this a decisive step and summarizes Hodgson's position as follows: "Feelings, no matter how intensely they may be present, can have no causal efficacy whatever, [Hodgson compared] them to the colors laid on the surface of a mosaic, of which the events in the nervous system are represented by the stones. Obviously the stones are held in place by each other and not by the several colors which they support" (1890, p. 130).

The question epiphenomenalism answers is understood in a specific way: when we ask whether mental events cause behavior we are asking whether consciousness plays a role in the initiation of bodily movement and motor control. This standard understanding of the question can be seen in the epiphenomenalist answer where causal efficacy is attributed to neural mechanisms but not to consciousness. Neural events cause bodily movement and consciousness, but consciousness cannot cause neural events or bodily movement. The question itself, however, had already been set by Descartes and involves the Cartesian concept of mind as a mental space in which I control my own thoughts and actions. Strictly speaking, for Descartes, only mental actions (thinking and volition) are free; actions of the body are not free, but they are governed by physical laws. On the Cartesian view, however, the problem is to explain how the mind directs the body, because what makes a certain bodily movement an action is the contribution of these mental processes. Descartes suggested that the mental events somehow interact with the brain, which then activates the muscles: "Now the action of the soul consists entirely in this, that simply by willing it makes the small [pineal] gland to which it is closely united move in the way requisite for producing the effect aimed at in the volition. . . . When we will to walk or to move the body in any manner, this volition causes the gland to impel the spirits toward the muscles which bring about this effect" (Descartes [1649] 1989, sects. xli, xliii). Concerning the will, he also writes, "Our volitions, in turn, are also of two kinds. Some actions of the soul terminate in the soul itself, as when we will to love God, or in general apply our thought to some non-material object. Our other actions terminate in our body, as when from our merely willing to walk, it follows that our legs are moved and that we walk" (1649, sect. xviii).

Without such interaction, we have mere behavior, the sort of thing possible for automata and animals. Unless the action is initiated in the mind—acted out, in some cases, explicitly in imagination—the external behavior is not really an action. Action on this definition is always voluntary or intentional action. If my bodily movement is not intentional, it is mere behavior, something like a reflex. If my bodily movement is determined by something other than my own reflective thought, it is involuntary movement, but not action.

The epiphenomenalist adopts the same Cartesian framework and simply answers "no" to the question of whether consciousness plays a causal role in action. Action is nothing more than motor behavior determined by processes other than conscious thought. The epiphenomenalist does not deny the existence of conscious thought or even necessarily that conscious thought appears to be something similar to what Descartes describes. But consciousness does not have causal efficacy in regard to the organism's behavior.

The Cartesian and the epiphenomenalist can agree on the phenomenology, but disagree on the etiology of action. The phenomenology that they can agree on is that when I act I reflectively experience having a desire or intention and then in some way I experience the generation of bodily movement. My action appears to be formed in these mental processes, and insofar as I am conscious of these mental processes along with my bodily movements, my actions appear to be under my conscious control. For the Cartesian, what appears to be the case is the case; for the epiphenomenalist, what appears to be the case is not the case. Both are answering the same question: do these mental processes cause the bodily movements that constitute my behavior? The idea of mental causation seems justified if the answer is yes: the movement that follows our mental intention is the result of our willing to do the action. If the answer is no, however, the intention is nothing more than a byproduct of brain processes and the brain processes control the action.

This is just the beginning of a long tradition that appeals to examples of bodily movements in discussions of mental causality and free will (such as "Look how I can freely raise my arm") (see, for instance, Chisholm 1964; Searle 1984).[2] Harry Frankfurt, for example, begins his account in this way: "The problem of action is to explicate the contrast between what an agent does and what merely happens to him or between the bodily movements that he makes and those that occur without his making them. According to causal theories of the nature of action . . . the essential difference between events of the two types is to be found in their prior causal histories. A bodily movement is an action if and only if it results from antecedents of a certain kind" (1978, p. 69). Although Frankfurt goes on to deny that the nature of action entails that they have causes, he nonetheless sticks to the conception that actions are certain kinds of bodily movements, albeit not mere bodily movements—that "a person must be in some particular relation to the movements of his body during the period of time in which he is presumed to be performing an action" (p. 70). Frankfurt believes that what is "not only pertinent but decisive, indeed, is to consider whether or not the movements as they occur are *under the person's guidance*. It is this that determines whether he is performing an action" (p. 72; original emphasis). He cites David Pears, who contends that there is no difference between mere bodily movements and actions except for the causal history. In either case, whether we reject or embrace causal theories of action, these theories seem to be centered on the idea that action is primarily or essentially controlled bodily movement.

Thus, Jonathan Lowe (1999, pp. 235–236), for example, claims that "in the case of normal voluntary action, movements of the agent's body have amongst their causes intentional states of that agent which are 'about' just such movements. For instance, when I try to raise my arm and succeed in doing so, my arm goes up—and amongst the causes of its going up are such items as a desire of mine *that my arm should go up.* The intentional causes of physical events are always 'directed' upon the occurrence of just such events, at least where normal voluntary action is concerned." Jing Zhu, who characterizes free will as "a mediating executive mental process, which somehow puts the bodily parts into action," thinks of motor control as the "prototype" of free action (2003, p. 64).

Within the discussion of mental causation, views of how consciousness relates to action are often cast in terms of a reflective theory of how movements are under conscious control. On this kind of theory, consciousness enters into the explanation of action just in so far as my action is controlled by my introspectively reflective choice-making, together with a self-monitoring of movement. The reflective theory holds that it is some form of reflection on some aspect of the intention or the action that gives me control over the bodily movement that constitutes the action. That is, attentional consciousness is directed at my inner intention and at how that intention is translated into bodily movement.

In contrast to reflective theories, perceptual theories state that it is some form of consciousness of the environment that gives me control over my movements. Naomi Eilan (2003) specifies this consciousness by explaining that perception plays two knowledge-yielding roles in regard to action. First, it delivers knowledge of the environmental objects or events that we target with the action. Second, perceptual feedback provides knowledge of whether the action was properly accomplished (see Eilan 2003, p. 190).

Consider the action of getting a drink. I'm thirsty and decide to get a drink. I get up from my desk and walk to the refrigerator, open it, and reach in for a drink. On the reflective theory, to simplify a little, my action originates in (is caused by) my conscious decision to get a drink, and this conscious decision is usually described in terms of becoming aware of my desire for a drink motivated by thirst sensations, having a belief that there is something to drink in the fridge, and then, for just these reasons consciously moving my body in the direction of the drink. The basic idea is that I initiate and control my action by consciously deciding on what I want and consciously causing my body to accomplish the goal. Consciousness, on this view, is self-attending or self-monitoring. On the perceptual theory, by contrast, my attention is primarily directed toward the world. I'm conscious of the thing that I want to get, where I'm moving and what I'm looking for—the fridge, the drink. This perception-for-action is complemented by perceptual feedback—proprioceptive and visual—that tells me, as I move along through my action, that I am accomplishing (or failing to accomplish) my goal. Perceptual consciousness seems important for controlling the action, and so plays a necessary and causal role in moving the action along.

From the point of view of epiphenomenalism, the perceptual theory of mental causality fares no better than the reflective theory, because the perceptual aspects described above can be causally explained in terms of third-person physical mechanisms. Indeed, if the kind of perceptual information described is precisely the kind of input required for motor control, most of the information useful for control is unconsciously processed (see, for example, Jeannerod 2003; Pockett 2006). If, for instance, I reach to grasp the drink, the grasping shape of my hand is not something that is consciously monitored by me; it is also clear that the initial motivation—my thirst—is itself reducible to nonconscious processes. Such processes may generate my conscious feeling of thirst, but the nonconscious processes themselves constitute a sufficient cause and I may find myself at the fridge and getting a drink while all my conscious attention is on the conversation that I am having with you. If consciousness keeps us informed about what we are doing in broad and general terms, it acts as a "dormant monitor" (Jeannerod 2003, p. 162), but it plays no role in the causal processes that move us. As conscious animals, we are seemingly just along for the ride.

Again, leaving aside whether interaction or epiphenomenalism, reflective theories or perceptual theories are correct or not, I want to call attention to the way the question is framed. This is clearly expressed by Joëlle Proust (2003, p. 202), who closely follows Frankfurt. "Standard philosophical approaches [to] action define action in terms of a particular psychological state causing a relevant bodily movement." She indicates that there is "now widespread convergence on this causal approach," even if there is some disagreement about the kind of psychological state involved. The best arguments both for and against mental causation are posed in these terms. Summing up what she calls the "standard philosophical approach," Proust states, "What is pertinent is whether or not the bodily movements tend to be under the agent's guidance. . . . Whatever the causal antecedents of a specific goal-directed movement may be, what makes it an action is the contribution of the corresponding agent to actively maintain the orientation of his bodily effort towards achieving a target event" (p. 207).

2. Experimenting with Free Will

The standard philosophical way of understanding the problem of mental causation also governs some recent psychological and cognitive neuroscientific studies of free will, and it is by considering these discussions that we will be able to get clear about precisely what is wrong with this standard. Experiments conducted by Benjamin Libet (1985, 1992, 1996; Libet et al. 1983), for example, are set up precisely in the framework that equates free will with the conscious control of bodily movement. Libet's experiments suggest that motor action and our sense of agency depend on neurological events that we do not consciously control and that happen before our conscious awareness of deciding or moving. In one experiment subjects with their hands on a tabletop are asked to flick their wrists whenever they want to. Their brain activity is monitored with special attention given to the time course of brain activity leading up to the movement, between 500 and 1000 milliseconds (0.5–1 seconds). Just before the flick, there is 50 milliseconds of activity in the motor nerves descending from motor cortex to the wrist. But this is preceded by several hundred (as much as 800) milliseconds of brain activity known as the readiness potential. Subjects report when they were first aware of their decision to move their wrists by referencing a large clock that allows them to report fractions of a second. It turns out that on average, 350 milliseconds before they are conscious of deciding to move, their brains are already working on the motor processes that will result in the movement. Thus, voluntary acts are "initiated by unconscious cerebral processes before conscious intention appears" (Libet 1985). The brain seemingly decides and then enacts its decisions in a nonconscious fashion but also inventively tricks us into thinking that our conscious decision matters.

The epiphenomenalist interpretation of these results is that mental causation is nothing more than an illusion (for example, Wegner 2002). Libet, however, suggests that consciousness can have an effect on our action because approximately 150 milliseconds remain after we become conscious of our intent to move and before we move. So, he suggests, we have time to consciously veto the movement (1985, p. 2003).

Patrick Haggard replicates and extends Libet's experiments to demon-strate the phenomenon of efferent binding—that is, the phenomenon that my intention, my movement, and its environmental effects are experi-enced closer in time than objective measurements indicate. He clearly in-dicates that these Libetarian experiments are set up within the standard philosophical understanding. "A further consequence of the efferent bind-ing approach is to reorder the traditional philosophical priorities in this area. The central philosophical question about action has been whether conscious free will exits. That is, how can 'I' control my body?" (Haggard 2003, p. 113). Haggard and Libet (2001) frame the question in exactly the same way, referring to it as the traditional concept: "How can a mental state (my conscious intention) initiate the neural events in the motor areas of the brain that lead to my body movement?" (p. 47). If we substitute "the pineal gland" for "neural events in the motor areas," this is precisely Descartes's question.

The problem with this approach is that it does not distinguish motor control issues from questions about mental causality and free will. For Libet, Haggard, Daniel Wegner, and other contemporary scientists, the question of free will remains a question about motor control, and in that sense, there is no reframing of the standard view. These experiments also help us to see how this standard view defines the temporal framework of mental causation. The exercise (or illusion) of conscious control is cir-cumscribed in the milliseconds of physiological signals of the readiness potential. Thus, consciousness of an action is "intertwined with the inter-nal models thought to underlie movement control" (Haggard 2003, p. 119).

Should these two questions—one of motor control and the other of mental causation or free will—be intertwined? I want to suggest that just as the question "Shall we go for a ride?" is different from "How does this car work?" so the question mental causation is different from the question of motor control—how we control our bodily movement. Just as one should think it strange if in response to the question "Shall we go for a ride today?" I start to describe in precise terms how the internal combus-tion engine in my car turns the wheels, so also one should think it odd if I start to discuss how body-schematic control of movement works if a per-son asks me what I'm doing. Developing a good answer to one of these questions is not the same as answering the other.

One way to see this is to consider cases where normal motor control mechanisms fail. In cases of deafferention, for example, many of the nonconscious, automatic body-schematic control processes are disrupted by the lack of proprioceptive peripheral feedback. Indeed, in such cases, the Cartesian reflective description of mental causation seems to be precisely the right description. Ian Waterman, a well-known subject who has lost proprioception and the sense of touch from the neck down, uses an alternative way to control his movement (Cole 1995; Gallagher and Cole 1995). To reach and grasp something, Waterman needs to consciously think about what he is doing. He has to first locate his hand, estimate the force necessary to move it to the right position for grasping, and then think about how to shape his hand to grasp the object. Similar considerations must be made in regards to walking, sitting, maintaining his posture, and so forth. The majority of his instrumental and locomotive movements are under his conscious control and depend on visual input that explicitly specifies where his body is in relation to the environment.

In a way that is unnecessary for those of us who have normal proprioceptive input, Waterman needs to cognitively control his movement. For him, it just is the case that, as Lowe (1999, p. 235) puts it, "movements of the agent's body have amongst their causes intentional states of that agent which are 'about' just such movements." He requires what Zhu (2003, p. 64) describes as "a mediating executive mental process, which somehow puts the bodily parts into action." He must take up an extremely "particular relation to the movements of his body during the period of time in which he is presumed to be performing an action" (Frankfurt 1978, p. 70), and the particular relation, in Waterman's case, is what Proust (2003, p. 202) calls a "particular psychological state causing a relevant bodily movement." In effect, the case of Ian Waterman requires a conception of mental causation that is completely in line with the philosophical standard that informs the recent experimental literature. The fact that this case is abnormal in regard to how the subject engages in action, however, should give us pause if we want to apply the philosophical standard to normal action.

The best answers we have to the question of normal motor control indicate that most control processes happen at a subpersonal, unconscious level. For example, the precise visual information that guides the shape of my grasp is not available to consciousness (Jeannerod 1997, 2003).[3] As we move through the world, we do not normally monitor the specifics of our motor action in any explicitly conscious way. Body schematic processes that involve proprioception, efference copy, forward comparators, ecological information, and so on do most of the work. Both phenomenology and neuropsychology support a combination of perceptual and nonconscious explanations of how we control bodily movements, and they rule out reflective theory in the normal case. That is, in the normal situation, we do not require a second-order representation of our bodily movement; we do not have to be reflectively conscious of the onset of the action or the course of the movement as we execute it. Rather, perceptual attention to the objects that we target, and nonconscious, or consciously recessive, perceptual-ecological feedback about our bodily performance contributes to motor control.

The experimental results in the studies of Libet and Haggard, then, are of no surprise unless we think that mental causation is about the conscious control of our bodily movements. The experiments are precisely about the control of bodily movement and in fact of an atypical involuted kind of control because in the experimental situation the subject is asked to reflectively pay attention to processes that we normally do *not* attend to and to move our body in a way that we do not usually move it (in a rough sense, the subject is asked to move in a way that is similar to the way that the deafferented subject is required to move). These experiments, however, and more generally the broader discussions of motor control, have nothing to tell us about mental causation per se.

3. A Pragmatic Phenomenology

The concept of mental causation does not apply primarily to abstract motor processes or even to bodily movements that make up intentional actions; rather, it applies to intentional actions themselves, described at the highest pragmatic level of description. I've offered a clarification of these points elsewhere (Gazzaniga and Gallagher 1998; Gallagher 2005, 2006). Specifically, there are three points that I will summarize here. First, as I suggested in the previous section, and consistent with a certain reading of the perceptual theory of action, when acting, one's intention is not focused on bodily movement; rather, it is focused on some aspect of the task to be accomplished. Second, mental causation is not something that can be squeezed into the time frame of milliseconds. Third, mental causation is best conceived on the highest available (and appropriate) pragmatic level of description.

First, if I am reaching to grasp anything, my focus is on the thing that I am reaching for, not on my bodily posture in preparation to lift the thing, the direction and thrust of the reach, the shaping of my hand for the grasp, and the rest—all of these practicalities are controlled for the most part by nonconscious body-schematic processes. Afferent proprioceptive-kinesthetic signals that register bodily position and movement are attenuated (see, for example, Tsakiris and Haggard 2005), and this kind of sensory suppression means that my body never gets in the way of my action. Such processes, in fact, free me to attend to things in the environment, or to think or daydream as the case may be.

Second, in regard to timeframe, neither intentions nor actions are made in the moment—they are not momentary and do not fit within the thin phenomenology of the milliseconds between the readiness potential and movement. For example, if I encounter something moving in the grass at my feet, my amygdala is immediately activated and within some hundreds of milliseconds I jump and move several yards away, and I enter into this behavior even before I am conscious of what is happening. Here, the entire set of movements can be explained purely in terms of nonconscious perceptual processes, neurons firing and muscles contracting, together with an evolutionary account of why our system is designed in this way. Such behavior does not involve mental causality in the proper sense; I did not, for example, consciously decide to jump away. Of course, what follows this reflex behavior is something different. I certainly noticed that I jumped, and why, as my consciousness catches up with my behavior and the fact of movement in the grass. If, for example, it turns out to be a snake in the grass, I can become conscious of that fact, and I can certainly act in a way that is informed by my thoughtful consideration of that fact. Several seconds after my automatic jump I may decide to catch the snake for my snake collection and I then take a step back and *voluntarily* make a quick reach for it, or I take my time and wait for the opportune moment to grab it.

Obviously, my action of catching the snake is different from my jumping reaction. What informs this action includes awareness of what has just happened—I would not have decided to catch the snake if I did not become conscious that there was a snake there—a thoughtful decision to collect that snake, which may include conscious realization that this type of snake is not poisonous or dangerous and so on. These conscious processes take place in a timeframe much larger than the milliseconds involved in the jump, or in anything like the motor control processes involved in reaching and grasping. Any reaching and grasping of the snake is already under the influence of the initial conscious decision to catch it. My bodily movement is, of course, intimately connected with my action, but my action is not well described simply in terms of making bodily movements.

This leads to the third point, namely, that the proper level of description when we are talking of mental causation, free will, or agency is not the level of description that pertains to motor control. And certainly the kinds of action that we freely decide are not the sort of bodily movements described by Libet's experiments (in which the subjects were required to turn their attention to a specific body movement that is normally subsumed within an intentional goal). If I am reaching to catch the snake and someone asks what I'm doing, I am not likely to say any of the following: "I am activating my neurons," "I am flexing my muscles," "I am moving my arm," or "I am reaching and grasping." These are descriptions appropriate for a discussion of motor control and bodily movement, but not for the action in which I am engaged. Rather, I would probably say, "I am trying to catch this snake for my collection." And this is a good description of what I decided to do.

In contrast to the kind of detached reflection described by the reflective theories of action, it seems possible to describe the situation in which I decide to catch a snake as one of *situated* reflection or deliberation. In such instances, my reflective regard is not focused on my beliefs and desires or on how to move my body in order to achieve a goal. When I am thinking and reaching for the snake, I am not thinking about my mental states or how to move my body; rather, I'm thinking about catching the snake, and, perhaps, how good this will be for my collection. My action is the result of a conscious practical reflection that is *embedded* or *situated* in the particular context that is defined by the present circumstance of encountering the snake and the fact that I have a snake collection. If I were not a snake collector, but I fancied eating a delicacy of barbequed snake, the movements involved in catching the snake for dinner could be absolutely identical with the movements involved in catching the snake for my collection.

At a higher and more appropriate level of description, however, my actions in the two situations—collecting a snake and catching one for dinner—are different. In either case, my action (and not merely my movement) involves a pragmatic deliberation, "a first-person reflective consciousness that is embedded in a pragmatically or socially contextualized situation.

It involves the type of activity that I engage in when someone asks me what I am doing or what I plan to do" (Gallagher and Marcel 1999, p. 294). This is neither introspection nor a reflection on my bodily movement; I do not reflect on my beliefs and desires as states within a mental space; nor do I reflectively consider how I ought to move my arm or shape my grasp. Rather, I start to think matters through in terms of the snake that I am attending to, the collection that I have, and the possible actions that I can take. This pragmatically situated deliberation shapes my actions. Granted, the thought "this snake would be excellent for my collection" does not necessarily cause me to reach for the snake in the same way that a billiard ball knocking into another billiard ball causes the second ball to move, but it certainly motivates my action in a way that, if I did not have this thought, I would likely not reach for the snake; and if I did reach for the snake but did not have this thought, or something similar in mind, I would certainly be hard pressed to say why I was reaching for the snake. Even for materialists, however, there is no reason to think that mental causation is equivalent to billiard ball causation, unless we are willing to think that persons are similar to billiard balls.

To the extent that consciousness and practical, situated deliberation enter into the ongoing production of action and contribute to the production of further action, even if significant aspects of this action rely on automatic nonconscious motor control, such mental events have an effect. By separating the issue of mental causation from the issue of motor control, however, I am not arguing for a disembodied notion of mental causality, as something that occurs in a Cartesian mind; nor do I mean to imply that the nonconscious brain events that make up the elements of motor control are simply irrelevant to action. Indeed, for two closely related reasons, such nonconscious embodied processes are essential to action that is specifically human. First, nonconscious body-schematic mechanisms of motor control subserve intentional action and are structured and regulated by relevant intentional goals. These processes are intentional, even if they are not intentional actions (see Anscombe 1957). They are structured and regulated by my intentional goals as much as they limit and enable my action. When I decide to catch a snake, or get a drink, all of the appropriate physical movements fall into place without my conscious monitoring of them (in clear contrast to the situation of the deafferented subject).

Second, precisely to the extent that we are not required to consciously deliberate about bodily movement or such things as autonomic processes, our deliberation can be directed at the more meaningful level of intentional action. Our possibilities for action are diminished to the extent that these supporting mechanisms fail. Proposals to answer questions about mental causation, free will, or agency in terms of mind-body or mind-brain interaction are looking in the wrong place. The kind of interaction that is relevant in this context is the interaction between a person situated in a physical and social environment, and some task that is set up in that environment, the kind of interaction found in the collecting of snakes, the helping of friends, and in the variety of deliberate actions that we engage in every day.

4. The Proper Sense of the Sense of Agency

Questions about how a sense of agency might be generated for an intentional action are directly related to these considerations about mental causality. Here a distinction between a sense of agency (the sense that I am the cause of an action) and a sense of ownership (the sense that it is my body that is moving) will be helpful (Gallagher 2000a, 2000b). In the case of involuntary action, for example, if someone pushes me from behind, I can say that it is my body that is moving or that I am moving, but I would not say that I am the agent of that action. I would properly attribute agency to the person who pushed me.

This distinction is related to the distinction made by George Stephens and Lynn Graham (2000), in their discussion of schizophrenic delusions of control. They distinguish between attribution of agency and attribution of subjectivity. Graham and Stephens's distinction is related to the level of higher-order cognition—they describe attribution as a product of a reflective, introspective act. In contrast, the distinction between sense of agency and sense of ownership applies to the first-order level of phenomenal experience. The subject lives through or experiences agency for an action, or experiences ownership for bodily movement at a prereflective level—at the level of "what it is like."

Schizophrenic symptoms of delusions of control and thought insertion may involve problems with both the *experiential sense* of agency and the *attribution* of agency. I have argued that the experience of involuntary movement has a similar experiential structure to delusions of control and thought insertion. In all of these cases (1) the subject experiences movement (or thinking) as movement of his body (or as taking place in his stream of consciousness rather than someone else's mind), thereby generating a sense of ownership for the movement or thinking experience; but (2) the subject does not experience a sense of agency for the movement (or thinking); and (3) the subject attributes agency to someone else. As part of a bottom-up account of the schizophrenic experiences I have claimed that the symptoms originate in some disruption at a neurological level, which generates a problem with the experiential sense of agency.

In contrast, Graham and Stephens propose a top-down account in which the problem originates at the higher-order cognitive level. For them attributions of agency are explained in terms of "our proclivity for constructing self-referential narratives," which allow us to explain our behavior retrospectively: "such explanations amount to a sort of theory of the person's agency or intentional psychology" (1994, p. 101; Stephens and Graham 2000, p. 161). In regard to the issue of thought insertion, they suggest, "Whether I take myself to be the agent of a mental episode depends upon whether I take the occurrence of this episode to be explicable in terms of my underlying intentional states" (1994, p. 93).

According to this approach, we reflectively make sense of our actions in terms of our beliefs and desires. So, if a subject does or thinks something but has no mental states (intentions, beliefs, or desires) that would normally explain or rationalize such actions, the first-order movements or thoughts would not appear to him as something he intentionally does or thinks. Thus, whether something is to count for me as my action "depends upon whether I take myself to have beliefs and desires of the sort that would rationalize its occurrence in me. If my theory of myself ascribes to me the relevant intentional states, I unproblematically regard this episode as my action. If not, then I must either revise my picture of my intentional states or refuse to acknowledge the episode as my doing" (1994, p. 102).

According to this approach, nonschizophrenic first-order phenomenal experience appears the way it does because of properly ordered second-order, reflective interpretations, and schizophrenic first-order experience appears the way it does because of second-order *misinterpretation*. "The subject's sense of agency regarding her thoughts likewise depends on her belief that these mental episodes are expressions of her intentional states. That is, whether the subject regards an episode of thinking occurring in her psychological history as something she does, as her mental action, depends on whether she finds its occurrence explicable in terms of her theory or story of her own underlying intentional states" (Graham and Stephens 1994, p. 102; see Stephens and Graham 2000, pp. 162ff).

Is there a way to adjudicate between bottom-up and top-down approaches? A bottom-up approach to schizophrenic symptoms would need to show how problems that develop at the neuronal level could lead to (1) the loss of the experiential sense of agency and (2) the generation of an experiential sense that one's movement or thought is caused by someone or something else. A number of neuroscientific studies have provided the relevant models for just this way of understanding the problem (Chaminade and Decety 2002; Farrer and Frith 2002; Farrer et al. 2003). These studies explicitly adopt the definitions and distinction that I suggested between the sense of ownership and the sense of agency (Gallagher 2000a, 2000b) and involve brain-imaging experiments designed to find the neural correlates for the sense of agency. A close reading of these experiments, however, motivate some important and interesting questions.[4] Specifically, the experiments raise questions about how we should understand the sense of agency, and they do so along the same lines that characterize the discussion of mental causation and free will. Does the sense of agency pertain to the realm of motor control and body movement, or does it pertain to the broader realm of the intentionality of intentional action?

In making the distinction between the sense of ownership and the sense of agency, I used the logic of involuntary movement to make the following suggestion. Because, in the case of involuntary movement, there is a sense of ownership but no sense of self-agency, and, likewise, my awareness of the sense of involuntary movement comes from afferent sensory-feedback (visual and kinaesthetic information that tells me that I'm moving), but not from efference or motor commands that I issue to generate the movement (because in fact there is no original efference in the case of involuntary movement), it seemed natural to suggest that in ordinary voluntary movement the sense of ownership might be generated by sensory feedback and the sense of agency might be generated by efferent signals. In a recent article, Manos Tsakiris and Patrick Haggard (2005) provide empirical evidence to support this division of labor: "the sense of agency involves a strong efferent component, because actions are centrally generated. The sense of ownership involves a strong afferent component, because the content of body awareness originates mostly by the plurality of multisensory peripheral signals" (p. 387; also see Marcel 2003; Tsakiris, Bosbach, and Gallagher, 2007).

This led them to criticize the set of experiments I have just mentioned because, in attempting to identify the neural correlates of the sense of agency, all of the experimental tasks involved in the experiments required the subjects to move their hands. Thus, according to what I'll call the *Tsakiris-Haggard objection,* the subjects would have experienced the sense of agency for their movement in each task and there would be no way to control for the sense of ownership. That is, because each task involved active, voluntary bodily movement, the subjects would experience a sense that it was their movement (sense of ownership) and that they were the ones causing it (sense of agency).

Let's take a close look at these experiments.

Chaminade and Decety (2002)

In the positron-emission tomographic study by Thierry Chaminade and Jean Decety (2002), subjects moved a joystick to control a circle on a computer screen to accomplish several tasks, the critical ones being task A and task B.

Task A: Subject moved the circle and observed another subject's icon following theirs (leader task)

Task B: Subject followed another subject's icon with their own circle (follower task)

The authors write, "Investigation of the neural basis of agency was performed using a paradigm in which the subjects either led (A) or followed (B) the other, in a computerized environment free of explicit reference to body parts. . . . The sense of ownership, related to motor control, and the sense of agency, related to the intentional aspect, can be segregated in the analysis" (p. 1977). The reason they made this latter claim is that movement was required in each case so the sense of ownership would be constant—the subject experiences her own movement in each case, but the sense of agency would be different for task A versus task B. One assumption here is that A (leading) would generate a sense of agency, while B (following) would not. The researchers found activation in the presupplementary motor area (SMA) and the right inferior parietal cortex (IPC) in task A, suggesting these areas as responsible for the sense of self-agency, and in contrast, activation of the left IPC and the right precentral gyrus as responsible for attributing agency to another. They also noted the relevance to schizophrenia—"abnormal increased activity in the right inferior parietal cortex has been observed in schizophrenic patients experiencing passivity phenomenon" (p. 1978, citing a study by Spence et al.).

One obvious objection is that in the experiment in both tasks (A and B) the subject may have a sense of agency for accomplishing the task. If asked to report (in fact, they were not asked to report), they might have said: "My task in A is to lead, and I have done so; and my task in B is to follow, and I have done so. I felt myself to be the agent of both actions." In that case, differential activation of the identified brain areas may be for something other than agency.[5] The Tsakiris-Haggard objection, however, is different. Rather, they suggest that the subject will have a sense of agency in both cases because in both A and B the subject moves his hand to control the joystick.

The difference between these two objections is the same difference at stake in the discussion of how to understand mental causation and free will—the difference between conceiving of agency (mental causality, free will) in terms of bodily movement/motor control and conceiving of it in terms of the intentional aspects of action (accomplishing the task). Tsakiris and Haggard, consistent with Haggard's previous work that focused on motor control and free will, understand agency to be directly tied to the efference signals involved in motor control. Thus, if the subject is actively moving in both A and B tasks, a sense of agency will be generated in both cases. In contrast, Chaminade and Decety, who carefully designed the experiment "in a computerized environment free of explicit reference to body parts" understand the sense of agency to be linked to the intentional aspect of action rather than to bodily movement. On their view, the sense of agency varies across the tasks as the intention changes across the tasks, while the sense of ownership remains constant because that is tied to afferent feedback from the consistent bodily movement.

Farrer and Frith (2002)

Chlöé Farrer and Chris Frith (2002), in their fMRI experiment, followed the same logic as Chaminade and Decety: "Subjects manipulated a joystick [to drive a colored circle moving on a screen to specific locations on the screen]. Sometimes the subject caused this movement and sometimes the experimenter. This paradigm allowed us to study the sense of agency without any confounding from the sense of ownership. To achieve this, subjects were requested to execute an action during all the different experimental conditions. By doing so the effect related to the sense of owner-ship (I am performing an action) would be present in all conditions and would be canceled in the various contrasts" (p. 597). So again, and for the same reasons, the claim is that the sense of ownership remains constant while the sense of agency changes. But again, the Tsakiris-Haggard objec-tion is that because in each case the subject is required to move the joy-stick, a sense of agency for that movement must result. Farrer and Frith, like Chaminade and Decety, however, are looking at the intentional aspect once again, and they consider the sense of agency to be tied to that rather than to motor control for the joystick.

In this experiment, however, things are complicated because in some trials the subject is informed ahead of each task whether the movement will be his or not his, and he is asked to perform the task regardless of whether what happens on the screen is known to the subject to be his ac-tion or the action of someone else. In those cases when the action repre-sented on the computer screen is not performed by the subject, because the subject knows it is not his action, then, one might suggest, his action short-circuits in the movement of the joystick—he knows that his move-ment doesn't accomplish anything on the screen. Even if he does not have a sense of agency tied to the intentional aspect of the task, his sense of agency may be redirected specifically to his bodily movement in a way that would be consistent with the assumptions behind the Tsakiris-Haggard objection. It turns out that in the case where he is not the agent for the task represented on the computer screen, the right IPC is activated. When he does know that he is causing the action on the screen, his ante-rior insula is activated bilaterally. Thus, the experimenters identify acti-vation in the anterior insula as the correlate of the sense of agency.[6]

Now, unfortunately, although Farrer and Frith want to link the sense of agency to the intentional aspect of the task, when it comes to their theory about why the anterior insula should be involved in generating the sense of agency they revert to a explanation more consistent with the Tskaris-Haggard objection—that is, they explain the involvement of the anterior insula in terms of motor control.

Why should the parietal lobe have a special role in attributing actions to oth-ers while the anterior insula is concerned with attributing actions to the self? The sense of agency (i.e., being aware of causing an action) occurs in the con-text of a body moving in time and space. Damasio (1999) has suggested that the sense of agency critically depends upon the experience of such a body. There is evidence that both the inferior parietal lobe and the anterior insula are representations of the body . . . the anterior insula, in interaction with limbic structures, is also involved in the representation of body schema. . . . One aspect of the experience of agency that we feel when we move our bodies through space is the close correspondence between many different sensory signals. In particular there will be a correspondence between three kinds of signal: somatosensory signals directly consequent upon our movements, visual and auditory signals that may result indirectly from our movements, and last, the corollary discharge associated with motor commands that generated the movements. A close correspondence between all these signals helps to give us a sense of agency. (601–602)[7]

If this is the case, the fact that for each task the subject is required to move does complicate things—as the Tskaris-Haggard objection seems to indicate.

Farrer et al. (2003)

We can turn to the third study to resolve some of these problems. One difference in this experiment is that the experimenters actually asked for the subject's report. In this study, however, all questions about agency were focused on bodily movement. Subjects were not given any intentional task to carry out other than making random movements using a joystick, and the focus of their attention was directed toward a virtual (computer image) hand that either did or did not represent their own hand movements, although at varying degrees of rotation relative to true position of the subject's hand. That is, they moved their own hand but saw a virtual hand projected on screen at veridical or nonveridical angles to their own hand; the virtual hand was either under their control, or not. Subjects were asked about their sense of agency for control of the virtual hand movements. The less the subject felt in control, the higher the level of activation in the right IPC, and this is consistent with Farrer and Frith (2002). The more the subject felt in control, the higher the level of activation in the right *posterior* insula, but this is in contrast with Farrer and Frith (2002), who associated the sense of agency with activation of the right *anterior* insula. Referencing this difference, Farrer et al. state: "We have no explanation as to why the localization of the activated areas differ in these studies, except that we know that these two regions are densely and reciprocally connected" (2003, p. 331). One possible explanation, however, is that the shift of focus from accomplishing a computer screen task (in Farrer and Frith) to controlling bodily movement (in Farrer et al.) might change the phenomenon that is being studied.

The Tskaris-Haggard objection seems to hold in regard to the work of Farrer et al. That is, if the sense of agency is generated by bodily movement rather than purposive action (at least a kind of purposive action that goes beyond the production of random movement)—and bodily movement seems to be the only thing at stake in this experiment—then the fact that the subject moves his own hand in all instances in this experiment certainly does not provide any way to discriminate the sense of ownership from the sense of agency. More than that, however, it suggests that, contrary to the previous experiments, the sense of agency is not construed in terms of intentional task. Again, complicating the issue, when it comes to a theoretical explanation of why the IPC is involved in the question of agency, the authors cite evidence that pertains to ownership rather than agency: "Lesions of the inferior parietal cortex, especially on the right side, have been associated with delusions about the patient's limb that may be perceived as an alien object or as belonging to another person" (Farrer et al. 2003, p. 329). Such delusions are clearly about ownership rather than agency.

5. Conclusion

Where does all of this leave us? First, as I have argued, the intentionality of intentional action is not about bodily movement. Consistent with phenomenological theories of embodiment, in everyday engaged action afferent or sensory-feedback signals are attenuated, implying a recessive consciousness of our body. We do not attend to our bodily movements in most actions. We do not normally stare at our own wrists as we decide when to flick them; we do not look at our feet as we walk, we do not attend to our hands as we engage the joystick. Most of motor control and body schematic processes are nonconscious and automatic. It still may be the case, however, that, because action is embodied, just such processes contribute to a sense of agency; indeed, without the experiential sense of embodied movement, our sense of agency would be very different. I also want to suggest, however, that the sense of agency is not reducible to just these embodied processes. Nor is it something that is constituted in a Cartesian mind. If our descriptions and explanations of what we are doing in action are cast at the highest possible pragmatic level of description— "I'm helping my friend" or "catching a snake" or whatever, rather than "I'm moving my hand"—then clearly our sense of agency for the action will be tied to that intentional aspect, and that aspect depends on where our attention is directed—in the world, in the project or task that we are engaged in. So clearly a form of *intentional feedback,* which is not afferent feedback about our bodily movements but rather some sense that my action is having an effect, must contribute to the sense of agency. I suggest that, if any of the contributory elements are missing—efferent signals, sensory (afferent) feedback, or intentional feedback—or if they fail to be properly integrated (for example, in brain areas like IPC or the insula)—we can get a disruption in the sense of agency. This also suggests that the loss of the sense of agency in various cases—including schizophrenia, anarchic hand syndrome, obsessive-compulsive behavior, or narcotic addiction-may, respectively—be different sorts of loss and that the sense of agency might be disrupted in different ways depending on what contributory element is disrupted.

The various ways that we can understand the sense of agency—as a first-order experiential sense that is linked to intentional aspect (task, goal, and so on) (Chaminade and Decety 2002; Farrer and Frith 2002); as a first-order experiential sense linked to bodily movement (Farrer et al. 2003; Tsakiris and Haggard 2005); or as the result of a second-order, reflective attribution (Stephens and Graham 2000)—suggests four possibilities for explaining the pathological loss of the sense of agency.

- *Top-down explanation:* disruptions in the sense of agency due to problems with introspective higher-order cognition (Graham and Stephens)—this may well be the case in advanced and involuted symptoms of schizophrenia where reflective cognition may be motivated by disruptions that occur on the level of first-order experience.
- *Bottom-up explanation:* disruptions in the sense of agency due to problems with motor control mechanisms—efference signals (Tsakiris and Haggard) or the integration of sensory and motor signals in specific brain areas (Farrer et al.).
- *Intentional theory:* disruptions in the sense that my action is having the intended effect on the world—problems caused by a perceived

lack of concordance between intention and effects of action (Chaminade and Decety; Farrer and Frith).

- *Multiple aspects theory:* disruptions of the integration of efferent, afferent, and intentional contributories.

The multiple aspects approach can integrate both the bottom-up explanation and the intentional theory and may thereby provide a more adequate account of how various disruptions at the first-order level of experience can motivate a top-down intervention by introspective or higher-order reflective consciousness.

One could go further to suggest that just this kind of involuted, introspective reflection, motivated by disruptions in first-order experience of agency—that is, just the kind of detached reflection that one finds in schizophrenia is opposite to the kind of situated reflection that characterizes intentional action and the exercise of free will. And within philosophical discourse about mental causation, the difference between these two kinds of reflection present, in part, a way to distinguish between the standard explanation and something much closer to an embodied and situated account.

NOTES

1. This is an idea that goes back to La Mettrie (1745), and was furthered by Cabanis (1802), Hodgson (1870), and Huxley (1874).

2. Even Aristotle offers an example like this: "An agent acts voluntarily because the initiative in moving the parts of the body which act as instruments rests with the agent himself" (*Nicomachean Ethics,* 1110a15).

3. Jeannerod (2003, p. 159) notes, "The shift from automatic to [consciously monitored] controlled execution involves a change in the kinematics of the whole [grasping] movement; movement time increases, maximum grip aperture is larger, and the general accuracy degrades." Also see Gallagher (2005).

4. One important question that I leave aside for purposes of this chapter is whether some of the experiments confuse the experiential sense of agency with the reflective attribution of agency. Although Farrar et al. (2002), for example, define the sense of agency in terms of first-order experience, the experimenters claim that they are testing for the neural correlates of the judgments of attribution.

5. Indeed, it is to be noted that the general results of this experiment do not fully match up with results found in other experiments, including the Spence experiment that Chaminade and Decety cite. According to Farrer and Frith, "In previous studies attribution of actions to another has been consistently associated with activity in the right inferior parietal lobe. Patients with delusions of control who er-

roneously attributed their actions to another showed abnormally high activation in this region (Spence et al. 1997). Subjects imagining someone else acting showed greater activity in this area than when they imagined themselves making the action (Ruby and Decety, 2001)" (2002, p. 597). The experiments in Farrer and Frith (2002) also suggested that the right IPC is activated for other-agency.

6. It is interesting to note that when the subject was not told that it was another person controlling the screen (finding out only in the last second when the circle moved differently from what he intended), no significant differences were found. Apparently, in that case his sense of agency for the task was intact, but this is not made clear by the experimenters.

7. To make things worse, they cite well-known evidence that the IPC, which they are associating with a sense of other-agency, is responsible for a sense of body ownership—"patients with right parietal lesion do not recognize their limbs as their own and perceive them as belonging to others" (p. 601).

REFERENCES

Anscombe, G. E. M. 1957. *Intention*. Oxford: Blackwell.
Cabanis, P. 1802. *Rapports du physique et du moral de l'homme*. 2 vols. Paris: Crapart, Caille et Ravier.
Chaminade, T., and J. Decety. 2002. Leader or Follower? Involvement of the Inferior Parietal Lobule in Agency. *Neuroreport* 13(1528):1975–1978.
Chisholm, R. 1964. Human Freedom and the Self. The Langley Lecture, 1964. University of Kansas. Reprinted in J. Feinberg and R. Shafer-Landau (eds.), *Reason and Responsibility: Readings in Some Basic Problems of Philosophy*, 11th ed. (pp. 492–499). New York: Wadsworth, 2002.
Cole, J. 1995. *Pride and a Daily Marathon*. Cambridge, MA: MIT Press.
Damasio, A. R. 1999. *The Feeling of What Happens: Body and Emotion in the Making of Consciousness*. New York: Harcourt Brace.
Descartes, R. (1649) 1989. *The Passions of the Soul*. Indianapolis: Hackett.
Eilan, N. 2003. The Explanatory Role of Consciousness in Action. In S. Maasen, W. Prinz, and G. Roth (eds.), *Voluntary Action: Brains, Minds, and Society* (pp. 188–201). Oxford: Oxford University Press.
Farrer, C., N. Franck, N. Georgieff, C. D. Frith, J. Decety, and M. Jeannerod. 2003. Modulating the Experience of Agency: A Positron Emission Tomography Study. *NeuroImage* 18:324–333.
Farrer, C., and C. D. Frith. 2001. Experiencing Oneself vs. Another Person as Being the Cause of an Action: The Neural Correlates of the Experience of Agency. *NeuroImage* 15:596–603.
Frankfurt, H. 1978. The Problem of Action. *American Philosophical Quarterly* 15:157–162. Reprinted in H. Frankfurt, *The Importance of What We Care About* (pp. 69–79). Cambridge: Cambridge University Press, 1988.
Gallagher, S. 2000a. Philosophical Conceptions of the Self: Implications for Cognitive Science. *Trends in Cognitive Science* 4(1):14–21.

————. 2000b. Self-Reference and Schizophrenia: A Cognitive Model of Immunity to Error through Misidentification. In D. Zahavi (ed.), *Exploring the Self: Philosophical and Psychopathological Perspectives on Self-experience* (pp. 203–239). Amsterdam: John Benjamins.

————. 2006. Where's the Action? Epiphenomenalism and the Problem of Free Will. In W. Banks, S. Pockett, and S. Gallagher (eds.), *Does Consciousness Cause Behavior? An Investigation of the Nature of Volition* (pp. 109–124). Cambridge, MA: MIT Press.

————. 2005. *How the Body Shapes the Mind.* Oxford: Oxford University Press.

Gallagher, S., and J. Cole. 1995. Body Schema and Body Image in a Deafferented Subject. *Journal of Mind and Behavior* 16:369–390.

Gallagher, S., and A. J. Marcel. 1999. The Self in Contextualized Action. *Journal of Consciousness Studies* 6(4):4–30.

Gazzaniga, M., and S. Gallagher. 1998. A Neuronal Platonist: An Interview with Michael Gazzaniga (Postscript on Free Will). *Journal of Consciousness Studies* 5:706–717.

Graham, G., and G. L. Stephens. 1994. Mind and Mine. In G. Graham and G. L. Stephens (eds.), *Philosophical Psychopathology* (pp. 91–109). Cambridge, MA: MIT Press.

Haggard, P. 2003. Conscious Awareness of Intention and of Action. In N. Eilan and J. Roessler (eds.), *Agency and Self-Awareness* (pp. 111–127). Oxford: Clarendon Press.

Haggard, P., and B. Libet. 2000. Conscious Intention and Brain Activity. *Journal of Consciousness Studies* 8(11):47–63.

Hodgson, S. 1870. *The Theory of Practice.* London: Longmans, Green, Reader, & Dyer.

Huxley, T. H. 1874. On the Hypothesis that Animals Are Automata, and Its History. *Fortnightly Review,* 16:555–580.

James, W. 1890. *Principles of Psychology.* New York: Dover.

Jeannerod, M. 1997. *The Cognitive Neuroscience of Action.* Oxford: Blackwell.

————. 2003. Self-generated Actions. In S. Maasen, W. Prinz, and G. Roth (eds.), *Voluntary Action: Brains, Minds, and Sociality* (pp. 153–164). Oxford: Oxford University Press.

La Mettrie, J. O. de. 1745. *Histoire naturelle de l'ame.* La Haye: Jean Neaulme.

Libet, B. 1985. Unconscious Cerebral Initiative and the Role of Conscious Will in Voluntary Action. *Behavioral and Brain Sciences* 8:529–566.

————. 1992. The Neural Time-factor in Perception, Volition, and Free Will. *Revue de Métaphysique et de Morale* 2:255–272.

————. 1996. Neural Time Factors in Conscious and Unconscious Mental Functions. In S. R. Hammeroff, A. W. Kaszniak, and A. C. Scott (eds.), *Toward a Science of Consciousness: The First Tucson Discussions and Debates* (pp. 337–348). Cambridge, MA: MIT Press.

Libet, B., C. A. Gleason, E. W. Wright, and D. K. Perl. 1983. Time of Conscious Intention to Act in Relation to Cerebral Activities (Readiness Potential): The Unconscious Initiation of a Freely Voluntary Act. *Brain* 106:623–642.

Lowe, E. J. 1999. Self, Agency, and Mental Causation. *Journal of Consciousness Studies* 6(8–9):225–239.

Marcel, A. 2003. The Sense of Agency: Awareness and Ownership of Action. In J. Roessler and N. Eilan (eds.), *Agency and Awareness* (pp. 48–93). Oxford: Oxford University Press.

Pockett, S. 2005. The Neuroscience of Movement. In S. Pockett, W. Banks, and S. Gallagher (eds.), *Does Consciousness Cause Behavior? An Investigation of the Nature of Volition* (pp. 9–24). Cambridge, MA: MIT Press.

Proust, J. 2003. How Voluntary Are Minimal Actions? In S. Maasen, W. Prinz, and G. Roth (eds.), *Voluntary Action: Brains, Minds, and Sociality* (pp. 202–219). Oxford: Oxford University Press.

Ruby, P., and J. Decety. 2001. Effect of Subjective Perspective Taking during Simulation of Action: A PET Investigation of Agency. *Nature Neuroscience* 4(5):546–550.

Searle, J. 1984. *Minds, Brains, and Science.* Cambridge, MA: Harvard University Press.

Spence, S. A., D. J. Brooks, S. R. Hirsch, P. F. Liddle, J. Meehan, and P. M. Grasby. 1997. A PET Study of Voluntary Movement in Schizophrenic Patients Experiencing Passivity Phenomena (Delusions of Alien Control). *Brain* 120:1997–2011.

Stephens, G. L., and G. Graham. 2000. *When Self-Consciousness Breaks: Alien Voices and Inserted Thoughts.* Cambridge, MA: MIT Press.

Tsakiris, M., S. Bosbach, and S. Gallagher. 2007. On Agency and Body-ownership. *Consciousness and Cognition* 16(3):645–660.

Tsakiris, M., and P. Haggard. 2005. The Rubber Hand Illusion Revisited: Visuotactile Integration and Self-attribution. *Journal of Experimental Psychology: Human Perception and Performance* 31(1):80–91.

Wegner, D. 2002. *The Illusion of Conscious Will.* Cambridge, MA: MIT Press.

Zhu, J. 2003. Reclaiming Volition: An Alternative Interpretation of Libet's Experiments. *Journal of Consciousness Studies* 10(11):61–77.

Comment: Disorders of Agency in Psychiatric Syndromes

Kenneth S. Kendler, M.D.

In his intriguing chapter, Shaun Gallagher first provides a general discussion of the nature of agency, which he considers to be the ability to initiate intentional actions. His broad point is that it is not in the details of the execution of an action (such as particular motor movements that are typically done automatically and off-line) that one should look for the effects of mind. Rather, it is in the planning—the development of the higher-order intentions that set the goals for an action that is then initiated and monitored—where we should look. In particular, the action is not that of an abstract Cartesian mind floating off in space but rather an embodied volitional agent where the entire experience of agency arises not only from the initial formulation of the intention but also from the subsequent efferent signals and sensory feedback. The second part of his chapter focuses on a description of a range of imaging studies that attempt to determine the brain regions that reflect agency.

My focus here is to take that account of agency and follow it into the arena of psychopathology. I give short shrift to the extensive prior philosophical writings on this subject going back to Plato and his concern in the Protagoras of how it could be that a person could judge action A to be the best course of action but then end up doing something other than A. It's clear that we have long recognized that two or more competing sources of agency can exist in the same individual—a state that has been termed *akrasia*.

Rather than try to comment on this rich literature, I will rather respond, as a psychiatric clinician, to Gallagher's closing challenge to begin to try to understand the nature of the sense of loss of agency in diverse psychiatric syndromes. I hope to infuse more psychiatrically relevant examples into the discussion of agency that might supplement some of the more typical prior examples in the philosophical literature such as the "anarchic hand syndrome" or "forgetting to turn left so as to stop off at the store when driving home" (Eilan and Roessler 2003). I will briefly examine five syndromes: schizophrenia, Obsessive Compulsive Disorder (OCD), bulimia, and both cocaine and Internet addiction. I will also add a personal experience of extreme thirst. I will try to explore how the sense of ownership of action or autonomy is altered in psychopathology. Finally, I will suggest that in addition to examining a "motoric" focus of our sense of agency—where the output is movement—from the perspective of psychiatric illness, it is useful to consider, as part of our sense of agency, our degree of control over what we might call roughly "thoughts" and "impulses."

Background

Aside from the rare monoclinic jerk that we might experience while falling asleep or the common "reflex action" (removing our finger from a hot stove or jumping back when seeing something move in the grass), individuals without major psychiatric illness rarely experience the feeling that their motoric movements are outside of their own control. When we get to thoughts and impulses, however, the questions are subtler. Most people would describe the general sense—through the capacity of attention—to control the focus and flow of their own thoughts, but this control is far from complete. We have all experienced the annoying tune that gets "stuck in our head" and that we cannot, by will power alone, banish from our minds. Most of us have experienced intrusive worries—Did I remember to lock the car? Maybe the airplane I am on will crash—that we would prefer not to have but that keep entering consciousness. Anyone who has ever tried to meditate will realize that the frequent admonition "Let your mind be cleared of thoughts" may sound easy to accomplish but in fact is difficult. In fact, meditation confronts us directly with what William James so aptly called the "buzzing, blooming confusion" of our own internal thoughts and experiences. The normative experience, however, is that while these thoughts are not always welcome into our mind, they are certainly "ours." We can also "turn down" our level of volitional control over our thoughts—daydreaming and the subjective experiences we have when falling asleep is partly a relaxation of attempts to exert agency about our own thoughts. Hence the feeling of one's thoughts "wandering" with no effort expended to try to focus them.

What about impulses? It would be a rare heterosexual male who would not have had the experience of standing close to an attractive woman on an elevator or subway and having the impulse to put his hands where they do not belong. This is often a slightly uncomfortable experience. Is the impulse ours? I think the response would most commonly be, "Well, I guess so." Like a badly behaving child, we are at least a bit hesitant to identify it as our own. Somewhat odder and more deviant would be the surprisingly common but uncomfortable impulses such as to shout out a profanity in the middle of a boring church service or to throw to the ground a crying baby who cannot be comforted despite all one's efforts. When describing such impulses, most people would make a face—showing an emotion of disgust—but begrudgingly admit, "I guess those came from me although I cannot understand why I would ever want to do something like that." One does not have to be seeped in psychoanalytic theory to come up with some commonsense ideas about why some impulses like these would enter our consciousness with a slight sense of "not-me-ness" about them. So, in thinking about disorders of agency, I would suggest a phenomenological continuum from thoughts to impulses to actions. With this background, let's look at some patients.

Loss of Agency

Let me begin with a clinical vignette of a patient whom I will call Bill I saw many years ago.[1] He was in his mid twenties and carried a new diagnosis of schizophrenia. I had just asked him a question about "thought insertion"—whether he had ever experienced thoughts put into his head that were not his own.

> *Bill:* Is that what you call it? Do you mean to say that other people have that experience too? It started happening just as I was falling ill.
> *KSK:* Can you tell me what it is like?
> *Bill:* Sure, Doc. You know the experience of listening to a radio in your car. Sometimes you are driving down the street and all of a sudden the voice of a police dispatcher cuts into your radio signal. That's what it is like.
> *KSK:* Do you mean the other thoughts just cut into your own?
> *Bill:* Yup, just like that.
> *KSK:* These are not your thoughts?
> *Bill:* Definitely not, and they confuse me when it happens a lot.

This patient conveys something that will be familiar with those who have dealt with schizophrenic patients: the subjective sense of the intrusion of a foreign agent into his own consciousness. The qualitative impression is clearly one of "otherness." Often this experience is delusionally elaborated—hence, the myriad forms of "influence machines" the sole purpose of which is to perform "thought projection" and other associated passivity phenomenon such as made feelings or impulses. I have seen many such patients who describe, with various degrees of insight and eloquence, the same phenomenon. More rarely, I have seen patients with schizophrenia who complained of experiencing "made actions." One young man upset a cart with dinner trays on it, making a horrendous mess. "They made me do it," he said. Of note, while the "they" were his persecutors whom he heard as auditory hallucinations, he did not, he claimed, hear a voice commanding him to upset the trays. Rather, they "took me over" "just like I was a robot."

OCD

Marsha was a part-time librarian at a small medical library in a community hospital. Every day she would come in, log in the new journals, and return to the shelves any books or journals that had been returned. Before she could leave, she developed the ritual of having to go through every one of the three or four hundred books and bound journals in her library to make sure they were all in order. She said, "What would happen if a doctor needed to find a journal when I wasn't there and they couldn't find it? Someone might die because of that." In the months before I saw her, she would find that the ritual—which took about ten minutes—would be nearly complete. She had her coat on and would just be ready to switch off the light and close the door when a doubt would enter her mind. The doubt was specific and predictable—it was that in a lapse of concentration, perhaps she misshelved a book, that it was not in its proper place. Along with this thought, she described the irresistible impulse to repeat the checking of all the volumes. So she would take off her coat and start again. At first she had to do it only twice but then three and then five times. Finally, she was there at nearly midnight and unable to leave the library having to review and re-review the books. She had to be forcibly removed in a panic and was hospitalized.

Marsha realized that the compulsion to recheck the books came from within her. In that sense, her experience was different from that of Bill. In retrospect, when I saw her in the hospital, she realized that these impulses were "crazy." (I was not convinced at the time that she believed that when she was in the middle of her ritual behavior. In fact, I suspect that she would have felt that she was performing a needed function—keeping all the books in her library in order.) However, she experienced intense anxiety if the ritual was not properly performed. She would relate this anxiety to her fear of "killing someone" if a doctor couldn't find the right article or book that was needed. She reported that the urge to recheck the books was typically "too strong for me" that she lacked the will power to resist it. She could only deal with her rising anxiety by starting the checking process again.

This was not black and white. As she recovered, she would describe a "tickle" of the obsessions coming back again—the rising sense of having to act, to straighten up—but she learned to "see them coming" and, with both medications and psychotherapy, her ability to resist grew and grew. What was once an authoritative urge that brooked no resistance became a slight annoyance that seemed to me little different from what I might experience when confronting a plate of chocolate chip cookies by our coffee machine that sometimes I can pass up—despite my desire for them. Shades of gray.

Addiction

I saw for several years a young man I will call Peter, who experienced, among other things, intermittent episodes of crack cocaine abuse. The pattern was always the same. He would sometimes be encouraged to use by friends in a social setting. Most commonly, he would want to have sex with a girl and the "price of admission" would be to buy crack for the two of them and use it together. He would always think he could take just one hit, but after his first dose he would, over the subsequent hours, go back again and again to the dealer until he had no money and the dealer would accept no more credit. It would take him weeks to recover from the post-binge depression, anxiety, and guilt. He often went months between episodes. A typical conversation with him about these episodes would run something like this:

> *KSK:* So you couldn't control it?
> *Peter:* That's right. When I start, I just can't stop. I should know better but that drug hunger, it just takes over. I want it so bad, I can't think of anything else. I have done all kinds of crazy things, including stealing from my own mother to get money for crack. You can't imagine how bad I feel the next day. My wallet is empty. I am depressed as hell and guilty.

If you pushed Peter on his motivation once he gets into an episode, he would usually say two things. First, the drug just made him feel so good that he wanted more. Second, as he was coming down from one dose, there was a terrible emptiness that he knew he could escape if he took more crack. While he would not deny that it was him doing the drugs, he would commonly use the phrase "the drugs" or "the crack" that "made me" do it. "I would want to stop but I couldn't." That is, he was unable to conform his actions to his "higher-order plans"—to stop his cocaine binge. I think that he was not only try to evade responsibility but also describing something at least a bit alien about how the drug hunger impinged on and eventually "took over" his volitional apparatus. This recalls the following quote from Sarah Buss's review article on autonomy:

> The puzzle at the heart of these questions is a puzzle about the relationship
> between the agent's power and the power of the forces that move her. . . .
> What distinguishes motives whose power is attributable to the agent herself
> from motives whose power is external to the agent's? What distinguishes
> motives on which the agent has conferred her authority from motives whose
> power has reduced her authorization to a mere formality? (Buss 2002)

Peter seemed to be describing motives that he did not fully authorize and
yet were not entirely foreign. More gray.

Bulimia

With one bulimic patient, let us call her Becky, I was able to obtain the
best description of what we came to call the "tipping point." She was a stu-
dent and, alas, a donut shop stood squarely on the corner of the best route
from school to her apartment. Donuts were her food of choice for binges.
Nineteen times out of twenty, when she was in a good state of mind, she
would pass the store without incident. There would be either no urge to buy
them or a passing thought, easily resisted, but given the right set of circumstances—a hard exam, a poor grade on an essay, a fight with boyfriend—her
response would be different. Now, she would stop to look in the window.
She would smell the donuts (their smell was an important cue for her crav-
ing), and then what was previously an easily resisted temptation became
an overwhelming urge. She would go into the shop, buy two dozen donuts,
go home, pull the window shades, and proceed to eat them all and then
purge. After the episode, hours of self-loathing with typically follow.

Over time, her level of impulsivity in these episodes varied. Typically,
she would not plan them and would hope to get by the store without incident (or she would take another way home to avoid the temptation).
Other times, however, she would reason to herself, "This was a bad day. I
deserve to do something nice for myself." And then she would plan the
binge. Thus, sometimes her binges were the result of a "reflective standpoint." She would accept her motives to binge and, literally, give herself
permission to have a "good binge episode." As might be imagined, I
viewed those episodes as less pathologic because I thought they would be
more amenable to intervention. They had a greater sense of "agency" about
them—more responsibility and autonomy—than did the more spontaneous impulsive binges. The level of agency in her binges clearly varied.

Sexual Addiction

The best description of the internal relationship with impulses came from an individual with an addiction to Internet pornography.[2] I will call him Devon. His job involved computers. He worked from home. The process that Devon described was as follows:

> I'd be working on a particular report. Then I would get this "little urge" to just take a "quick look." Sometimes I would feel like one of those Disney cartoon characters who would sometimes experience two little versions of themselves sitting on each shoulder. One would be the "angel me" with wings and a harp and always counsel to do "good things"—in this case, get on with the report. The other would have a pitchfork and a long red tail, "the devil me," and provide contrary advice to be "bad." I would struggle for a few minutes. But once I had a quick look, I usually couldn't stop. I would look up and sometimes 30 minutes, sometimes 2 hours would have gone by. Only by jerking off could I easily get out of these. That would relax me and I could then get back to work.

If he was pushed about the specific experience of looking up the sex sites, he would say,

> Devon: It's weird. Typically, I would almost watch my hands doing it. I'd go to the browser and then my bookmarks looking down the list of which to click on.
> Therapist: But wasn't it you doing it?
> Devon: Sure, but it didn't always feel that way. It was almost like it was the little devil in me.

My impression was that he would, at that moment, experience a gentle sense of derealization. He did not convey a full sense of agency in these actions. Had he "authorized" them? Only sort of. Gray.

Thirst

Having never been addicted or had OCD, bulimia, or schizophrenia, I want to convey one personal experience that I have often pondered in considering the concept of agency. Through a series of adolescent misadventures, along with two friends I had spent an entire day hiking in the hot California sun up a ridge in Big Sur with a single small canteen of water among the three of us. We expected that by nightfall we would be able to get down to the stream some 500 feet below. We started down in the late afternoon but badly misjudged the time and the steepness of the ridge. It was pitch black by the time we were 100 feet above the stream. It was so steep that further attempts to get down were too dangerous, and we spent the night huddled in a bush hearing the sounds of running water below but unable to get a drink.

I was intensely thirsty and found—as I moved between waking and sleep through the night—that the desire to drink consumed my consciousness. All I could think about was water. I heard it. I visualized it. I could almost taste it. My body called out for it with a deep primordial yearning. I was consumed by thirst. At the first light of dawn, I made my way carefully down the creek. Few things in my life tasted as good as those first gulps of cool water.

What can I say about that experience? The feeling of thirst was certainly "my" thirst. It was not imposed on me from the outside but arose within me. It had a very physical feeling to it; however, was it within my power, my will, or my volition to suppress the thirst? Could I distance myself from my thirst and assume a "reflective standpoint"? With great effort, I could think about something else for a minute or two, but as soon as I relaxed my focus, the urges would rise again and flood my consciousness. Could I have not drunk water at the first opportunity? I suppose so, but it was clearly beyond my ability even to contemplate such a plan of action. Did I authorize the emergence of these feelings and urges? Clearly not. In that sense, they were imposed on me by my internal state.

How was my thirst different from Peter's cocaine hunger? My thirst arose out of a natural biological process. Hydration levels in mammals are tightly regulated, and our bodies function within only a small window of cation and anion concentrations. It had no sense of oddness or irrationality, but, like Peter, my general sense of self was consumed by this urge. Was my sense of agency compromised? Certainly, this was a qualitatively different experience from having a tune stuck in my head.

Reflections

The sense of agency is not black or white. Although most normal people have a pretty tight sense of intentional control over their own planned motor actions, that control is a bit less tight when it comes to impulses and a good deal more lax when it comes to thoughts. The attribution of agency may be clear in neurological conditions such as Huntington disease, in which motoric actions are entirely involuntary, but less clarity emerges when we examine the range of disturbances of agency that arise in psychiatric disorders.

With respect to the disorders examined, it is tempting to lump them into three broad groups of schizophrenia, OCD, and the addictions (roughly including bulimia in this category). Schizophrenia seems the "most different." Here the disruptions of the sense of agency are cleanest with the crucial subjective distinction being the sense of otherness of the intruding thoughts, impulses or actions.

The qualitative feeling of the disturbance of agency in OCD is different from the addictive states. This difference is difficult to capture. At the simplest level, the addictive states involve positive affective motivations— Peter liked the effect of cocaine. Devon—at some level—enjoyed and sought for the sexual tension and release associated with his Internet porn. Becky found at least the first phase of her binge-purge cycle to be enjoyable. Marsha, however, did not want her obsessions. What she wanted was to "escape" the rising sense of panic that resulted from her obsessional fears. This was more like the second of Peter's motivations—a sense of being willing to "do anything" to avoid the terrible feeling of the postcrack depression and emptiness.

Unlike OCD, the addictions involve biological hedonic processes. Cocaine directly stimulates brain dopamine systems commonly thought to subserve a sense of pleasure. Sex and food are among our strongest reinforcers. Nothing of the sort is at work in OCD. No pleasure pathways are driving motivation. OCD feels much more like a disturbance of "planning and checking functions" (which, as noted above, occasionally annoy all of us) than the appetitive functions that are disturbed in addictions.

What do we learn about my experiences with extreme thirst? For evolutionary reasons, it makes sense that strong survival systems, like thirst, have the capacity to take over our sense of agency and focus it toward the specific organismic need. From this perspective, the ability of sexual impulses—through the wide variety of deviations—from paraphilias to Internet porn addiction—to "override" our normative sense of agency also makes sense. Current biological theories of drug addiction often speak of the "hijacking" of brain pleasure systems (Koob and LeMoal 1997). An analysis of the dysfunction of agency in addiction may be the subjective consequences of those brain stage changes.

Challenges

We know that we are consciously aware of only the tip of the iceberg of our actions. That is, we are not, as agents "active all the way down." In fact, I am aware now only of typing the words of this sentence and have no awareness of the extraordinary level of coordination required of my arm, forearm, and finger muscles to perform the actions of striking the keys on my keyboard in a moderately coordinated fashion, let alone how I access the particular spelling of words as they pour forth from my thoughts via the keyboard into an electronic file. My consciousness seems much more potent at selecting the target of a behavior than governing the precise way in which that target behavior is implemented. Empirical work summarized by Naomi Eilan and Johannes Roessler (including the famous studies with blindsight) (2003) provides further indications that we are not as consciously aware of all aspects of our own motoric behavior as we are naturally inclined to believe. We attribute more of a sense of ownership to our actions than they always deserve.

What relevance does this work have for some of the psychopathological manifestations of disorders of agency noted above? When Devon watches his hands stop what they are doing and strike the keys needed to get to a sex website, the subjective sense is not that the hand motions are foreign, but they do not have a full sense of conscious control—of agency. Once Becky has bought her donuts, she watches the subsequent binge unfold before her.

These behaviors are reminiscent of the automatic actions we all make extensive use of in our everyday life—of being able to drive home on automatic pilot. We don't have to intend them. We just "set" the general goal—to get home—and our brain takes care of the rest. But in addictions in particular there is one important difference. My goal of driving home is entirely consistent with my intentions. My subvolitional mechanisms are operationalizing an intent that is entirely congruent with my wishes. This is not the case for addictions. Here the individual is clearly in a state of *akrasia*—experiencing multiple conflicting volitional states. It is tempting to interpret the semiautomatic behavior in a psychological manner. That is, at some level these individuals want what they regard as unacceptable—

the state of a cocaine high, the pornography-induced state of sexual arousal. By "distancing" these impulses to a semiautomatic volitional mechanism, they can stand by and watch these deflected wishes be fulfilled and yet escape the full sense of responsibility for their fulfillment.

How much should we view an addicted patient as being what Buss (2002) calls a "weak-willed self-governor?" In a well-turned phrase, she states that "human agents have the capacity to govern themselves in a way that they themselves take to be unjustified." In what ways would Peter, Becky, and Devon differ from an obese individual who couldn't stop eating chocolates or an individual who always buys a sport club membership each new year with firm resolve to exercise regularly but, despite the "best of intentions," always manages to put off planned exercise to another day? To what extent should all the patients I describe be seen as helpless victims of their own impulses?

My highly preliminary conclusion is that there is at least one broad continuum of a sense of agency. One end is rooted in the clearly involuntary behaviors associated with a number of neurological conditions. The other end reflects the endless give and take of daily urges and our editing of those—which we choose to fulfill and which deny—in the course of our psychologically healthy daily lives. Toward the "neurological" end of things are the experiences of the schizophrenic: thought insertion and made feelings and impulses. Somewhere in the middle are the highly disordered signals of a dysfunctional planning and checking module (probably in our frontal cortices) in OCD. Then, occupying a broad range are the addictions, which I suggest, by my example of thirst, might closely mimic how our volitional behaviors are evolutionarily shaped by the primitive urges that are necessary for survival.

We humans rather often fail to govern ourselves properly, and these failures can be central to certain psychiatric disorders. From a psychopathological perspective, disorders of choice making come in many shades of gray.

NOTES

1. The cases I describe here are disguised, and sometimes I combine information from several different patients.

2. This case was the only one I did not personally see but was described carefully by a colleague over several conversations.

REFERENCES

Buss, S. 2002. Personal Autonomy. In *Stanford Encyclopedia of Philosophy* (March). http://plato.stanford.edu/entries/personal-autonomy.

Eilan, N., and J. Roessler. 2003. Agency and Self-awareness: Mechanisms and Epistemology. In J. Roessler and N. Eilan (eds.), *Agency and Self-Awareness: Issues in Philosophy and Psychology* (pp. 1–47). Oxford: Clarendon Press–Oxford University Press.

Koob, G. F., and M. Le Moal. 1997. Drug Abuse: Hedonic Homeostatic Dysregulation. *Science* 278:52–58.

PART III

NOSOLOGY

Real Kinds but No True Taxonomy

An Essay in Psychiatric Systematics

PETER ZACHAR, PH.D.

In chapter 8, Peter Zachar focuses on two deceptively simple inter-related questions: *What kinds of things are psychiatric disorders?* And *By what principles should we classify them?* His chapter focuses only briefly on the first question and then reviews in more detail the second. To frame his discussion, it might be helpful to consider two hypotheses about the kinds of things that psychiatric disorders could be. First, they could be what some philosophers have called "natural kinds." The paradigmatic example of natural kinds is chemical elements. They reflect a deep structure in our universe that exists independently of any human effort. They are discovered and not invented. Any advanced civilization anywhere in the universe would have to end up describing the same kinds of elements, albeit with different names. Second, at the other end of the spectrum, psychiatric disorders could be what have been called "social constructs." Roughly, a social construct is something that does not exist in nature but, rather, is a concept that humans impose on their world. Consider a particular fashion in clothing—the "hip look." Although there may be a bit of consistency in this definition across small social cliques, across time and space the "hip look" would be variable because it is, at its essence, a highly malleable social convention that does not reflect any constancies of the world in which we live. These two different visions of what psychiatric disorders are have a wide range of contrasting implications for what psychiatry is about.

Zachar does not settle for either of these two hypotheses but, instead, strives for a thoughtful and probably more realistic middle ground. In his earlier writing, he proposed a concept that he calls "practical kinds" (Zachar 2003), which reflects a pragmatic approach to developing diagnoses that best achieves the things we need from them both as scientists and practitioners. He approaches this issue a few times in his chapter. When he notes that what might be considered the best psychiatric disorder would depend on the particular validator that is emphasized (for example, genetics, outcome, treatment, or neurobiology), he writes, "Based on some of the ideas put forth in this chapter, one possible way to think about this problem is that the conditions classified by different validators might be considered to be real kinds, but none is *the* real kind. This could be called realism without literalism."

Later, he concludes, "Kinds in psychiatry can be 'real,' or 'genuine,' or 'legitimate,' or 'valid.' It's a matter of degree, but standards for making these evaluations can be specified." So, his ultimate approach is a pragmatic one—one that suggests we focus less on metaphysical speculation about the ultimate nature of diagnoses and more on the practical problems associated with our various reasons for classifying. This chapter adds to his previous work by making clear why kinds in psychiatry can also be considered to be "real."

The bulk of the chapter addresses the equally difficult and related task of pondering how we ought to organize our disorders. He calls this effort, appropriately, "psychiatric systematics." He makes the critical point that psychiatry and psychology are not the only disciplines that have worries about how to classify. In fact, biology has been struggling with this problem long before there was anything remotely resembling the medical specialty of psychiatry or clinical psychology. Zachar provides a helpful review of how biology has approached this problem contrasting it with the approach taken by chemistry to the periodic table.

Zachar notes the deep appeal of chemical-like taxonomy, so neat and tidy. It would make us feel like real scientists, as good as the infectious disease specialists. Alas, as he points out, this simply isn't going to work well for the multifactorial psychiatric disorders. Zachar ponders whether the "biological taxonomy model" has more lessons for psychiatry and psychology—a question he answers in the affirmative. One of his main points is that biologists accept that scientific classification is, in some way, patched together and not uniform throughout. He thinks psychiatrists and psychologists should accept this as well.

Although the nature of the issues involved—classifying biological organisms into species, genus, family, and so on versus constructing a structure for *DSM* and *ICD*—are rather different, there are a surprising number of similarities. One good side effect of this chapter would be if psychiatric nosologists studied more closely the approaches to classification in biology that has had a longer and more sophisticated history for these debates than has psychiatry.

Particularly illuminating is the long debate between numerical taxonomy and cladistics (Hull 1990), which illustrates the struggle between those who want to classify based on external appearances versus those who want to use scientifically technical criteria (in this case, objective evidence for common descent—but this has obvious parallels to those in psychiatry would might advocate the use of genes or magnetic resonance imagine findings to answer issues about where disorders should be placed).

Zachar points out the obvious problems with the simple clinical or phenotypic approach. This is still the commonsense approach, used for example by Kraepelin when he sorted his famous index cards with the histories of his patients. But, as Zachar notes, classification by phenotype could lead to problems that parallel early biological models in which dolphins were classified with fish and bats with birds, neither of which we currently consider to be correct.

Zachar generally avoids a highly doctrinaire approach. There is not, he argues, a single right or wrong way to address the deep problem of psychiatric classification. Different approaches have strengths and limitations. He, for example, reviews the strengths of possible dimensional approaches, now much discussed especially with respect to the personality disorders. His is not a call for despair but should blunt, at least a bit, the zeal with which some are approaching the needed to "remake" our nosologic systems in *DSM-V* and *ICD-11* to "truly" reflect what psychiatric disorders "really are." In contrast, Zachar proposes that all good classifications inevitably both reveal and conceal realities about the objects being classified.

If I were attempting a "folksy" summary of what I think Zachar is trying to say, it might come out something like this:

We need diagnoses. Just can't do without them. There might not be (and probably isn't) a real structure out there that can ground all our diagnoses. But that shouldn't stop us from trying to improve our classifications. However, we should avoid spin and not oversell our efforts claiming them to be better than they actually are.

Kenneth S. Kendler, M.D.

REFERENCES

Hull, D. L. 1990. *Science as a Process: An Evolutionary Account of the Social and Conceptual Development of Science*. (Science and Its Conceptual Foundations series). Chicago: University of Chicago Press.

Zachar, P. 2003. The Practical Kinds Model as a Pragmatist Theory of Classification. *Philosophy, Psychology, and Psychiatry* 9:219–227.

* * *

Deciding whether mental disorders are real requires asking, "A real what"? A real disease? A real illness? A real syndrome? An equally relevant question is "Are they really mental?" Although these questions deserve careful scrutiny, I will focus on another problem, specifically, are mental disorders *real kinds?* After offering a definition of real kinds, I will explore how such kinds are to be related to each other systematically.

1. Kinds: Real or Natural

What counts as a real kind? Exemplars of real kinds include chemical elements such as *gold* and biological species such as *tigers.* In contrast, *white things* and *drugs* probably don't name real kinds. As John Stuart Mill ([1843] 1973) noted, the only property that most white things have in common is being white, whereas real kinds, such as tigers, supposedly have an inexhaustible number of properties in common regardless of whether we have identified those properties. White things can be lumped together into a logically definable category, but that category is not a real kind in Mill's sense of the term.

I do not favor labeling psychiatric disorders *natural kinds* (Zachar 2000a, 2000b, 2002, 2006). My claim that psychiatric disorders are not natural kinds expresses skepticism about the tradition of natural kinds rather than suspicions about the scientific legitimacy (or reality) of psychiatric disorders.

Natural kind is an abstract concept encompassing a diverse range of properties. These properties include the following:

1. Being naturally occurring.
2. Being categorical or discrete.
3. Having an internal casual structure.
4. Operating according to rules.

To give some examples, water is *naturally occurring,* while computers are not. Things that are naturally occurring can be said to exist independently of human practices. They would still be a part of the structure of the universe whether or not human beings existed.

The collection of even numbers such as 2, 4, 6 is *categorical.* Even numbers form a proper class with unambiguous defining properties. Any particular number either is or is not an even number. The class is discrete; there are no interforms. The construct of weight, in comparison, is continuous rather than categorical. Everything has a value on the dimension of weight. Categorical distinctions with respect to this dimension, such as "heavy," are stipulated rather than discovered. To illustrate, any 42-year-old male whose weight in kilograms divided by his height in meters squared is 25 or greater is considered by physicians to belong to the category of overweight or heavy. Such categorical distinctions are made using variables external to the dimension of weight.

The stable properties of a chemical element such as gold are related to its *internal causal structure,* namely, the number of protons in the nucleus; change the number of protons, and the properties change. Being a parent, by contrast, is a relational property and is not caused by a person's internal structure. With in vitro fertilization and egg donation, a woman can be a child's birth parent but not be the biological parent proper. In cases of adoption, being a parent may not even be related to one's biological history.

An important quality of natural kinds is that the internal causal properties are also sortal properties—meaning properties that can be used to sort individuals into groups (Gelman and Hirschfeld 1999; Zachar and Bartlett 2001). Internal structure defines whether a particular individual is a member of the class of things named by that kind—so any substance having exactly 79 protons in the nucleus is gold. Biologists and philosophers of science working in a Darwinian framework, however, have long argued that biological species can't be sorted only with respect to a fixed internal causal property such as DNA, especially because the relevant internal property changes over time (Ghiselin 1974, 1999; Hull 1976). An alternative method of sorting species is by a relational property, namely, descent. "Same species" means having the same set of ancestors.

Operating according to rules means that kinds behave in a regular and predictable way and their behavior can be understood in a causal framework. For example, gold will melt if heated to a temperature of 1,948 degrees Fahrenheit. The strongest types of rules in sciences are called laws, which often connote necessity and even universality. Lawful regularities are supposed to be necessary for natural kinds.

As Mitchell (2000) points out, a majority of regularities in biology and the social sciences are neither universal nor necessary. They tend to be context dependent. The relationship between sexual abuse and Borderline Personality Disorder is an example of such a regularity. Sexual abuse is often present in the histories of people with Borderline Personality Disorder, but not always (Zanarini et al. 2006).

Because the four properties of naturalness, discreteness, internal causal structure, and predictability can exist in different combinations and do not necessarily co-occur, it may be better, scientifically, to evaluate the presence and scientific desirability of these properties individually. To illustrate, something can have an internal causal structure and be discrete but not naturally occurring. Examples include all elements with an atomic number higher than 94 (such as curium, einsteinium). In other cases, things can be naturally occurring and operate according to rules, but not discrete, even if they appear that way; for example, ionic bonds and covalent bonds are better considered two endpoints on a continuum. Finally, many naturally occurring processes operate according to rules but lack an internal causal structure, for example, dominance hierarchies and seasons of the year. Strictly speaking, curium, covalent bonds, and seasons are not natural kinds.

Two additional attributes are often added to the concept of natural kind, and these attributes are often considered to be fundamental:

5. Carving nature at the joints
6. The presence of a real essence

Identifying these abstract properties requires an evaluative judgment. The attribute of carving nature at the joints is often mentioned in its putative absence. If a distinction is difficult to draw or to agree on, or if it leads to inconsistent, vague, and overlapping categories, it is often said, metaphorically, that nature is not being carved at the joints. A good example in psychiatry is the distinction between normal and abnormal, where no definitive "joint" appears to exist.

Often, the assumption of a correct inherent structure of the universe is lurking in the background when the phrase *carving at the joints* is used. The problem with the inherent structure approach is that there are many different kinds of structure. It comes in multiple forms and is not a single thing. For example, although there is no single point that demarcates normal from abnormal on the continuum of blood pressure, there are clearly zones that are associated with increased risk to health. Such zones count as structure—they are not arbitrary.

The term *essence* is more straightforwardly evaluative, referring to the most important and/or necessary property. Essentialist thinking is philosophically suspect to thinkers schooled in the Darwinian perspective because it has a strong association with Platonism or the view that what is really real are abstract forms that exist independently of the material world. For Platonists, true knowledge is not to be gained by studying nature as is done by scientists, but by understanding a transcendent reality. Essentialism in all its various guises has not been able to eliminate the taint of Platonism.

Although a part of the tradition of natural kinds, the attribute of carving nature at the joints and the possession of a real essence are not necessary for understanding what Mill calls real kinds. Because of the baggage associated with these two attributes, they should be dispensed with in scientific discourse, and along with them the concept of a natural kind.

2. Why Kinds?

Understanding kinds is important because kinds, not individual persons, are classified in the *DSM* and the *ICD*. As described by Peter Zachar and Kenneth Kendler (2007), kinds refer to groups of cases about which generalizations can be made. If we can group cases together and name something they share (for example, depression) and also gain information about depression by studying that group of cases, depression is a legitimate kind in science. For example, mental health professionals have learned that people with a Major Depressive Disorder are at the highest risk for suicide in the early phases of recovery.

A real kind has what Nelson Goodman (1983) refers to as *projectibility*. Although he discussed projectibility with reference to general statements such as "all emeralds are green," Goodman also stated that the concept of projectibility could also be used to make distinctions between "genuine" and "merely artificial" kinds (p. 122). In Mill's terms, kinds that are more real would be more projectible.

Projectibility has two dimensions: inferential power and entrenchment. Turning first to inferential power, the question is what inferences do we want to make with respect to psychiatric disorders?

1. We want to make inferences about the past and how the psychiatric disorder came to be (causal understanding).

2. Many statements true about one instance of the psychiatric disorder should be true about other instances (generalizability).

3. We want to make inferences about what is going to happen in the future or how the disorder might manifest (or behave) in new situations (predictability).

Three empirical facts also need to be acknowledged as important limiting factors to making inferences about psychiatric disorders:

First, psychiatric disorders have complex etiologies; their pasts are varied. As noted, a history of sexual abuse is common among those with borderline personality, but not necessary. Furthermore, causality in psychiatry can be understood on multiple levels of analysis. Genetics, neurochemistry, personality traits, and trauma can all be part of the causal story. There are many "causes."

Second, the manifestation of a psychiatric disorder can vary by context—so instances differ from one another. Anorexia, a compulsion to maintain an abnormally low body weight, will present differently in a well-controlled and disciplined patient than in an impulsive patient who has difficulty delaying gratification. In the latter case, binging and purging is more common.

Third, psychiatric disorders can have multiple developmental trajectories; the future is not written in stone. A sizeable collection of variables— including level of social support, inherent talents and abilities, quality of treatment, and random events (good or bad luck)—can alter how a case of depression or schizophrenia develops over time.

It is tempting to increase inferential power by defining the construct for a disorder narrowly to enhance uniformity among the cases. The strategy of maximizing internal consistency is an important one, but it invariably leads to either marginalization of individuals that lie outside the narrow boundaries of the homogeneous cases, or, more likely, it leads to a slow steady increase of the number of kinds recognized (that is, classificatory splitting).

The second dimension of projectibility, *entrenchment,* is more difficult to explain, especially in terms of kinds. One way of explaining it is to say that entrenchment is analogous to the notion of repeatability in a scientific experiment. Results that can be replicated are considered to be more valuable. Like good experimental findings, entrenched kinds can or potentially will stand the test of time. In explaining it this way, I am filtering

Goodman's ideas through Ian Hacking's (1983) analysis of scientific realism. According to Hacking, scientists interact with things or "intervene in the world" and then use those interactions to talk and theorize about their objects of study. Entrenched kinds can withstand the systematic tests of experience and are more than things with which we are familiar.

Entrenchment is more secure if the inductions we make about a kind are coherent with other well-established generalizations. In psychiatry, these would include generalizations in genetics, pharmacology, cognitive science, psychometry, and psychodynamics.

3. A System of Kinds

Psychiatrists and psychologists not only classify kinds but also organize them in relation to each other. This project could be called *psychiatric systematics*. For example, Bipolar Affective Disorder and Unipolar Affective Disorder are placed in the same section of the diagnostic manual because they are considered to be related. Generalized Anxiety Disorder (GAD) is placed in a different section of the manual because it is considered to be more related to conditions such as the phobias and Obsessive Compulsive Disorder (OCD). In this sense, both the *DSM* and *ICD* are systems that model relationships between various disorders.

Several strategies are available to scientists for organizing their domain of study. I will now explore two strategies that correspond to exemplary real kinds, namely, the causal-structural model of the chemical taxonomy and the nested hierarchical model of biological taxonomies.

Chemical Taxonomy

Chemical elements are organized via a causal-structural model called the periodic table of the elements. The relevant casual factor is atomic number—which represents the number of protons in the nucleus. Organizing the elements with respect to atomic number results in a relatively complete ordinal structure, beginning with element number 1, hydrogen, and proceeding upward.

Implementing a periodic table strategy in psychiatry would require identifying some internal causal structure and using that structure to sort disorders. The most obvious choice would be to demarcate disorders by means of a specific genetic or biological etiology.

The problems with basing classificatory distinctions on etiology have been discussed by Kenneth Schaffner (2002), Kendler (2005), and Zachar and Kendler (2007). Rather than a single problem, there is a diverse concatenation of problems associated with giving priority to bottom up causal factors. For purposes of this chapter, I want to discuss only one issue—relating to classification and kinds. The main idea, borrowing some phraseology from Rebecca Bryant (2000), is that we can *discover* a lot of important etiological facts about the conditions studied in psychiatry, but we have to *decide* how to classify them.

Alzheimer Disease, a condition with both early-onset and later-onset versions, is a good example of a psychiatric disorder with diverse etiologies. As discussed by both Schaffner (2002) and Irving Gottesman (2002), there are at least three genetic pathways for an early-onset type of Alzheimer Disease—these pathways begin with genetic variants on, respectively, chromosome 21, chromosome 14, and chromosome 1. There are most likely multiple genetics pathways for the later-onset versions of the disorder. One confirmed pathway begins with chromosome 19, which contains a susceptibility gene. People who inherit a copy of this gene from one or both parents are at increased risk.

If one adopts a robust causal-structural model, then different cause equals different disease. That means that there are at least four disorders in the Alzheimer family, not one. The problem with the four disease model is that these distinct causal pathways appear to have a common anatomic-biochemical outcome and grouping cases with the same outcome together and studying what they share can still be informative. For instance, all four of these genes may be producing aberrant copies of the amyloid precursor protein resulting in neural degeneration in the entorhinal cortex. That *final common pathway* is also a causal variable.

Alzheimer Disease defined via genetic etiology indicates one set of boundaries—similar to the boundaries of the earlier onset condition identified by Emil Kraepelin and classified in *DSM-I* and *DSM-II* (American Psychiatric Hospital Service 1952; American Psychiatric Association 1968). Defining the condition with respect to anatomic etiology (tangles and plaques) suggests different boundaries, paralleling the current, broader boundaries in which Alzheimer Disease refers to a condition not limited by time of onset. In addition to discovering facts about etiology, what we call Alzheimer Disease requires a classificatory decision about what counts as the same kind of condition.

Biological Taxonomy

A second organizational strategy is the tree of life strategy used to organize biological species. The metaphor of a tree refers to a nested hierarchy with earlier groups branching off to form later groups. Elizabeth Flanagan and Roger Blashfield (2000) made an interesting and illuminating comparison between biological and psychiatric taxonomies. Although they focused on folk biological taxonomies, a similar comparison with scientific biological taxonomies can also be made.

In the tree of life, all subgroups descended from a common ancestor are related to each other like twigs on a branch. For example, on the primate branch biologists place prosimians (such as lemurs), New World monkeys (such as spider monkeys), Old World monkeys (such as macaques), the lesser apes (gibbons), the great apes (gorillas), and the hominids (*Homo sapiens*). According to the branching pattern, humans and chimps share a more recent common ancestor with each other than they do with gorillas (Dodson and Dodson 1985; Futuyma 1998).

Near the end of this chapter I will discuss some claims that, although a treelike or bushlike metaphor is the best model we have for understanding the relationships among biological species, the structure of species can only be partially represented in any single tree diagram. One conclusion to draw is that, if treelike, hierarchical models are inadequate in biology, then treelike models of psychiatric disorders are likely to have even greater flaws because, unlike species, it is not plausible to hypothesize that all psychiatric disorders have a common origin. Species are continuous via descent from common ancestors, while the "kingdom" of psychiatric disorders is probably a rather motley assortment of different kinds of things.

4. Traditional Organizational Strategies in Psychiatric Nosology

The primary strategy used to organize psychiatric taxonomy has been clinical observation, which gives priority to presentation—or shared phenotype. By this I mean that conditions that look the same with respect to having shared symptoms and similar time courses are identified as the same disorder. This strategy is common to Kraepelin, Sigmund Freud, Karl Jaspers, Robert Spitzer, and the authors of the Feighner criteria.

There are multiple problems with organizing the manual based on clinical presentation or "phenotypic" similarity. The three problems to be discussed here are (a) that observed similarity may be superficial, (b) that deciding which characters can be used to justify classifying two conditions as "similar" is not always obvious, and (c) that observations of similarity can be and have been overridden by theoretical preferences.

The first problem is that the observed similarity and dissimilarity between disorders may be superficial and elide deeper connections with other disorders. One example of this problem is that Bipolar Disorder and Major Depressive Disorder both share episodes of severe anhedonia and vegetative symptoms, so they are classified together as mood disorders in the *DSM* and the *ICD*. Research in psychology and psychiatric genetics, however, indicates that Major Depressive Disorder and GAD may share a closer relationship (Kendler et al. 1992; Krueger 1999). Susan Mineka, David Watson, and Lee Anna Clark (1998) even claimed that Major Depressive Disorder and GAD are genetically indistinguishable. This alternative approach to classifying disorders receives additional support from evidence that antidepressants are useful treatments for unipolar depression and GAD but recommended only with caution for Bipolar Disorder (such as the alternative classification has some entrenchment value) (Allgulander et al. 2004; Ghaemi et al. 2004).

A second problem with classifying disorders based on phenotypic similarity is deciding which observable characters should be used to define a group or used to differentiate between groups. As noted by both Goodman (1972) in philosophy and Douglas Medin (1989) in psychology, the number of similarities that exist between two or more groups of cases usually outnumbers the similarities that are afforded classificatory importance. For example, if depression and anxiety were to be classified together in the *DSM-V*, one could argue that shared irritability, insomnia, rumination, fatigue, and pessimism were not properly weighted by earlier generations of classification experts.

It is not easy to decide when differences in presentation signal distinct groups and when they merely signal variety within a larger group. For example, symptoms such as impulsiveness, grandiosity and being melodramatic are shared between several personality disorders (and manic episodes), but in the current nosology, psychiatrists are asked to pick one or more discrete categories. Let's say a diagnostician chooses Antisocial Personality Disorder for a particular patient. If this patient is also grandiose and melodramatic, a potential comorbidity problem exists between antisocial personality, narcissistic personality, and histrionic personality. If, however, psychiatry was to follow W. John Livesley's (2003) recommendation and make the target diagnostic category *personality disorder,* these traits would be expected to co-occur. The comorbidity of three distinct disorders would no longer exist. What counts as the same and different is partly prescribed by the classification system.

A third criticism of organizing disorders based on shared presentation, ironically, claims that the phenotypic similarity model has not been followed consistently, sometimes being overridden by theoretical preferences. One example of ignoring phenotypic similarity in favor of theoretical preferences is the placement of schizotypy in the *DSM* as a personality disorder rather than as a schizophrenia spectrum disorder. Symptomatic homogeneity with respect to the schizophrenic spectrum was downplayed in favor of classifying personality pathology as a group. In the *DSM,* the schizophrenic spectrum is fragmented.

In the *ICD,* by contrast, Schizotypal Disorder is classified with schizophrenia. When schizotypy is classified with schizophrenia, the schizophrenic spectrum is unified but the personality disorders are fragmented. This creates a problem as well because Schizotypal Disorder is a traitlike condition that shares the general features of personality disorders such as inflexibility, pervasiveness, and adolescent onset.

Schizotypal personality is also closely related to a normal personality trait that has been referred to variously as *psychoticism, cognitive distortion, and eccentric perceptions* (Harkness, McNulty, and Ben-Porath 1995; Clark et al. 1996). This personality trait emerges in studies that assess psychiatric symptoms. It is also trait to which the currently popular five-factor model of personality appears to be blind (Shedler and Westen 2004). Understanding the role of psychoticism illuminates not only personality pathology but also the schizophrenic spectrum.

I am not claiming that the *DSM* got it right and the *ICD* got it wrong; rather, I am claiming that this is an unresolvable classificatory dilemma. Right and wrong isn't how we should evaluate this kind of problem. It is helpful for the authors of the two systems to have made different choices regarding the placement of schizotypy: having alternative models better reflects the domain of psychiatric disorders. Certain types of information about schizotypal personality may emerge in the study of personality disorders and other types of information emerge in the study of schizophrenia-related disorders. Both types of information might have practical importance, but it would not be available to someone who is too literal about any one system. One implication of this analysis is that there might be some scientific benefit if the classifications of the World Health Organization and the American Psychiatric Association were more free to vary than they seem to have been for *ICD-10* and *DSM-IV.* The still extant political pressure to integrate the two taxonomies is based on reasonable goals, but it is not scientifically advantageous *tout court.*

The domain of psychiatric disorders is myriad. The structure that exists occurs on many overlapping levels and in many forms. Which aspects of that structure we decide to classify depends on our goals for classification. Dominic Murphy's work on levels of analysis in psychiatry (chapter 3 in this volume) presents a more philosophically satisfying exposition of this situation than I have been able to, particularly his argument that reductive explanations may complicate rather than simplify psychiatry (namely, provide new kinds of generalizations without eliminating previously discovered generalizations).

Let me note that these considerations do not warrant the adoption of either radical constructionism or "whatever goes" relativism. Classification is more than a matter of preference and/or ideolology. Classifications can be invalid. One example is involutional melancholia (IM)-supposedly a type of depression that begins after age 50. In the *DSM-I,* implicitly, and *DSM-II,* explicitly, IM was identified as a separate category of depression that was not a reaction to life stress, had an anxious presentation, had psychotic features, and occurred in patients with no previous episodes of depression. So it was like a psychiatric time bomb that went off later in life. Over time, the construct increasingly emphasized first episode agitated-psychotic depressions in women during menopause.

Is IM a real kind? Being 50 years old does not have the same biological significance today that it did in the early twentieth century, so comparisons between past and present are difficult to make. Let's focus on IM only as a disease contingent upon menopause. There is good evidence that rates of depression for women are not higher during menopause, that cases of depression occurring during menopause often have precipitants, and that an anxious presentation is related to past histories of depression (Weissman 1979; Berrios 1991; Becker et al. 2001).

In reference to some conclusions that will be presented at the end of this chapter, IM does not appear to be a very good psychiatric disorder. The inferences made about women diagnosed with prototypical IM do not provide relevant information beyond what would be provided if they were diagnosed with *Major Depressive Disorder, single episode, severe with psychotic features.* Some of the inferences formerly associated with IM probably wouldn't be validated unless the diagnostic specifier was recurrent rather than single episode.

To summarize, I have just explored the strategy of grouping disorders by using observable features. This important strategy has some shortcomings. Conditions that look alike may sometimes be different, and different-looking conditions may actually be the same thing. Also, what counts as an important feature can be influenced by theoretical preferences. Clinically observable similarity by itself does not do very much classificatory work.

5. An Alternative Strategy: The Dimensional Model

A different strategy for organizing the disorders systematically is to implement a numerically derived phenotypic classification.

> It is clear to all but the most conservative workers in the field that the taxonomy of the future will be greatly aided if not entirely carried out by computers. (Sneath and Sokol 1973, p. xiii)

When people make decisions about how to carve up the world, their ability to do so is limited by how much data they can attend to and organize in their heads. In contrast to the clinical observation approach, the quantitative approach uses computers and bases classificatory decisions on a consideration of thousands of data points. Factor analysis, which provides a computer-derived structural model for representing the phenotypic variation found in the domain of psychiatric disorders, is the basis of the dimensional model revolution that is being proposed for *ICD-11* and *DSM-V.*

The factor-analytic approach can be briefly explained by examining one of its uses in the development of psychological tests, in this case, a test called the *Personality Assessment Inventory (PAI),* developed by Leslie Morey (1991). The *PAI* measures eleven psychopathological constructs such as depression, anxiety, somatization, mania, and borderline features. These scales are all correlated with each other—in statistical terms they share variance.

One of the axioms of psychometry is that a correlation between two subtests indicates that they are measuring a similar construct. The higher the correlation, the more overlap between what is being measured. A perfect correlation would mean two tests are measuring the same thing. With factor analysis, a test developer can, for example, determine how much of the shared variation among the eleven *PAI* scales can be "explained" by a smaller number of underlying (latent) dimensions. The goal is to find a reasonable number of dimensions that model the shared variance and can thereby account for the pattern of similarities and differences between people on these eleven scales. Factor analysis is clearly a scientifically important tool—enabling researchers to look behind clinical observation to discover hidden patterns.

With respect to Morey's own factor analysis of the *PAI,* a three-factor solution appears to be most consistently relevant to understanding psychopathology. The first factor is a distress factor defined by anxiety and depression. The second factor is an externalizing or acting out factor defined by antisocial features and substance abuse. The third factor is more difficult to characterize. It seems to involve excessive confidence and energy. Morey describes it as narcissism-callousness.

I mentioned earlier that the five factor model of personality appears to be blind to the personality trait of psychoticism. The general principle involved here is that structural models don't account for all the patterns that exist in any domain. One consequence of these limitations for classification is that factor analysis and related strategies do not eliminate classificatory conundrums. Similar to psychoactive drugs, new organizational strategies always have unwanted side effects.

To illustrate, a large body of research has pointed to the possibility of organizing selected psychiatric disorders with respect to two latent factors. The two groups would be called internalizing disorders and externalizing disorders (Krueger 1999, 2002; Achenbach 2002). Internalizing disorders include anxiety and depression. They are about feeling distress. Externalizing disorders include Antisocial Personality Disorder, alcohol abuse, and drug abuse. They are about acting out distress. The theory is that the disorders in each group are the result of shared vulnerability factors. As Watson (2005) notes, an advantage to organizing the manual in this way is that it would better represent actual patterns of comorbidity. It could eliminate many conundrums regarding the anxiety and depression and psychopathy-substance abuse overlap.

The problem is that any single factor summarizes a lot of information and tends to represent a fairly broad construct. This is especially true with the internalizing factor. To be clinically meaningful the overly inclusive group of people who score high on internalizing usually has to be split up, and in this process classificatory anomalies inevitably appear.

Let's explore some problems that arise. There is persuasive evidence that the anxiety-depression domain is statistically more powerful if it is decomposed into two subgroups. According to Robert Krueger (1999) and Wilma Vollebergh and colleagues (2001), the two subgroups are anxious-misery (such as depression, dysthymia, generalized anxiety) and fear (such as panic, phobias).

As stated, with new organizational strategies, new conundrums inevitably appear. Some conundrums regarding internalizing and the classification of anxiety disorders are discussed by Watson (2005). The first is that panic has a high correlation with fear and moderate correlation with the misery group, but it is typically classified with the fear facet. Post-traumatic Stress Disorder (PTSD), by contrast, is classified as a misery-based disorder, although it has only a moderate correlation with misery. Watson speculates that PTSD's correlation with misery can probably be traced to its dysphoria dimension, whereas the hyperarousal and avoidance dimensions of PTSD are likely to be more associated with fear. Another anxiety disorder, Obsessive Compulsive Disorder, may be better grouped with fear than with misery, but its loading onto the fear group is also moderate. Some psychiatrists have argued for placing OCD on a completely separate dimension referred to as the obsessive-compulsive spectrum. Other disorders in this spectrum might be Trichotillomania and Tourette Syndrome (Phillips et al. 2003).

The internalizing dimension offers improved nosological clarity when major depression and generalized anxiety are being classified, but it becomes increasingly opaque as additional disorders are considered. The number of factor loadings is considerably increased as more conditions are placed under internalizing's classificatory lens. Other conditions loading onto an emotional distress factor include borderline, paranoid, histrionic, and dependent personalities, plus anorexia and schizophrenia (Morey 1991; Trull 1992).

The breadth of the internalizing factor is confirmed by Thomas Achenbach's (1995, 2001) rigorous empirical analysis. According to Achenbach, internalizing disorders include not only anxiety/depression, but somatic complaints and withdrawal. Social immaturity, attention problems and thought disorder also load onto the internalizing factor. Internalizing and externalizing are also positively correlated in samples of children. In other words, there may be one broad thing there (emotional distress).

Returning to the notion of having to decide what counts as similar, unless internalizing was used to group every disorder that is accompanied by the experience of distress, classifiers have to make some judgments about which similarities are to be weighted as important and which similarities are to be ignored or minimized. As Goodman (1978) notes, deleting, supplementing and smoothing out are normal aspects of classification. Nosologists can discover a lot of facts about the dimension of internalizing, but they have to decide what counts as an internalizing disorder.

In terms of psychometric theory, an underlying dimension such as internalizing may be homogeneous, but the real kinds associated with the dimension such as depression, GAD, and borderline personality usually have additional attributes that are not homogenous with respect to the target dimension. To the extent that these additional attributes are a central feature of the construct for that kind, the underlying dimension does not contain all of the relevant information about that kind.

So where do these complications regarding dimensional model organizational strategies leave us? Understanding the overlap that occurs among different groups of cases (kinds) is important. The advantage of dimensional models is that they offer a better solution to this problem than the current system. Empirically demonstrated relationships between disorders should not be ignored by classifiers. The relationships that exist between kinds, however, are not simple. They exist on many levels of analysis and in varying degrees. Which relationships will be afforded recognition in the classification system is a matter of decision. Mere discovery is inadequate.

6. Classification in Biology

For several years now, I have hypothesized that scientists describe their classifications to students, lay persons, and scholars from other disciplines in simplified terms, knowing all the while that the "reality on the ground" is more complicated than these cleansed summaries indicate (Zachar 2000b). Students and others often take these descriptions literally and, therefore, don't conceptualize things such as *the constants of nature, chemical bonds,* or *species* as the experts conceptualize them. My specific concern has been the extent to which psychiatrists and psychologists adopt these summaries as standards by which their own classifications are to be judged and thereby disavow classificatory recognition of "reality on the ground" because it doesn't seem scientifically rigorous enough. In the following section I explore this territory by examining scientific classification in biology. I begin by examining three approaches to the classification species and then describe three models for organizing species together systematically.

The Species Problem (What Counts as a Real Kind)

The computer-based quantitative approach to the classification of psychiatric disorders has a close cousin in biology, called numerical taxonomy. In biology, numerical taxonomy has traditionally referred to a procedure called cluster analysis. As described by Mark Aldenderfer and Roger Blashfield (1984), in cluster analysis observed characteristics are measured and then submitted to a computer program. The program calculates an index of overall similarity and places similar individuals together into dyads. Dyads are then combined and the process continues until a certain level of coherence is reached.

Clusters tend to be heterogeneous, which is a virtue for Darwinians but a problem for those committed to the natural kind perspective. Similar to Wittgenstein's notion of family resemblance categories, members in the center of a cluster are fairly similar to each other with respect to the properties being measured, but as one moves out toward the boundary of the cluster, members become more diverse. Peter Sneath and Robert Sokol (1973) describe clusters as a polythetic categories—a term also used in the *DSM* to describe psychiatric disorders.

Clustering methodologies can be used to define species and to group species into higher-order taxa. The general problem with cluster analysis is that the groups constructed by the algorithms are sensitive to the information one enters into the program. In statistics this is referred to as the garbage-in, garbage-out problem. Both the choice of characteristics and the specific algorithm chosen by the researchers to define similarity affect the outcome.

Another problem with *"phenotype-based"* approaches such as cluster analysis, as mentioned earlier, is that observed similarity and dissimilarity between entities may be superficial and elide deeper connections with other entities. To illustrate, there are species of fruit flies that are morphologically indistinguishable but cannot interbreed (Dodson and Dodson 1985). There are also dramatic instances of unexpected hybridization between phenotypically distinct species, including lions and tigers, sheep and goats, and dolphins and false killer whales (Short 1997).

An alternative to the phenotypic similarity approach is called the *biological species concept,* which is most closely associated with Ernst Mayr (1988, 1991). According to Mayr, a species is a population of individuals that can interbreed and is reproductively isolated from other populations. In contrast to the pre-Darwinian species concept, which claimed that members of a "species class" share a common essence, the biological species concept states that members within a "population" vary. For Darwin, variation is part of the nature of species that evolve—it is not an accidental deviation from some ideal type.

The biological species concept, however, has problems attributing species status to organisms that do not reproduce sexually. Bacteria are the primary example. Proponents of the biological species concept have had to grit their teeth and assert that asexually reproducing organisms are not species. Technically, sterile hybrids such as mules can not breed either— and are therefore not a proper biological species.

A third approach to understanding species is called the *phylogenetic species concept.* According to Brent Mishler and Robert Brandon (1987), being the same species means having the same set of ancestors. Proponents of this model believe that the facts of descent should determine which organisms can be placed together. Groups defined by descent may vary in size and coherence, but they can be objectively described.

There is also a problem with the phylogenetic species concept. Because higher order taxa may be heterogenous collections spanning millions of years, deciding what counts as a group called a "species" is not straightforward. This is particularly true for plants, which can widely hybridize— for example, oaks and hawthorns. In some parts of the United States there are a multitude of fertile oak hybrids. Some of these oaks look like trees, others look like shrubs, and biologists do not agree on how to rank them in the taxonic hierarchy (that is, classify them as genus, species, incipient species, variety, form, and so on). Descent alone cannot be the determining factor for categorizing species.

In a defense of species pluralism, Marc Ereshefsky (1992) notes that evolution works in complex ways, and there is no single criterion that can be used to identify a species. Sometimes the presence of isolating mechanisms is adequate, but not always. Occupying the same ecological niche (bacteria, Emory oaks) or having a particular line of descent (mules, peppermint) might work in some instances. In other instances, however, various criteria for "ranking" species may conflict. For example, three populations of salamanders distributed over a range may count as three different "ecological species," two "interbreeding species," but only one phylogenetic species. Paralleling what I earlier noted about psychiatric disorders, the plurality of species concepts makes the species category a motley assortment of different kinds of things.

The Taxonomy Problem (Organizing Kinds)

The major focus of numerical taxonomy has not been to identify species themselves, but to understanding how species are related to each other. As is true elsewhere, similarity can be deceptive. For example, the presence of wings in bats and wings in birds should not be used to classify them into the same phylogenetic group. The "wings" evolved independently, a process called convergent evolution. Bats have more in common with cats than they do with birds.

Because they rely on computerized algorithms, numerical taxonomies such as those based on cluster analysis are somewhat atheoretical—they churn out structural models if provided data. Such mathematically derived models have to be integrated with the rest of biology post hoc. Sometimes, theoretical considerations from other areas of biology such as evolutionary theory and genetics cast doubt on a proposed structural model (that is, the model lacks entrenchment value). For example, although various species of zebra can be classified together according to shared phenotype, some zebras (mountain zebras) bear a much closer historical relationship to horses than they do to other zebras.

A second taxonomic theory is termed the *cladistic model,* which uses phylogeny or shared ancestry to group species. Cladism is inspired by the writings of Willi Hennig (1966). As described by Mark Ridley (1986), the idea behind cladistics is that phylogenetic groups or clades should contain an ancestor and all of its descendants, referred to as a monophyletic group. In order to map clades, taxonomists make the assumption that evolution occurs by a parental group being split up into two or more lines of descent.

A cladistic species will therefore always be identified relative to a sister species. Two sister species will be identified relative to a group that lies outside the clade. In this triad, the two sister species are identified by traits each inherited from their most recent common ancestor and that they do not share with the outgroup. These shared derived character states are considered to have evolved in that ancestor and are unique to its line.

For example, scientists have convincingly demonstrated that birds and crocodiles are sister groups relative to an ancestor lizard called archosaurs, and turtles are an outgroup. The shared derived characters for birds and crocodiles include the design of the ankle, a four-chambered heart, and caring for their young.

One problem with cladistic classification is its self-imposed limits. Cladists are interested in modeling only branching patterns, nothing else. *When* the branching occurred is not important. According a cladist, "reptile" is not a real taxon because it excludes birds. Crocodiles are cladistically more related to birds than other "reptiles." "Fish" is also not a real taxon either—it excludes lizards. Salmon are cladistically more similar to lizards than they are to other fish. At one point in time, however, reptiles and fish were cladistically real taxa and served as ancestors to birds and lizards. Cladism does not recognize evolutionary history in this sense.

A more troubling problem in cladistics is that it may not be possible to accurately represent evolutionary history in a tree or cladogram. The reason is lateral gene transfer, which is the exchange of genes between different organisms independently of the process of reproduction. Among prokaryotes, genes are not just passed on to descendants via reproduction; they are passed on to other organisms via lateral gene transfer. Lateral gene transfer may have been so common early in evolutionary history that prokaryotes such as bacteria are descendants of multiple and disparate branches (that is, separate lines on the phylogenetic tree have been repeatedly combined) (Doolittle 1999). The discovery of lateral gene transfer has at least complicated cladistic analyses that use gene sequences as characters, and, depending on how extensive it is, may make the goal of mapping the "one true tree of life" highly improbable.

A third approach to taxonomy is called *evolutionary systematics.* Both the numerical taxonomists and the cladists seek objective, algorithmic methods for classifying groups. Once a method is outlined, they follow it rigorously. In contrast, the proponents of evolutionary systematics such as Mayr (1982) hold that classifiers should be free to attend to all the empirical information available and not ignore certain kinds of information because it isn't accounted for in one's classificatory algorithm. They also recognize that scientific classification serves multiple purposes and are unwilling to reduce it to any single goal.

Evolutionary systematists do not dispute that birds and crocodiles share a recent common ancestor, but they would be more willing to take into account the degree of divergence between birds and crocodiles. The number of changes between extant birds and the reptilian archosaur is likely large, whereas crocodilians evolved and stabilized long ago—the amount of change for crocodiles is more limited. In addition to the derived traits birds share with crocodiles, they also possess nonshared derived traits. They include feathers, warm bloodedness, and bipedalism. Such traits may have taxonomic value, thereby justifying grouping birds as a distinct taxon relative to "reptiles."

One forceful criticism of evolutionary systematics is that it contains subjectivist or value elements. Sometimes branching alone is used and at other times degree of divergence is used to draw taxonomies. Deciding that sister species are too different to be classified together recapitulates all the problems endemic to similarity judgments. From a cladistic perspective, the unique traits of birds are taxonomically relevant for classifying different kinds of birds, but not for understanding the phylogenetic position of birds in the tree of life.

7. The Biologist's Concept of a Good Species and Its Implications for Psychiatry

The dual issues of what counts as a species and how to relate them cannot be neatly segregated. A taxonomist cannot group kinds of things together until the kinds are defined, but one's theory about the organization of a domain can alter one's theory of what counts as a legitimate kind.

To live with the frustrating problem of competing models for understanding species and their relationships, many biologists accept the value of having multiple models—realizing that different models have their own advantages and disadvantages. Groups that meet most requirements of the various models are called *good species.* For many (not all) entities, numerical taxonomy, the biological species concept, and the phylogenetic species concept give a similar answer regarding what species exist and how they are to be related.

As noted above, one of the problems faced in biological taxonomy not faced in chemical taxonomy is the problem of hybridization among basic entities—a consequence of the fact that species have evolved. For example, lions and tigers can interbreed to form both ligers and tigons. A liger is the offspring of a female tiger and a male lion; it the largest kind of cat in the world. A tigon is the offspring of a female lion and a male tiger and is smaller than both parental species. Such *interforms* are outlawed in the tradition of natural kinds.

Ligers and tigons notwithstanding, lions and tigers are still pretty good species. Hybridization between the two has a low base rate because isolating mechanisms are present and they don't breed in the wild. Furthermore, their lines of descent can be traced and separated and they are morphologically and behaviorally distinct. It is therefore, important to not be rigid in defining real kinds in biology. Classification systems in biology are not made up, and they have objective bases but are still coddled together.

Could there also be an analogous concept of a *good psychiatric disorder?* Some ideas discussed by Kenneth Kendler (1990) might suggest that the answer is "yes." According to Kendler, psychiatry has the important task of validating psychiatric disorders, but researchers pick validators based on some construct or model of what counts as a legitimate psychiatric disorder. The validators indicate how good a diagnostic category is relative to the construct. For example, if researchers hypothesize that schizophrenia is a genetically based disorder that runs in families, then they are going to validate that construct by examining base rates in various family groups compared to the base rate in the general population. Conditions whose base rates rise as the genetic overlap in the family groups rise get one check in the good disorder column.

Different constructs for what counts as a disorder, however, might suggest examining alternative validators. Researchers who conceptualize schizophrenia as a major mental illness with a poor prognosis might examine outcome data. Because it is important to identify the major mental illnesses, the criteria for a disorder can even be altered to isolate cases with poor outcome.

Kendler then asks what nosologists should do if one validator, such as family history, suggests one set of boundaries for a category and another validator, such as poor prognosis, suggests another? This seems to be the case with respect to the schizophrenia family. The genetically validated condition is broader, the prognosis validated condition is more narrow. Which one is really schizophrenia?

Kendler's analysis suggests that deciding between different constructs for a disorder is not only an empirical question. This means that there is no crucial experiment that psychiatrists can design to tell them what construct to pick. It does not mean that there are no reasons for picking a particular construct for a disorder or that empirical evidence can be ignored. When nosologists have to decide which of several possible classifications is better, however, theoretical and pragmatic considerations gain classificatory weight. On the basis of some of the ideas put forth in this chapter, one possible way to think about this problem is that the conditions classified by different validators might be considered to be real kinds, but none is *the* real kind. This could be called realism without literalism.

Like *natural kind* and *species, psychiatric disorder* is an abstract concept. It may not refer to a uniform thing. The important validators for a good disorder can be present in varying degrees and in different combinations depending on the condition being studied. Like the concept of a species, it is important to have empirically supported criteria for what counts as good disorder, but it is also important to not be too rigid in listing what qualify as "real kinds" in Mill's sense.

The requirement for flexibility is even greater if the task is understanding how the different kinds studied by psychiatry are to be related to each other. For example, Major Depressive Disorder is similar to both GAD and the Bipolar Disorders, but GAD and the Bipolar Disorders are clearly distinct. A host of factors are relevant in deciding how to organize these conditions relative to each other and relative to other conditions such as the personality disorders, alcoholism, and conduct disorder.

As in biology, a disciplined flexibility would be a virtue. Scientists can at least hope that sets of different validators might converge or triangulate on a common answer regarding what kinds of conditions exist in the domain and how they can be organized. As argued by Kendler and Zachar (this volume), understanding where this stability lies is an important task. Once various stabilities are mapped out, the question of how to classify them will still require nosological decisions.

8. Conclusion

I am mindful of Guy Scadding's (1993) caution against making too close an analogy between independent entities such as organisms/species and processes that occur in organisms, such as diseases. The differences are important. For example, diseases are processes that have no existence independent of organisms. Another difference is that the *ICD* and *DSM* are manuals of (1) conditions that (2) require treatment. Deciding what conditions exist is not the same as deciding what needs to be treated, but both are necessary for deciding what counts as a psychiatric disorder. All the same, both biologists and psychologists study and classify kinds and the relationships between kinds. In biology and psychiatry, kinds are groups of entities/processes that share a variety of properties about which we can make inferences.

Although the analogy between the problems of biological taxonomy and the problems of psychiatric nosology is limited, like species, both personality traits and psychiatric disorders are the products of the evolutionary processes and are therefore subject via selection to the same kinds of multilevel structures/causes, convoluted histories, widespread variability, and classificatory conundrums. We should not expect more clarity in a psychiatric nosology that we can achieve in a biological taxonomy. Failure to appreciate the complexity of biological taxonomies leads to unrealistic standards for what counts as an adequate psychiatric nosology.

Kinds in psychiatry can be "real," or "genuine," or "legitimate," or "valid." It's a matter of degree, but standards for making these evaluations can be specified. Because it is a matter of degree, like biology has for species, psychiatry needs the concept of a good psychiatric disorder. It should adopt some flexibility in applying that concept. Furthermore, because "real kind" partly refers to inferential power, and what inferences one can make about kinds depends on how classifiers group them together, psychiatrists shouldn't be too literal about any single organizational strategy. Those who expect to find the true system tend to settle on one eventually and thereby compromise their ability to learn more about what is really there.

ACKNOWLEDGMENTS

Helpful commentary on this chapter was provided by Andrea Solomon, Rosine Hall, Kenneth Kendler, Jared Keeley, Kenneth Schaffner, and Dominic Murphy.

REFERENCES

Achenbach, T. M. 1995. Empirically Based Assessment and Taxonomy: Applications to Clinical Research. *Psychological Assessment* 3:261–274.

————. 2001. Empirically Based Assessment and Taxonomy across the Life Span. In J. E. Helzer and J. J. Hudziak (eds.), *Defining Psychopathology in the Twenty-first Century* (pp. 155–168). Washington, DC: American Psychiatric Publishing.

Aldenderfer, M. S., and R. K. Blashfield. 1984. *Cluster Analysis.* Newbury Park, CA: Sage.

Allgulander, C., A. A. Dahl, C. Austin, P. L. P. Morris, J. A. Sogaard, R. Fayyad, S. P. Kutcher, and C. M. Clary. 2004. Efficacy of Sertraline in a 12-week Trial for Generalized Anxiety Disorder. *American Journal of Psychiatry* 161:1642–1649.

American Psychiatric Association. 1968. *Diagnostic and Statistical Manual of Mental Disorders,* 2nd ed. Washington, DC: American Psychiatric Association.

American Psychiatric Association Mental Hospital Service. 1952. *Diagnostic and Statistical Manual of Mental Disorders.* Washington, DC: American Psychiatric Association Mental Hospital Service.

Becker, D., J. Lomranz, A. Pines, D. Shmotkin, E., Nitza, G. BennAmitay, and R. Mester. 2001. Psychological Distress around Menopause. *Psychosomatics* 42:252–257.

Berrios, G. E. 1991. Affective Disorders in Old Age: A Conceptual History. *International Journal of Geriatric Psychiatry* 6:337–346.

Bryant, R. 2000. *Discovery and Decision.* London: Associated University Presses.

Clark, L. A., J. W. Livesley, M. L. Schroeder, and S. L. Irish. 1996. Convergence of Two Systems for Assessing Specific Traits of Personality Disorder. *Psychological Assessment* 8:294–303.

Dodson, E. O., and P. Dodson. 1985. *Evolution: Process and Product.* Belmont, CA: Wadsworth.

Doolittle, W. F. 1999. Phylogenetic Classification and the Universal Tree. *Science* 2284:2124–2128.

Ereshefsky, M. 1992. Eliminative Pluralism. *Philosophy of Science* 59:671–690.

Flanagan, E., and R. Blashfield. 2000. Essentialism and a Folk-taxonomic Approach to the Classification of Psychopathology. *Philosophy, Psychiatry, and Psychology* 7:183–189.

Futuyma, D. J. 1998. *Evolutionary Biology,* 2nd ed. Sunderland, MA: Sinauer Associates.

Gelman, S. A., and L. A. Hirschfeld. 1999. How Biological Is Essentialism. In. D. S. Medin and S. Atran (eds.), *Folkbiology* (pp. 403–446). Cambridge, MA: MIT Press.

Ghaemi, S. N., K. J. Rosenquist, J. Y. Ko, C. F. Baldassano, et al. 2004. Antidepressant Treatment in Bipolar versus Unipolar Depression. *American Journal of Psychiatry* 161:163–165.

Ghiselin, M. T. 1974. A Radical Solution to the Species Problem. *Systematic Zoology* 23:536–544.

————. 1999. Natural Kinds and Supraorganismal Individuals. In D. S. Medin and S. Atran (eds.), *Folkbiology* (pp. 447–460). Cambridge, MA: MIT Press.

Goodman, N. 1972. Seven Strictures on Similarity. In N. Goodman (ed.), *Problems and Projects* (pp. 23–32). Indianapolis: Bobbs-Merrill.

————. 1978. *Ways of Worldmaking.* Indianapolis: Hackett.

Gottesman, I. I. 2002. Defining Denetically Informed Phenotypes for the DSM-V. In J. Z. Sadler (ed.), *Descriptions and Prescriptions* (pp. 291–300). Baltimore: Johns Hopkins University Press.

Hacking, I. 1983. *Representing and Intervening.* New York: Cambridge University Press.

Harkness, A. R., J. L. McNulty, and Y. S. Ben-Porath. 1995. The Personality Psychopathology Five (PSY-5): Constructs and MMPI-2 Scales. *Psychological Assessment* 7:104–114.

Hennig, W. 1966. *Phylogenetic Systematics.* Urbana: University of Illinois Press.

Hull, D. L. 1976. Are Species Really Individuals? *Systematic Zoology* 25:174–191.

Kendler, K. S. 1990. Toward a Scientific Psychiatric Nosology. *Archives of General Psychiatry* 47:969–973.

———. 2005. "A Gene for . . . ": The Nature of Gene Action in Psychiatric Disorders. *American Journal of Psychiatry* 162:1243–1252.

Kendler, K. S., M. C. Neale, and D. Walsh. 1995. Evaluating the Spectrum Concept of Schizophrenia in the Roscommon Family Study. *American Journal of Psychiatry* 152:749–754.

Krueger, R. F. 1999. The Structure of Common Mental Disorders. *Archives of General Psychiatry* 56:921–926.

Livesley, W. J. 2003. Diagnostic Dilemmas in Classifying Personality Disorder. In K. A. Phillips, M. B. First, and H. A. Pincus (eds.), *Advancing DSM* (pp. 153–189). Washington, DC: American Psychiatric Association.

Mayr, E. 1988. *Toward a New Philosophy of Biology: Observations of an Evolutionist.* Cambridge, MA: Harvard University Press.

———. 1991. *One Long Argument: Charles Darwin and the Genesis of Modern Evolutionary Thought.* Cambridge, MA: Harvard University Press.

Medin, D. L. 1989. Concepts and Conceptual Structure. *American Psychologist* 44:1469–1481.

Mill, J. S. (1843) 1973. A System of Logic. In J. M. Robson (ed.), *Collected Works of John Stuart Mill,* vol. 7. Toronto: University of Toronto Press.

Mineka, S., D. Watson, and L. A. Clark. 1998. Comorbidity of Anxiety and Mood Disorders. *Annual Review of Psychology* 49:377–412.

Mitchell, S. D. 2000. Dimensions of Scientific Law. *Philosophy of Science* 67:242–265.

Mishler, B. D., and R. N. Brandon. 1987. Individuality, Pluralism, and the Phylogenetic Species Concept. *Biology and Philosophy* 2:397–414.

Morey, L. C. 1991. *The Personality Assessment Inventory: Professional Manual.* Lutz, FL: Psychological Assessment Resources.

Phillips, K. A., L. H. Price, B. D. Greenberg, and S. A. Rasmussen. 2003. Should the DSM Diagnostic Groupings Be Changed? In K. A. Phillips, M. B. First, and H. A. Pincus (eds.), *Advancing DSM* (pp. 57–84). Washington, DC: American Psychiatric Association.

Ridley, M. 1986. *Evolution and Classification: The Reformation of Cladism.* New York: Longman.

Scadding, G. 1993. Nosology, Taxonomy, and the Classification Conundrum of the Functional Psychoses. *British Journal of Psychiatry* 162:237–238.

Schaffner, K. F. 2002. Clinical and Etiological Psychiatric Diagnoses: Do Causes Count? In J. Z. Sadler (ed.), *Descriptions and Prescriptions* (pp. 271–290). Baltimore: Johns Hopkins University Press.

Shedler, J., and D. Westen. 2004. Dimensions of Personality Pathology: An Alternative to the Five-factor Model. *American Journal of Psychiatry* 161:1743–1754.

Short, R. V. 1997. An Introduction to Mammalian Interspecific Hybrids. *Journal of Heredity* 88:355–357.

Sneath, P. H. A., and R. R. Sokol. 1973. *Numerical Taxonomy.* San Francisco: W. H. Freeman.

Trull, T. J. 1992. DSM-III-R Personality Disorders and the Five-factor Model of Personality: An Empirical Comparison. *Journal of Abnormal Psychology* 101:553–560.

Vollebergh, W. A. M., J. Iedma, R. V. Bijl, R. de Graf, F. Smit, and J. Ormel. 2001. The Structure and Stability of Common Mental Disorders: The NEMESIS Study. *Archives of General Psychiatry* 58:597–603.

Watson, D. 2005. Rethinking the Mood and Anxiety Disorders: A Quantitative Hierarchical Model for *DSM-V. Journal of Abnormal Psychology* 114:522–536.

Weissman, M. M. 1979. The Myth of Involutional Melancholia. *Journal of the American Medical Association* 242:742–744.

Zachar, P. 2000a. Psychiatric Disorders Are Not Natural Kinds. *Philosophy, Psychiatry, and Psychology* 7:167–182.

———. 2000b. Folk Taxonomies Should Not Have Essences Either. *Philosophy, Psychiatry, and Psychology* 7:191–194.

———. 2002. The Practical Kinds Model as a Pragmatist Theory of Classification. *Philosophy, Psychiatry, and Psychology* 9:219–227.

———. 2006. Les troubles psychiatriques et le modèle des espèces pratiques. *Philosophiques* 33:81–98.

Zachar, P., and S. Bartlett. 2001. Basic Emotions and Their Biological Substrates: A Nominalistic Interpretation. *Consciousness and Emotion* 2:189–221.

Zachar, P., and K. S. Kendler. 2007. Psychiatric Disorders: A Conceptual Taxonomy. *American Journal of Psychiatry* 164:557–565.

Zanarini, M. C., F. R. Frankenburg, J. Hennen, D. Bradford Reich, and K. R. Silk. 2006. Prediction of the 10-year Course of Borderline Personality Disorder. *American Journal of Psychiatry* 163:827–832.

Comment: A Tail of a Tiger

Kenneth F. Schaffner, M.D., Ph.D.

Peter Zachar tackles major, difficult, and perennial issues in his chapter. He referred to both gold and tigers, and I'd like to start by noting that he has a tiger by the tail with his topic in addressing the issue of real kinds and his skeptical thesis of the possibility of discovery of a true taxonomy for psychiatry.

As Zachar notes, these issues of real kinds go well beyond the concerns of just psychiatrists and psychologists, where the issue is usually framed in terms of validities and typically as one of construct validity. In the general sense of these questions, those issues have been central for philosophers, at least since Plato proposed the existence of eternal forms, which most of us experience only as derivative shadows of reality. Fundamental reality has been previously been characterized as unknowable in any direct sense by Kant, with his distinction between the noumenal and the phenomenal. Thus, by raising the questions he has, Zachar points toward key and foundational questions, including the nature of reality. Readers of his chapter will appreciate the subtlety that Zachar approaches these issues within the psychiatric context—this is good philosophy, not soundbite or short-answer philosophical analysis.

In the interest of full disclosure, I should note that my general philosophical orientation is pragmatic, in the tradition of James, Pierce, and Dewey, but also has Aristotelian, as well as analytic, aspects. My reliance on the pragmatic tradition should become more evident toward the close of my comments.

Areas of Agreement

There is much to think about in the material presented in Zachar's chapter. I will focus on just a few points, some of which I fully agree with, some on which I take a different contrary position and several ideas around which I'd like to propose an alternative view—or maybe an extension of Zachar's positions.

Regarding the issue of where we might search for models of successful kind terms that may be of help with analyzing the nature of psychiatric kinds, Zachar says do not look to physics or chemistry (for example, with gold in terms of its atomic number as a sortal), but rather look to biology, with its species concept, such a tiger, its tree of life, and in classifying an entity into a species kind and organizing species in terms of descendents. I will return to this biological analogy and its pros and cons shortly.

I also think Zachar is right about taxonomy—in his arguing *against* a view that the goal of an analogue of Mendeleev's periodic chart is where

psychiatry should be heading. Zachar suggests that this kind of clear taxonomy is not possible because of diverse etiologies for disorders and the
uncertainty as to which characteristics of a disorder we should focus on
for identifying similarities. The periodic chart model has, however, been
seductively attractive, even to biologists and excellent geneticists, such as
Eric Lander. Lander argued that this type of biological classification was
where the new genomics of microarrays would help take us, albeit there
would need to be 100,000 boxes, not a hundred plus, as in the chemical
elements chart (Lander 1999).

Zachar also proposes that we best look to biology—and at least consider the tree of life metaphor to organize mental disorders, as analogues
of species, into a taxonomy. Zachar thinks the tree of life model is suggestive, though he says that it too has problems and that the model is somewhat flawed because psychiatric disorders have "no common origin."
Zachar also notes both Ernst Mayr's approach to species, as well as the
cladists and the numerical taxonomists, as useful biological approaches.
Ultimately, however, Zachar suggests that all of these have flaws and that
the best we might do is work with multiple models simultaneously.

Some Concerns with Zachar's Approach

The distinction between Mayr's proximal (current) causation versus ultimate (evolutionary) causation has not been fully appreciated in discussing the origin of psychiatric disorders (see Mayr 1961). We do invoke
various proximate causes in psychiatry, such as stressful life events
influence the likelihood of depression. Much less securely, we could appeal to evolutionary (Mayr's ultimate) causes, such as in Tim Crow's speculative proposal (2000) that schizophrenia is the price we pay for being
able to use language. It is not fully obvious to me what kind of "origin"
Zachar is considering here in comments about the utility of the "tree of
life" as a model for classification in psychiatry. I particularly doubt that
evolutionary (ultimate cause) arguments are ever going to be that useful in
psychiatric classification—there are no fossils of schizophrenia.

A related issue is that biological organism and species relations are
much more likely to resemble a multirooted bush, with multiple origins
and intertwining, than a tree with branches originating from a common
trunk and ending in smaller branches and then twigs. At places Zachar ac-
knowledges the possibility of bushiness in biology but seems not to offer

ways to take those complications into account in a classification system. Even here, that bushiness will be encountered largely in the proximal cause sense. The intuition is that both developmentally and in terms of classifying common mechanisms accessible in the present day, one encounters a bushy set of cross-connections and relations. This intuition uses biology but not evolutionary biology—at least in any direct sense.

Zachar notes the attractiveness of dimensional accounts in psychiatry as better than categorically discrete analyses. On this point I agree with him, and *DSM-V* and *ICD-11* probably will begin to acknowledge dimensionality more, especially in the area of personality disorders. (For comments on this prospect in connection with *DSM-V,* see First et al. [2002].) For implementing the dimensional approach, Zachar suggests that factor analysis (FA) might help. I think it can, and the best example I know is W. John Livesley's FA empirical derivation of four of the five-factor model's (FFM) superfactors from a patient population (Livesley et al. 1998). (They comprise the CEAN components, Conscientiousness, Extraversion, Agreeableness, and Neuroticism, but not the O—Openness—superfactor.) Zachar also cites some of Livesley's work on personality disorders, but he does so more critically, because Zachar suggests that such FFM models may miss an important psychoticism category. Livesley also defends a spectrum approach to normal personality and personality disorders.

But FA has limitations, is linear (because it is a specialization of the general linear model), and applications do not always agree. One area of application has been to the dimensions of schizophrenia, where a threefold model (involving positive, negative, and disorganization dimensions) seems the most popular. A final consensus about the methods and number of dimensions, however, is yet to be attained (see Peralta and Cuesta 2001). Possibly more complex models, maybe Bayesian nets, maybe neural network classification or numerical taxonomy (NT) would do better, but they do not have as developed in the literature to date. The remaining sections of Zachar's chapter explore biological classification in an attempt to find a deeper approach to classification than the psychologists and psychiatrists have been able to develop.

Echoing some issues that arise in dimensional approaches to psychiatric disorders, Zachar first considers the numerical taxonomic position of Peter Sneath and Robert Sokal (1973) as one way to approach defining a species. NT, with its application of cluster analysis and its polythetic groups, is attractive for psychiatry, as Zachar notes. (In the interests of philosophical fairness, however, I want to add that Morton Beckner [1959] anticipated this important notion years before the NT work, calling it "polytypic," in his classic philosophy of biology book.) Cluster analysis or any phenotype-based approach is risky, as Zachar mentions, because it may capture only superficial similarities, and Zachar suggests that the biological species concept might be a useful corrective to this. The biological species concept does, however, have its own problems, and yet another notion, the phylogenetic species concept, which appeals to the ancestors of a group, may be needed to help clarify the issue. Actually, all three approaches might be needed, which suggests that a species pluralism is the best one can do. These three ways of approaching species—NT, biological, and phylogenetic—have also been used do describe ways of approaching larger classification issues (ones above the species level, including the genus level, and so on), as well as the general issue of the underlying principles of the tree of life. Thus, Zachar then moves to another section of his chapter, where he discusses the taxonomy problem, summarizing the numerical taxonomists, the cladists, and evolutionary systematics (a cousin of the biological species approach).

Zachar provides interesting potential parallels in the biological world that could be exploited as models for sharpening and deepening psychiatric classification, but I suspect that the enterprise is fundamentally flawed. This is not because there has not been extensive research and debates developing each of the three biological approaches mentioned—on this issue, compare David Hull's account of the debate between the numerical taxonomists and cladists in Hull (1988), and the overview of the interrelations of these various approaches to species and taxonomy in the work of Kim Sterelny and Paul Griffiths (1999, chapter 9). The issue, rather, is that each of these different approaches to species and to taxonomy had as a critically important backdrop *a rich history of the evolutionary record.* Added to this backdrop are current developments involving DNA sequences, which attempt to fine tune lineages based on similarities of key genetic features of currently available primitive model organism descendents, such as bacteria, worms, flies, mice, and humans (Schaffner 1998b).

In psychiatry, though, we have no such evolutionary record—as already noted, there are no fossils that allow us to capture ancestral forms of depression or schizophrenia. Moreover, with the possible exception of mice and rats, the use of animal models is not likely to provide us with any kind of empirical control over lineages of mental disorders. Thus, a key feature of what Zachar is searching for—something that will provide the grounds for an entrenchment—is not present to ground and control psychiatric parallels to biological classification.

I suspect that the weakest of the approaches that Zachar mentions, NT, will paradoxically be the most useful for psychiatrists, because it is anchored in the present. But NT has, as Zachar and many other commentators have discussed, serious methodological weaknesses.

I would take a different tack—looking more at the possibility of underlying biological explanations of psychiatric disorders and hoping to find ways of defining disorders and interrelating disorders by an analysis in the present day, not by appealing to ancestors and evolutionary history. This approach, however, is itself currently limited, as I point out in my chapter in this book and as other contributors to this conference also have noted.

How might we begin to make additional progress on the topics of disorder definition and disorder interrelations that can clarify whether both enterprises are valid? In a commentary I can provide only the barest of outlines, but even this may have some value in a volume of this nature.

An Alternative Approach to Clarifying Kinds
Clinical Validity

For the in-progress revisions of *ICD-11* mental disorders, however, as well as the *DSM-V* revision scheduled for 2012, I believe the major work will involve various aspects of *clinical validity,* a notion that I shall reexamine further below. This clinical validity concept carries forward both the classical suggestions of Eli Robins and Samuel Guze (1970), as well as Kenneth Kendler's multifaceted and multilevel approaches (1985, 1990), more than it does several reductive programs proposed Nancy Andreasen and Steven Hyman (Andreasen 1995; Hyman 2002), which may achieve success for future *ICD-12* and *DSM-VI* versions.

To assess the proper way that reductive etiopathogenic validity may figure in diagnostic classification, and also to motivate the notion of clinical validity, I want to begin from a provocative 2003 article by Robert Kendell and Assen Jablensky. Kendell and Jablensky proposed two strong conditions for validity. First they wrote, "We suggest . . . that a diagnostic category should be described as valid only if one of two conditions has been met. If the defining characteristic of the category is a syndrome, this syndrome must be demonstrated to be an entity, separated from neighboring syndromes and normality by a zone of rarity [i.e., interforms would be very rare]." They also proposed another condition, writing, "Alternatively, if the category's defining characteristics are more fundamental—that is, if the category is defined by a physiological, anatomical, histological, chromosomal, or molecular abnormality—clear, qualitative differences must exist between these defining characteristics and those of other conditions with a similar syndrome" (p. 8).

Although Kendell and Jablensky argue persuasively, I want to take a different approach. In my view, studies of simpler organisms such as regulatory mechanisms in bacteria and behavioral traits in the worm (*Caenorhabditis elegans*) and the fly (*Drosophila*) suggest that such traits will *not* resolve into discrete forms at the molecular level (Kendler and Greenspan 2006). I think the evidence demonstrates that there are numerous interforms and *quantitative* traits: *this is dimensionality all the way down.* A good example of this is found in the operon model of gene regulation in bacteria, where there are many interforms—what Benjamin Lewin, the author of a major textbook on molecular genetics, called "a panoply of operons" (Lewin 1994). Expecting discreteness because of fundamentality is, I think, a "Platonic" prejudice. It can be satisfied in chemistry, as in the periodic chart, but it is rare in biology.

A Prototype Approach

Variation and dimensionality can still be made tractable, by using an approach that identifies the most robust categories as prototypes, related to other prototypes by similarity; also compare Dominic Murphy's chapter in this volume. Some, such as Juan Mezzich (see Cantor et al. 1980), think that a related fuzzy set, grade of membership, analysis will also assist a prototype approach representation schema. I would argue that the prototype approach is supported by the deep structure of biology, and I develop such a prototype approach to biology, including genetics and the neurosciences, in my 1993 book (Schaffner 1993). In that 1993 book, I contrast the structure of the physical sciences, such as in mechanics, electromagnetic theory, and quantum mechanics, with an alternative theoretical structure for biology.

In my view, we do not have what Lee Cronbach and Paul Meehl, in their 1955 validity article, called a simple "network of [universal] laws" that constitutes a theory, either in biology, psychology, or psychiatry, though we do find such networks frequently in physics, and occasionally in chemistry (Cronbach and Meehl 1955). Rather, in biology, and I would argue eventually in psychiatry, we have families of models or mechanisms with, in any given subdiscipline, a few prototypes. These prototypes are typically interlevel: in biology they *intermingle* ions, molecules, cells, cell-cell circuits, and organs, in the same causal/temporal process—an issue I shall return to in a moment. The prototype models are related to each other by dimensional similarity, and there are many interforms. The prototypes in this view are narrow classes, but do allow for lawlike/causal predictions, and explanations, sometimes just for individuals. Extensive variation among the models and mechanisms is a natural consequence of the result of how evolution operates: by replicating entities with many small variations, and assembling odds and ends—thus "tinkering," as François Jacob has written about evolution.

A prototype approach—again see Cantor et al. (1980), for an early discussion of this approach in psychiatry by Mezzich's group—can conform well to a polythetic categorical approach in the limiting case, but a prototype approach can also permit a dimensional representation. A dimensional approach coupled with a prototype analysis may, in point of fact, be emerging in *DSM-V* and *ICD-11,* particularly for the personality disorders. We may see a dimensional approach as a parallel analysis to a standard categorical definition—see First et al. (2002) and Helzer et al. (2006)—or we may see some hybrid approaches (Paul Pilkonis, personal communication, 2004). Such an approach, whether it be dimensional or hybrid, will have to be carefully developed and rigorously tested for clinical validity and user friendliness. An evidence-based psychiatry is key here. And the prototype-dimensional approach may also be more consistent with etiopathogenic validations to come in the future, perhaps in *ICD-12.*

Reductive versus Interlevel Approaches to Neurobiology

A close inspection of the disciplines of molecular genetics and neuroscience, including their research articles and textbooks, will indicate that the prototypes that are used in these sciences are actually and typically interlevel, and *not* unilevel and simply reductionistic (that is, one does not *only* use molecules in describing the results of studies in these areas).

These levels include atoms and molecules at the smallest level, but can range up through organisms and social groups and also include internal (subjective) monologue and intersubjective dialogue, as well as values, at the upper levels.

Recent work on how molecular geneticists explain the difference between social and solitary feeding in the worm, C. *elegans,* shows an interlevel example of a circuit in the worm controlling social feeding (see Schaffner, this volume, and de Bono et al. [2002] for details and Schaffner [1998a, 1998b] also, for background on the worm). That work suggests that important information, and generalizations, might be obtained at any level of aggregation—in fact, the molecular level may not be the best place to identify such information, intervene, and predict. Paying attention to interrelations and possible integrations among different levels of aggregation, often in the "same process," is an important feature of the biomedical sciences, and also for any science that depends on the basic biomedical sciences.

Clinical Utility and Clinical Validity

With these considerations as background, let us again return to Kendell and Jablensky's seminal 2003 paper to consider what type of validity might be feasible in the area of psychiatry. In that article, Kendell and Jablensky also sharply distinguish diagnostic *validity* from diagnostic *utility:* "In our view, it is crucial to maintain a clear distinction between validity and utility, and at present these two terms are often used as if they were synonyms." At this point in their article they cite Robert Spitzer's classic writings in connection with *DSM-III.* Kendell and Jablensky then add, "We propose that a diagnostic rubric may be said to possess utility if it provides nontrivial information about prognosis and likely treatment outcomes, and/or testable propositions about biological and social correlates" (p. 9).

Although the Kendall and Jablensky definition of utility is excellent, *it is also what has traditionally been called "predictive validity,"* as has been recently noted by First et al. (2004). To a philosophical pragmatist such as myself, such *utility* is constitutive of what we think of as *reality,* and thus such utility is an indicator of an appropriate form of validity (as predictive validity) in the realm of clinical reality.

How might we best try to think further about this complicated notion of "reality"? From my perspective, a philosophical pragmatist does not think we can directly access an independent reality. Rather, we can only "triangulate" or converge on it through multiple useful indicators and interventions in the world. There is no simple "gold standard" waiting "out there." The great American pragmatist Charles Saunders Peirce suggested we would only get to true reality at the end of time or when we had a completed science. Some of these triangulating indicators and interventions that help us toward a pragmatic reality do involve sophisticated technologies and long chains of inference (for example, gene action and functional magnetic resonance imaging results; see Mirnics et al. [2006]). But information from all levels, including high levels such as interpersonal experience—which may be "more real" for many purposes for a pragmatist than molecular pathways—will continue to be key for psychiatry.

A related issue has been discussed in both the philosophical and the psychiatric literature. This is whether, as we go forward with our more sophisticated understanding of molecular genetics and neuroscience, what we take to be reality, especially involving the standard set of mental disorders such as schizophrenia and depression, might radically change? The multilevel "reality" that we commit to as a result of this on-going (scientific) process is, I think, always provisional. Thus, it could be subject to major modifications via scientific revolutions of a Kuhnian sort, as described by Thomas Kuhn in his extraordinary *Structure of Scientific Revolutions* (1970). It is thus *possible* that our current classification categories will radically change and be replaced as a result of advancing genetics and neuroscience, a thesis that I have speculated on along with Herbert Harris (see Harris and Schaffner 1992).

My best guess at present, however, is that current *ICD-10* and *DSM-IV-TR* categories will *slowly* evolve etiopathogenically and, at the margins, rather than suffer a catastrophic collapse and replacement with some as yet unforeseeable psychiatric classification system. But we should also keep in mind yet another possibility—that our "Ptolemaic" *ICD-10/DSM-IV* classification system may continue as mainly *clinically valid,* while an etipathogenic, but horrendously complex and virtually *clinically useless* "Copernican" system, slowly emerges.

I have described this view changing view of reality as "conditionalized realism" in my 1993 book, and I will not go into this technical notion in the present chapter. In the book, I also show how two different senses of universal can be distinguished, a distinction that allows for universal-like causal predictions for individuals (the idea here is that "same conditions yield the same effects" can work for particulars). This analysis is a response to worries that we do not have any "laws" in biology, such as we do in physics. Pragmatism tolerates considerable flexibility, but it also prizes stable classifications and strong predictability.

In summary, I think that "reality," and attempts to validate our constructs and determine the real kinds in this reality, will take the form of provisional multilevel prototypes that interrelate dimensionally. I believe we will encounter these both in the clinical validity area, as well as ultimately—but perhaps not for many years to come—in the etiopathogenic area, because we do not have sound etiopathogenic reductionist prototypes, even in such well-plumbed areas as schizophrenia, as yet (see, for example, Harrison and Weinberger [2005] and my chapter in this volume).

Conclusion

On major substantive issues, I think I am in more agreement than disagreement with Zachar; we are triangulating together on a set of goals that are difficult to navigate toward, but are valuable destinations nonetheless. My largest disagreement with Zachar was over the fact that I tend to think evolutionary theory guidance is valuable only as a source for motivating proximate prototype thinking in psychiatry—but I am a Darwinian in biology. Ontogenetically, I argued that life is a bush, not a tree; and psychiatry will likely be likewise. Finally, I sketched a way that I think prototype thinking and refinements in the notion of clinical validity, what type of kinds we can discover or develop in psychiatry, as well as how rapidly etiopathogenic validity will be helpful, as psychiatry struggles on with its meanings of validity and their interrelations. Dealing with reality concepts is terribly difficult, as Zachar has shown us, but we cannot give up, and must continue to try and hold that tiger.

REFERENCES

Andreasen, N. C. 1995. The Validation of Psychiatric Diagnosis: New Models and Approaches. *American Journal of Psychiatry* 152(2):161–162.
Beckner, M. 1959. *The Biological Way of Thought*. New York: Columbia University Press.
Cantor, N., E. E. Smith, R.S. French, and J. Mezzich. 1980. Psychiatric Diagnosis as Prototype Categorization. *Journal of Abnormal Psychology* 89(2):181–193.

Cronbach, L. J., and P. E. Meehl. 1955. Construct Validity in Psychological Tests. *Psychological Bulletin* 52(4):281–302.

Crow, T. J. 2000. Schizophrenia as the Price That *Homo sapiens* Pays for Language: A Resolution of the Central Paradox in the Origin of the Species. *Brain Research: Brain Research Reviews* 31(2–3):118–129.

de Bono, M., D. M. Tobin, L. Davis, and C. I. Bargmann. 2002. Social Feeding in *Caenorhabditis elegans* Is Induced by Neurons That Detect Aversive Stimuli. *Nature* 419(6910):899–903.

First, M. B., C. C. Bell, B. Cuthbert, J. Krystal, et al. 2002. Personality Disorders and Relational Disorders: A Research Agenda for Addressing Crucial Gaps in DSM. In D. J. Kupfer, M. B. First, and D. A. Regier (eds.), *APA Research Agenda for DSM-V* (pp. 123–199). Washington, DC: American Psychiatric Association.

First, M. B., H. A. Pincus, J. B. Levine, J. B. Williams, et al. 2004. Clinical Utility as a Criterion for Revising Psychiatric Diagnoses. *American Journal of Psychiatry* 161(6):946–954.

Harris, H. W., and K. F. Schaffner. 1992. Molecular Genetics, Reductionism, and Disease Concepts in Psychiatry. *Journal of Medicine and Philosophy* 17(2):127–153.

Harrison, P. J., and D. R. Weinberger. 2005. Schizophrenia Genes, Gene Expression, and Neuropathology: On the Matter of Their Convergence. *Molecular Psychiatry* 10(1):40–68.

Helzer, J. E., H. C. Kraemer, and R. F. Krueger. 2006. The Feasibility and Need for Dimensional Psychiatric Diagnoses. *Psychological Medicine* 36:1–10.

Hull, D. L. 1988. *Science as a Process: An Evolutionary Account of the Social and Conceptual Development of Science.* Chicago: University of Chicago Press.

Hyman, S. E. 2002. Neuroscience, Genetics, and the Future of Psychiatric Diagnosis. *Psychopathology* 35(2–3):139–144.

Kendell, R., and A. Jablensky. 2003. Distinguishing between the Validity and Utility of Psychiatric Diagnoses. *American Journal of Psychiatry* 160(1):4–12.

Kendler, K. S. 1985. Diagnostic Approaches to Schizotypal Personality Disorder: A Historical Perspective. *Schizophrenia Bulletin* 11(4):538–553.

———. 1990. Toward a Scientific Psychiatric Nosology: Strengths and Limitations. *Archives of General Psychiatry* 47(10):969–973.

Kendler, K. S., and R. J. Greenspan. 2006. The Nature of Genetic Influences on Behavior: Lessons from "Simpler" Organisms. *American Journal of Psychiatry* 163(10):1683–1694.

Kuhn, T. S. 1970. *The Structure of Scientific Revolutions.* Chicago: University of Chicago Press.

Lander, E. S. 1999. Array of Hope. *Nature Genetics* 21(1 Suppl.):3–4.

Lewin, B. 1994. *Genes V.* New York: Oxford University Press.

Livesley, W. J., K. L. Jang, and P. A. Vernon. 1998. Phenotypic and Genetic Structure of Traits Delineating Personality Disorder. *Archives of General Psychiatry* 55(10):941–948.

Mayr, E. 1961. Cause and Effect in Biology. *Science* 134:1501–1506.

Mirnics, K., and P. Levitt. 2006. Critical Appraisal of DNA Microarrays in Psychiatric Genomics. *Biological Psychiatry* 60(2):163–176.

Peralta, V., and M. J. Cuesta. 2001. How Many and Which Are the Psychopathological Dimensions in Schizophrenia? Issues Influencing Their Ascertainment. *Schizophrenia Research* 49(3):269–285.

Robins, E., and S. B. Guze. 1970. Establishment of Diagnostic Validity in Psychiatric Illness: Its Application to Schizophrenia. *American Journal of Psychiatry* 126(7):983–987.

Schaffner, K. F. 1993. *Discovery and Explanation in Biology and Medicine*. Chicago: University of Chicago Press.

———. 1998a. Genes, Behavior, and Developmental Emergentism: One Process, Indivisible? *Philosophy of Science* 65:209–252.

———. 1998b. Model Organisms and Behavioral Genetics: A Rejoinder. *Philosophy of Science* 65:276–288.

Sneath, P. H. A., and R. R. Sokal. 1973. *Numerical Taxonomy: The Principles and Practice of Numerical Classification*. San Francisco: W. H. Freeman.

Sterelny, K., and P. E. Griffiths. 1999. *Sex and Death: An Introduction to Philosophy of Biology*. Chicago: University of Chicago Press.

CHAPTER 9

The Incredible Insecurity
of Psychiatric Nosology

KENNETH S. KENDLER, M.D.,
AND PETER ZACHAR, PH.D.

It is highly likely that this chapter will be judged the most accessible
in this volume, especially by those readers with stronger backgrounds
in mental health than philosophy. This introduction will, therefore, be
brief, providing some additional background information and a short
summary of the main points.

One of the themes running throughout this book is that even if the
generalizations discovered by scientists do not rise to the level of universal scientific laws, it is still important that they have a high degree
of stability. Stability, however, seems to be a particular problem in
psychiatry.

Psychiatrists have had to endure intense criticism for declassifying
homosexuality as a mental disorder by taking a vote of the membership. Is psychiatric nosology a scientific endeavor or the expression
of shifting political winds? Psychiatry's troubles in this regard are
not limited to sexual orientation. Is cross-dressing a disorder? Are
oppositional-defiant adolescents mentally ill? Should subthreshold
conditions be medicated? It helps psychiatry's case that astronomers
held a vote in 2006 to decide whether Pluto is really a planet, but the
astronomer's decision to rewrite the definition of a planet has not removed lingering doubts about the scientific legitimacy of psychiatric
nosology.

What about geographically limited diagnoses, such as amok, latah,
and koro? Are they unique medical conditions, cultural variants of
other *ICD* and *DSM* disorders, or perhaps social roles, but not actually
psychiatric disorders? In retrospect, the conversion disorders studied
by Freud and Charcot could have been late-Victorian versions of
(mostly) culture-bound syndromes. The concept of a culture-bound

syndrome also suggests that psychiatric disorders that do not currently exist could appear at some future date as social conditions evolve.

Finally, there is the more subtle but equally important issue of the relationship between researchers and the operationalized diagnostic categories of the *DSM*. If psychiatry is a progressive discipline and each new edition of the manual is an improvement on the past, does that mean that studies using old criteria are outdated? Did latent schizophrenia, neurasthenia, and inadequate personality cease to exist when the *DSM-III* was published? Did they ever really exist? Will borderline and narcissistic personality disorders be judged never to have existed if the *DSM-V* adopts a thoroughgoing dimensional model?

An understandable impulse on reading James Woodward's notion of explanatory invariance and Sandra Mitchell's ideas about the continuum of stability is to say that psychiatry should evolve in the direction of valuing increased stability in the same way that Dominic Murphy claims it should develop in a more etiological direction. Perhaps psychiatrists have been too tolerant of diagnostic fads and should be more minimalist with respect to future revisions of the manual. Raising the bar in this way might attenuate destabilizing political influences. Science is a community project and politics exist in all communities, but it is a little unseemly when putative scientists become determined advocates and wage spirited campaigns for their favored changes in the manual or against unwanted changes.

The arguments in this chapter are inspired by an honest acknowledgment that there is something seductive about putting psychiatry on a more secure path to being the kind of science that studies what philosophers call natural kinds, or objective entities whose reality is not influenced by shifting political winds and that exist regardless of whether we recognize them. A careful reading of various claims made in this book, however, also leads to the conclusion that we should not allow ourselves to be so easily seduced. Neither should we deny the value of stability in a psychiatric nosology or be pessimistic about potential progress in this area. One can seek increased stability without making a religion of it.

This chapter, therefore, explores different strategies for establishing greater degrees of stability in psychiatry. Some of Kenneth Kendler and Peter Zachar's proposals suggest that increased resources should be devoted to studying all aspects of conditions such as major depressive disorder and schizophrenia, not merely those symptoms that the *DSM* enumerates to signal their presence. Psychiatry and psychology should pay more attention to content validity and not confuse the diagnostic criteria chosen to efficiently detect a disorder with the disorder itself. Two ways to be more comprehensive are to expand (or develop) structured clinical interviews to assess a broader range of data, including phenomenological data, and use psychological tests to collect information about normal and abnormal personality traits.

Another key idea offered in this chapter examines stability in the context of evolutionary theory. Although his claims are not without critics, Paul Ekman's notion of basic emotions also suggests some avenues for seeking increased stability in psychiatry. Ekman's basic emotions (namely, fear, anger, sadness, joy, disgust, and surprise) are supposed to be evolutionary homologues shared widely throughout the mammalian line and across cultures among *Homo sapiens*. Is it possible that there could also be basic psychiatric disorders?

Kendler and Zachar do not have an answer to that question, but it seems that, if the evolutionary clock could be set back and allowed to run multiple times, things like dominance hierarchies and broken bones would always emerge. Why not certain psychiatric disorders as well? This chapter is mostly a thought experiment, so the authors don't nominate any candidate disorders, but they do suggest that achieving increased stability may not always be a matter of developing more fine-grained and precise categories; rather, stability may be found in studying broader categories. The internalizing and externalizing dimensions constitute two possible pathways in this direction. They may even reveal some unity to the history of psychiatry that is hidden by visible but shifting diagnostic categories.

Peter Zachar, Ph.D.

*   *   *

While we have many reasons to feel excited about the future of psychiatric science, we have a critical point of vulnerability: the instability of its diagnostic system. After a brief introduction to the nature of this problem, we illustrate this liability with a fictional story. We then describe a series of practical ways to manage this problem in the short term. The next section raises a longer-term problem about the nature of the diagnostic categories we are trying to describe. We then view our current nosology from the perspective of two frameworks drawn from the philosophy of science: concepts of "explanatory invariance" and "levels of conditionality." We then explore the possibility of anchoring diagnoses in constants of the human condition. We conclude that, although nosologic instability in psychiatry is beyond a full resolution, the adverse effects on the progress of scientific psychiatry can be reduced.

1. Classification and the Conceptual Status of Psychiatric Nosology

Classification is fundamental to any scientific discipline. Particle physicists rely on the current classification of quarks and neutrinos. Chemists depend on their periodic table. Molecular biologists cannot proceed without distinguishing among different kinds of amino acids and proteins, and field biologists require their catalog of animal and plant species.

Classification is equally fundamental to the science of psychiatry. Whether we are doing epidemiologic studies, searching for genes, tracing neural circuits, or describing the pain and suffering of psychiatric patients, our results are typically organized and communicated through diagnostic categories. Yet how secure are these diagnoses? Is psychiatric nosology more akin to the periodic table of elements (a stable, objective feature of our universe) or to the stages of European history (social constructions, endlessly debated and shifting inevitably from one generation of historians to the next)?

2. Nosological Insecurity

Empirical researchers who study psychiatric illness potentially live in a state of nosological insecurity. Let us illustrate this with a story.

Starting in 1994, a psychiatric researcher begins accumulating detailed data on the genetics, natural history, and treatment response of disorder X. In all this research, she has used the *DSM-IV* criteria as assessed by one of the specifically developed diagnostic interviews. She awakes one morning in 2012, after eighteen years of detailed research, to find that the newly released *DSM-V* has proposed adding several new criteria for disorder X and eliminating others. She searches frantically through the structured interview and the rest of her data base and finds that she did not collect the information needed to rate these new criteria. She is in despair, anticipating that the value of her work will substantially decline. The diagnostic category she has been using will be viewed as "out of date" and "old fashioned." It will be more difficult, she concludes, to publish her work in the best journals or to obtain additional grant support to continue her investigations.

Although this story may seem overly dramatic, past revisions have introduced major changes in criteria and eliminated disorders. Editors and referees also complain about studies that use older criteria. Two reasons for these complaints come to mind. First, it has been said that the *DSM* is the psychiatrist's bible (Kutchins and Kirk 1997). As with bibles, some thinkers tend to take the *DSM* descriptions literally. *Diagnostic literalists* will be particularly concrete about current editions of the manual.

Second, psychiatry, like any science, is supposed to be progressive. Editors and referees who focus on the progressive nature of each new edition of the manual may be uncomfortable publishing studies that use what they see as the imperfections of the past.

Although these two groups may torment our fictional researcher for different reasons, the outcome of each set of reasons seems equally problematic with respect to long-term research programs. Can anything be done to prevent the occurrence of such problems and increase the stability of psychiatry's diagnostic categories?

3. Responses to Nosologic Insecurity—Part I
Don't Build Castles on Sand; Or, Avoid Planned Obsolescence

Most data-collection projects in psychiatry use structured psychiatric interviews as the major method of data collection. These interviews are typically designed to operationalize one or a small number of specific diagnostic systems. That is, the goal in most clinical and epidemiologic work is not to gather a detailed historical and symptomatic evaluation of psychiatric disorders. Rather, it has become "to collect data sufficient to assess all the diagnostic criteria for a particular condition in *DSM*." This represents a form of institutionalized tunnel vision.

Our structured psychiatric interviews are like animals evolved to function in a specific ecological niche. With a slight shift in the environment, they are vulnerable to extinction. By collecting only data specific to one *DSM* (or *ICD*) version and using the different combinations of those criteria to make a decision on the presence or absence of a disorder, we make our research especially vulnerable to shifts in diagnostic criteria.

Become Phenomenologists (Again)

There was a time in psychiatry when the careful study of phenomenology of psychiatric illness was highly valued. Since the introduction of various editions of the *DSM* and the demands of managed care, this skill and orientation—the careful observation and recording of the signs and symptoms exhibited by our patients—has been devalued. It has now become standard, in both clinical and research evaluations, to limit assessments to the determination of the presence or absence of the needed *DSM* diagnostic criteria.

Ironically, although the DSM institutionalizes the approach called *descriptive diagnosis,* it is actually remarkably thin, descriptively. The operationalized criteria for the various disorders have become the phenomenal universe of what is assessed. The actual phenomenal universe of any family of conditions is considerably larger, as exemplified in thicker descriptions by authors such as Emil Kraepelin (1907) and Aubry Lewis (1967).

Furthermore, because they are descriptively impoverished, our current diagnostic classifications are unlikely to be optimal for mapping onto the results of studies in many research areas such as imaging, neurobiology and genetics. By restricting our clinical evaluations to *DSM* criteria, we reduce the chances of better understanding the etiologic pathways to psychiatric illness.

Specific diagnostic criteria will always represent a compromise between economy and depth. They are not designed to and never will be able to represent the full richness of the conditions we study. Structured interviews will necessarily be limited, but it would be better to have diagnostic interviews that provide a richer assessment of the key dimensions of psychopathology rather than being tied, in lock-step, to the latest diagnostic criteria.

This approach will come at a cost. It will take more time and money to assess carefully a range of psychiatric signs and symptoms. For some research questions—where "counting" or quantity of subjects assessed will be most important—we may have to use a "stripped-down" set of *DSM* criteria, but this should be the exception rather than the rule.

Avoid Presentism and Be Realistic about What Has Been Accomplished

Although pride in the "*DSM* revolution" is justified, the accomplishments of U.S. psychiatric nosology since *DSM-III* are often exaggerated. We have improved the reliability of psychiatric diagnoses, but there is little evidence that the validity of our major categories has substantially improved. Therefore, it is hard to claim that *DSM-IV* criteria are superior to those found in *DSM-III-R* or *DSM-III*. Just because a set of diagnostic criteria is from the "latest" *DSM* edition does not, in and of itself, mean that it is better than what has come before.

It is critical to avoid the "presentism" so prominent in American culture at large. To avoid resembling the world of fashion, where only the latest "styles" are valued, reviewers of submitted articles and grants should be cautious in criticizing research work solely because it utilizes diagnostic criteria other than the most recent *DSM* edition.

Study Traits as Well as Disorders

Psychiatric disorders are currently conceptualized as complex syndromes made up of a collection of more basic symptoms and signs. These symptoms and signs are, in turn, often reflections of underlying psychobiological traits such as neuroticism and impulsivity (Krueger 1999; Kendler et al. 2003). In addition to an appropriate focus on diagnostic categories, another way for researchers to protect themselves from the effects of diagnostic instability at the level of syndromes is to also study these underlying traits. Assessing traits will throw a wider net descriptively and formal measures of traits will not change according to a programmed schedule like the *DSM* and the *ICD*. They are potentially stable across versions, and differences between new and older trait models can be easily assessed.

Don't Make Small Changes in Diagnostic Criteria

The human desire to tinker is nearly irresistible, but logic suggests that small changes made to diagnostic criteria are more likely to be harmful than helpful. Small changes are unlikely to affect substantially reliability and validity while also requiring a retooling of previously collected data sets. In light of the adverse effects of diagnostic change on ongoing research, our nosologic process should have a rigorous set of "criteria for changing criteria" (Rounsaville et al. 2002) and enforce them strictly. Such an effort is needed to counter-act the often strong desire of members of *DSM* workgroups to leave their imprint on the *DSM* criteria.

For example, to increase the distinction between generalized anxiety disorder (GAD) and panic disorder, criteria assessing arousal were eliminated from the assessment of GAD in the *DSM-IV.* The resulting change led to an emphasis on distress criteria, which increased the overlap with depression (Watson 2005). Similar problems occurred in the *DSM-III* definitions of histrionic and borderline personalities. Making "hysteria" more pathological by transforming it into histrionic personality and reducing the overlap between borderline personality and psychotic disorders resulted in histrionic and borderline personalities being difficult to distinguish. This led authors of the *DSM-III-R* to alter criteria to better distinguish the two disorders (Gunderson et al. 1995; Pfohl 1995). In each of these cases, and unbeknownst to diagnostic literalists, the world didn't change; only the criteria did.

Study History to Dampen the Swings

The past century has seen massive changes in the basic paradigms of the field. The changes from psychoanalysis to biological psychiatry have been particularly wrenching. Such shifts and the associated prophesies that the new method (be it neuropathology, psychoanalysis, neurochemistry, imaging, or genetics) will solve all the major problems of psychiatry are a symptom of our scientific and philosophical immaturity. Just as we hope that further maturation will dampen affective instability in our adolescent patients, we should hope that our field learns to keep its center and avoid large and dramatic shifts in the future. A balanced understanding of history is usually a partial antidote to the passions that fuel some of our more contentious debates.

4. A Deeper View of the Problem
Surviving "Tape Rewinds"

The evolutionary biologist Stephen J. Gould (1990) wondered what would happen if we could repeatedly rewind the tape of history and begin evolution anew. He argues that it is improbable that anything like human life would have evolved on earth because it was too dependent on a host of random, unrepeatable influences such as an asteroid hitting the earth 65 million years ago and wiping out the dinosaurs.

For our purposes, we suggest rewinding the tape for only about 10,000 years—to the end of the last ice age. At this point, modern *Homo sapiens* had completely evolved and agriculture and cities were soon to develop. Waiting long enough, something like our modern medicine would, we assume, develop from which a field somewhat like psychiatry would eventually emerge. At some point, this field would want a formal nosology and would create one. The key question is, *How much would that nosology resemble the current DSM?* There are too many random factors to be confident that a "tape rewind" would produce something closely resembling our current system. But would it be completely different?

Because basic human biology has changed little in 10,000 years, such afflictions as broken bones, diabetes, and strokes are likely to appear after every rewind. Some features of human social organization such as dominance hierarchies and pair bonding would also likely be relatively constant. What about psychiatric disorders? How often would we find syndromes resembling schizophrenia, autism, major depression, dysthymia, panic disorder, or narcissistic personality on these "tape rewinds"?

Good Scientific Theories, Good Scientific Categories

Philosophers of science have carefully thought about the criteria by which to judge the quality of scientific theories and the objects and processes modeled by these theories. Two concepts developed by these philosophers can illuminate the instability problem faced by psychiatric nosology. These are the concepts of *explanatory invariance* and *conditionalities.*

Explanatory Invariance

James Woodward (2003) argues that explanatory invariance is a central characteristic toward which scientific theories strive (see also his chapter in this book). Traditionally, explanations or *causal generalizations* that are stable and apply to a wide range of conditions have been called laws. Also traditionally, science is supposed to seek laws. Causal generalizations that only apply some of the time have not been considered to be true laws.

The problem is that many explanations in biology and the social sciences are true in only a limited set of background conditions. Consider, for example, two statements: (1) p*sychoanalytic psychotherapy is an effective treatment for personality disorders* and (2) *the proper administration of a vaccine cures rabies.* Statement 1 has a low level of explanatory invariance because, although it might be true for a patient with a particular social background (for example, Western, college-educated, psychologically minded, and articulate), it is unlikely to apply to individuals with very different cultural or educational backgrounds (for example, New Guinea tribesperson, Peruvian highland coca farmer). By contrast, statement 2 has high explanatory invariance because the treatment works for individuals across all cultural and social groups.

This principle can also be applied to the generalizations we make about psychiatric diagnoses. Those diagnoses with low explanatory invariance permit generalizations that are applicable in only limited historical or cultural contexts and would infrequently arise in "tape rewinds." Those with high degrees of explanatory invariance permit generalizations that can be observed across the wide range of human conditions and would be expected to emerge reliably from most "tape rewinds."

Conditionalities

In her evaluation of scientific theories, Sandra Mitchell (2003) introduces the closely related concept of *conditionalities.* By this we mean What are the things that have to be true in order for the world to exist as it does?

For example, the existence of fundamental entities of physics and chemistry (subatomic particles, elements) are conditional on particular physical constants of our universe. If certain of these values differed, stable atoms could not exist. But, given these constants, which apply uniformly throughout our universe, these entities are invariant and will always be found.

The entities of biology such as species share all the conditionalities of physics, and then some. They are all dependent on the emergence of life on Earth. Species are also conditional on historical events because evolution is an historical process in a way that is not true of physics or chemistry. Species come and go over time. This is not true of the periodic table.

Where in this framework of conditionalities do psychiatric diagnoses sit? Certainly, they have all the conditionalities of biology because psychiatry primarily studies only one species as evolved on one planet, but psychiatric nosology has a host of other conditionalities. Our current nosology is conditional on the existence of certain historical individuals such as Kraepelin, Schneider, and Spitzer, without whose influence the nature of our manual would surely be different.

Our diagnostic system has also been influenced by major historical events (for example, the Vietnam war leading to increased interest in post-traumatic stress disorder), the development of new treatments (for example, the interest in panic disorder following the discovery that it was an antidepressant responsive form of "anxiety neurosis" [Klein 1964]), changing social values (which have affected our approach toward homosexuality and the premenstrual syndrome), broad cultural influences (such as the rising prevalence of bulimia in non-Western cultures due to increased acceptance of "Western" standards canons of feminine beauty [Keel and Klump 2003]), and diagnostic fads within the mental health community (for example, multiple personality disorder).

Even for the same class of disorder, signs and symptoms tend to vary from patient to patient. As the concept of *pathoplasticity* suggests (Birnbaum 1974), psychological and cultural conditions can so strongly influence the presentation of disorders that the same underlying diagnostic entity can appear in diverse ways.

5. Responses to Nosologic Insecurity—Part II
Can Psychiatric Disorders Be Nonconditional and Can Causal Generalizations about Them Be Invariant?

One way to increase the stability of psychiatric diagnoses would be to give priority to the classification of disorders that might survive multiple tape rewinds. These disorders could be expected to have *low conditionality*—their existence and recognition is not dependent on a particular historical, individual, or social movements, and they are likely to be recognized across most historical and cultural milieus and *high explanatory invariance*—and the generalizations we make about them can be applied to most cases in most situations.

If pursued, this strategy would prescribe anchoring psychiatric diagnoses in human constants. These constants would include basic aspects of our neurobiology or relatively stable aspects of our social and cultural life. We could even be encouraged in this venture by evidence that the emotional aspects of human facial expressions (Ekman et al. 1969) and the structure of personality (McCrae and Terracciano 2005) appear to be cross-culturally stable and would likely replicate well over multiple tape rewinds. Perhaps some psychiatric disorders would as well.

A Conflict

Ian Hacking (1998) describes the rise and fall of a psychiatric syndrome termed "automatisme ambulatoire" that was characterized by compulsive wandering in a fugue state with associated loss of memory. He suggests that this syndrome was a "niche diagnosis" because it arose in a geographically limited area—being common in France, rarely seen in Germany, and nearly unknown in Great Britain and the United States. It was temporally limited and was commonly diagnosed for only a twenty-two-year period from 1887 to 1909. Finally, it arose in and was influenced by a temporally and culturally specific set of social and psychological factors.

Niche diagnoses will be unlikely to appear on "tape rewinds" because of their high degree of conditionality on specific historical, social, and cultural factors. To the extent that nosological stability is a legitimate goal for psychiatric classification, a high threshold should be applied to the acceptance of "new" psychiatric disorders, especially those that arise in specific cultural and social contexts.

However, and here is the rub, new disorders do appear. The past 100 years have seen, for example, the rise of bulimia, phencyclidine abuse, and post-traumatic stress disorder, conditions that, in different ways, have been influenced by recent cultural, pharmacological, and historical developments. Would we want to argue that, because of their recency, they are not legitimate psychiatric disorders?

We have here an open conflict between the needs of psychiatric science for nosologic stability and the practical need of the psychiatric clinician to be able to have diagnoses that reflect the syndromes that present for treatment. This conflict illustrates clearly the tensions between competing needs of our nosologic system. Our research enterprise will be best served by focusing on disorders that are largely independent of social and historical forces. Clinicians might, by contrast, argue that they can ill afford that luxury if it leaves them without good categories with which to classify their patients.

A Possible Way Out: Levels of Analysis and Hierarchical Structure

The reliability of psychiatric diagnosis is typically higher for broader classes of disorders than it is for individual disorders. For example, two diagnosticians will agree that a particular patient has an anxiety disorder more often than they will agree on what specific anxiety disorder the patient has.

This finding raises the possibility that we might seek constancy at levels in our nosology higher than that of the specific diagnosis. The question becomes what levels in the diagnostic hierarchy have the highest degrees of stability, being recognized throughout the world and throughout history?

For example, a range of recent studies have suggested a clear, empirically supported higher-order structure for common psychiatric disorders of adolescence and adulthood, captured by the two underlying dimensions of internalizing and externalizing disorders (Krueger et al. 1998; Krueger 1999; Kendler et al. 2003). Studies in genetically informative samples have shown genetic and environmental risk factors that are shared across phobia subtypes (Kendler et al. 2001) and personality disorder clusters (Kendler et al. 2006). Broader diagnostic classes such as externalizing disorders or odd, eccentric personality disorders are likely to be less conditional and higher on explanatory invariance than individual disorders. This would be particularly plausible for phobias because some phobic stimuli (for example, tall buildings, airplanes, needles, and public speaking) will be rare or entirely absent in certain cultures and historical epochs.

Focusing on broader diagnostic classes is not likely to resolve nosological insecurity, but it could dampen it. Indeed, the conflict between the scientific need for nosologic stability and the clinical need for a diagnostic system sensitive to changing social and cultural conditions reflects deep tensions inherent in a field like psychiatry with divergent constituencies.

When our fictional researcher wakes up in 2012 to find that the diagnostic criteria have changed, it is unlikely that the broader diagnostic class that she is studying has been entirely eliminated. As long her specific disorder can be associated with the still existing diagnostic class, her research will still be of relevance. Her situation would be more secure if structured diagnostic interviews, in addition to assessing criteria specific to an individual disorder, routinely assessed broader aspects of psychopathology at the level of the class.

An obvious corollary of our position is that nosologists should be considerably more accepting of new or "niche" diagnoses that reflect variations of a broader class than on those with no resemblance to other conditions in the current or past diagnostic manuals. For example, although simple deteriorative disorder (simple schizophrenia) was a "new" diagnosis introduced into the appendix in *DSM-IV,* it in fact had an extensive historical pedigree and both clinical and research findings suggesting a close relationship with the accepted more classical schizophrenic syndromes (Kendler et al. 1994).

The approach we are suggesting here could attenuate the effect of diagnostic literalism. We see no value to such literalism at any level of analysis, but its presence is an unavoidable reality. In the approach we are suggesting, a preference for stable kinds can be fulfilled by the devoting diagnostic attention to the higher-order classes—the constants of psychiatry. The conditions further down in the hierarchy might be more readily seen as variations.

What about the proponents of scientific progressivism? According to the progressive viewpoint, our fictional researcher is using an outdated category. There is something important in the progressive viewpoint that needs to be respected. In the approach we are suggesting, the constants of psychiatry are often going to be rather broad constructs, and they can be instantiated in various forms. Although it is important to identify and study the most typical forms, it should still be possible to learn something about the constant itself by studying older categories, especially if an older category is a direct ancestor of a current category.

6. Conclusion

We live at a time of great promise for research into the etiology and treatment of psychiatric disorders. Because of its potential instability, our diagnostic system represents a weak link in our science. We are truly at risk for *building castles on sand.* This chapter suggests that we can limit the damage from our nosologic insecurity by a few practical steps. Informed by approaches to evaluate the quality of scientific theories, we then explore the deeper issue of the conditionalities of our diagnoses. We suggest that our field should strive for diagnoses that would survive multiple "tape rewinds," trying to improve the explanatory invariance of the disorders we study and treat by grounding them in constants of the human condition. We close by noting that the pathoplastic features of psychiatric disorders need to be recognized. One potential way to compromise between the need of psychiatric science for stable entities and the need for clinical psychiatry to have classifications for the diverse and culturally influenced syndromes is to permit variation at the lowest level of the diagnostic species, but at the genus level to focus on maximally invariant conditions.

ACKNOWLEDGMENTS

This work has been supported in part by National Institutes of Health grants DA-011287 and MH-068643 and by the Rachel Brown Banks Endowment Fund.

REFERENCES

Birnbaum, K. 1974. The Making of a Psychosis: The Principles of Structural Analysis in Psychiatry. In S. R. Hirsch and M. Shepherd (eds.), *Themes and Variations in European Psychiatry: An Anthology* (pp. 199–238). Charlottesville: University Press of Virginia.

Ekman, P., E. R. Sorenson, and W. V. Friesen. 1969. Pan-cultural Elements in Facial Displays of Emotion. *Science* 164:86–88.

Gould, S. J. 1990. *Wonderful Life: The Burgess Shale and the Nature of History.* New York: W. W. Norton.

Gunderson, J. G., M. C. Zanarini, and C. L. Kisiel. 1995. Borderline Personality Disorder. In W. J. Livesley (ed.), *The DSM-IV Personality Disorders* (pp. 141–157). New York: Guilford Press.

Hacking, I. 1998. *Mad Travelers: Reflections on the Reality of Transient Mental Illnesses.* Charlottesville: University Press of Virginia.

Keel, P. K., and K. L. Klump. 2003. Are Eating Disorders Culture-bound Syndromes? Implications for Conceptualizing Their Etiology. *Psychological Bulletin* 129:747–769.

Kendler, K. S., N. Czajkowski, K. Tambs, S. Torgersen, et al. 2006. Dimensional Representations of *DSM-IV* Cluster A Personality Disorders in a Population-based Sample of Norwegian Twins: A Multivariate Study. *Psychological Medicine* Aug 8 [epub], 1–9.

Kendler, K. S., M. McGuire, A. M. Gruenberg, and D. Walsh. 1994. An Epidemiologic, Clinical, and Family Study of Simple Schizophrenia in County Roscommon, Ireland. *American Journal of Psychiatry* 151:27–34.

Kendler, K. S., J. Myers, C. A. Prescott, and M. C. Neale. 2001. The Genetic Epidemiology of Irrational Fears and Phobias in Men. *Archives of General Psychiatry* 58:257–265.

Kendler, K. S., C. A. Prescott, J. Myers, and M. C. Neale. 2003. The Structure of Genetic and Environmental Risk Factors for Common Psychiatric and Substance Use Disorders in Men and Women. *Archives of General Psychiatry* 60:929–937.

Klein, D. F. 1964. Delineation of Two Drug-responsive Anxiety Syndromes. *Psychpharmacologia* 5:397–408.

Kraepelin, E. 1907. *Clinical Psychiatry: A Text-Book for Students and Physicians.* Abstracted and adapted from the 7th German edition of Kraepelin's *Lehrbuch der Psychiatrie,* by A. Ross Diefendorf, MD. New York: Macmillan.

Krueger, R. F. 1999. The Structure of Common Mental Disorders. *Archives of General Psychiatry* 56:921–926.

Krueger, R. F., A. Caspi, T. E. Moffitt, and P. A. Silva. 1998. The Structure and Stability of Common Mental Disorders (*DSM-III-R*): A Longitudinal-epidemiological Study. *Journal of Abnormal Psychology* 107:216–227.

Kutchins, H., and S. A. Kirk. 1997. *Making Us Crazy—DSM: The Psychiatric Bible and the Creation of Mental Disorders.* New York: Free Press.

Lewis, A. 1967. Melancholia: A Clinical Survey of Depressive States. In A. Lewis (ed.), *Inquiries in Psychiatry: Clinical and Social Investigations* (pp. 30–72). New York: Science House.

McCrae, R. R., and A. Terracciano. 2005. Universal Features of Personality Traits from the Observer's Perspective: Data from 50 Cultures. *Journal of Personality and Social Psychology* 88:547–561.

Mitchell, S. D. 2003. *Biological Complexity and Integrative Pluralism.* Cambridge: Cambridge University Press.

Pfohl, B. 1995. Histrionic Personality Disorder. In W. J. Livesley (ed.), *The DSM-IV Personality Disorders* (pp. 173–192). New York: Guilford Press.

Rounsaville, B. J., R. D. Alarcon, G. Andrews, J. S. Jackson, et al. 2002. Basic Nomenclature Issues for *DSM-V.* In D. J. Kupfer, M. B. First, and D. A. Regier (eds.), *A Research Agenda for DSM-V* (pp. 1–29). Washington, DC: American Psychiatric Association.

Watson, D. 2005. Rethinking the Mood and Anxiety Disorders: A Quantitative Hierarchical Model for *DSM-V. Journal of Abnormal Psychology* 114:522–536.

Woodward, J. 2003. *Making Things Happen.* New York: Oxford University Press.

Comment: Psychiatric Diagnosis

Josef Parnas, M.D., Dr. Med. Sci.

Although I almost fully agree with the picture that Kenneth Kendler and Peter Zachar draw of the psychiatric nosology and its problems, I nonetheless have a couple of comments and supplements.

Kendler and Zachar take the contemporary operational psychopathology, with its diagnostic categories based on a specific number of criteria, as an unquestioned starting point for future improvements, which they propose, such as assessing psychopathological features that are themselves not the diagnostic criteria. Yet it is perhaps thinkable (and possible) that the impasse of psychiatric diagnosis is not independent of the basic assumptions of psychiatric operationalism (see also the section on phenomenology): (a) that grasping and describing experience (that is, symptoms and consciousness) is analogous to describing a physical object or a thing, (b) that is possible to define operationally the majority of psychiatric terms and concepts, and (c) that a membership of a diagnostic class is most optimally assured by fulfilling the number of required criteria, without any *prototypical considerations,* that is any considerations of how much the patient *resembles the typical exemplars* of the diagnostic category in question (see a classic, instructive article by Schwartz and Wiggins [1987]). I think that none of these three assumptions can resist a critical analysis.

This type of critique is often dismissed as being subjectivistic and therefore useless but such dismissal does not eliminate the root problems. The situation is like in a joke: a man is searching under a street light for his lost keys; asked where he lost the keys, he answers, "On the other side of the street, but there is such a good light here."

The possibility of "tape rewind" reminds us of the immense contingency of human existence. I also think that it should dampen the scientific appeals to evolution, especially in the context of psychiatry, if only, because cognition is too soft to leave a paleontological record (Fodor 1998).

To Kendler and Zachar's list of concrete proposals of steps aiming at improving the stability of psychiatric nosology, we could perhaps add two measures. First, there are all reasons to believe—as forcefully articulated by Immanel Kant—that human experience or subjectivity is not amorphous but has certain invariant structures. We should study potential alterations of these structures in various psychopathological conditions. This is the task of phenomenological psychopathology, the task of *basic psychopathological research.* Second, a closer collaboration of psychiatry with psychology, neuropsychology, developmental psychology, and the cognitive sciences may expand the repertoire of aspects, dimensions, or facets of human behavior that could be useful in improving the explanatory invariance of psychiatric concepts.

REFERENCES

Fodor, J. 1998. *In Critical Condition: Polemical Essays on Cognitive Science and the Philosophy of Mind.* Cambridge, MA: MIT Press.

Schwartz, M. A., and O. P. Wiggins. 1987. Diagnosis and Ideal Types. *Comprehensive Psychiatry* 28:271–291.

Epilogue

JOSEF PARNAS, M.D., DR.MED.SCI.

In this epilogue I highlight a few issues that have clearly emerged in the main contributions and arguments of this volume. I also mention some other aspects, only marginally addressed in this volume, but which naturally belong to the field of philosophy of psychiatry, and provide some further introductory reading suggestions, in case we have whetted the appetite of any of our readers to delve further into this fascinating field.

Philosophy

This volume testifies to Kenneth Kendler's claim in the introduction that there is an intimate and, indeed, fundamental link between psychiatry and philosophy. At each step of her working life, a scientist and a mental health professional is confronted with the issues all of which have important, if only potential or implicit, theoretical, and philosophical implications.

Psychiatrists encounter patients who are real people inhabiting specific cultural and social contexts and who have, for one reason or another (and sometimes, by what almost seems "a chance"), crossed the locally prevailing threshold of contact with treatment facilities. We classify their sufferings, experiences, beliefs, and actions, seek explanations for these descriptive categories, and offer therapeutic measures. One important, perhaps even crucial, difference between psychiatry and other branches of medicine is the pivotal role of experience or consciousness in defining the very subject matter of psychiatry. From that, it is therefore only a small step to facing up to a variety of philosophical questions, ranging from describing experience, classifying phenotypes, discussing the notions of causality, explanation, and understanding and the accompanying views on the building blocks of reality, its segmentation into constituents or "levels," and the place of consciousness in nature. Just to try analyzing the concept of "belief" risks losing oneself in endless ruminations.

Naturally, the editors and contributors of this volume did not invent the link between psychiatry and philosophy. This link was always somehow, even if often marginally, present in psychiatry from its beginnings. It was clearly and forcefully articulated by Karl Jaspers in the first half of the twentieth century. In our own time, we are witnessing a new and steady surge of philosophical interest in psychiatry, perhaps as a sign of certain intellectual and professional dissatisfaction with the continuing absence of magic etiological bullets and the limitations of the modes of thinking that are now prominent in the field.

The World Psychiatric Association, as well as the British, American, and other national associations, have established specific sections on philosophy of psychiatry, and a similar trend is visible in psychology. The Johns Hopkins University Press publishes *Philosophy, Psychiatry, and Psychology,* a journal devoted to philosophical issues in psychiatry and psychology, with many articles of direct clinical or scientific relevance. The Oxford University Press publishes a book series on philosophy and psychiatry. Earlier, yet still valuable publications in psychiatry and philosophy include John Sadler and colleagues' 1994 volume focusing on the nosological issues, and two other collections focusing on psychopathology, both edited by Manfred Spitzer (Spitzer et al. 1988; Spitzer and Maher 1990).

This volume addresses many and diverse issues, with a dominant focus on the philosophy of science and with a lesser emphasis on the philosophy of mind and the metaphysical questions ("metaphysical" means here pertaining to the nature or essence of what exists). What the presented arguments achieve—spelled out on a concrete scientific background—is

a sensitization of the reader against dogmatism (that is, any rigid conviction that one particular doctrine or perspective on the nature of and causes
for psychiatric illness is true and nearly complete and therefore the only
one worth seriously entertaining). Our knowledge is always partial, our
arguments are always played out within a certain framework of overarching, often tacit assumptions, and we are rarely aware of the full range of
sociological or cultural influences shaping our beliefs—all that despite our
deliberate careful strivings for objectivity. What we consider as knowledge of facts or as an adequate frame of reference for gaining such knowledge is, or at least should be, open to critical questioning and reflection,
including the questioning of underlying conceptual foundations of our
scientific claims and activities. This is neither an invitation to relativism
where "anything goes" nor a misplaced echo of postmodernism. Rather, it
is a call for a certain intellectual modesty, an openness to other and new
ideas, and a willingness to engage in a critical self-reflection. We don't
have to put up with artificial dichotomies that are often foisted on us. One
has to consider either only the frequently wonderful advances in systems
and molecular neuroscience or only the psychological and social context
often so important in the etiology and development of psychiatric illness.
One is either a "hard-nosed" true scientist in your pursuit of the causes of
mental illness or a soft-headed and soft-hearted advocate of the subjective
and the mental.

A helpful and instructive volume for psychiatrists and scientists to
consult in this context is Maxwell Bennett and Peter Hacker's *Philosophical Foundations of Neuroscience* (2003). The authors, a neuroscientist
and a philosopher, critically examine the main, often highly renowned,
neuroscientific explanatory models for the phenomena of perception, cognition, experience, and volition.

Causation

As doctors, raised in biology, we wish to uncover the causal chain of
(molecular) biological events to which more complex phenomena may be
reduced and to specify the mechanism of causal transition from the cause
C to the effect E, say, a pathological tendency to blood clotting as a cause
of an occlusion of a blood vessel and the ischemic changes in the affected
tissue. An *ideal cause* is thus understood as a spatiotemporal specification of the transition mechanism from C to E. All other relations are seen

as only causal *approximations,* a view strongly reinforced by the paradigm of biological reductionism and physicalism.

Yet what we learn from contemporary philosophy is *a less mechanism-bound view of causation:* the "interventionist view." For a variable A to be a cause, with the full dignity of this designation, is that a change in A produces a certain invariant effect on variable B. We uncover a causal relation if, taking potential confounders into consideration, a modification of A by an intervention I makes a stable difference in B. Mental health professionals are rarely familiar with such view of causation. We know it, for example, from the controlled randomized double-blind studies of therapeutic interventions. What is important in the interventionist view is that it deletes the "mechanic-substantial" component from the *definition* of causality, which in this way becomes less metaphysically burdened. That is, these interventionist models of causality are agnostic with respect to the specific mechanism involved. The models can apply—given the needed experimental rigor—to variables ranging from atoms to culture. Causality *as such* appears to some as enigmatic, perhaps matched only by the enigma of consciousness or experience. Freeing causality concept from the need to specify its mechanisms transforms this concept into a more pragmatic direction and makes it legitimately applicable to studying relations between variables from different regions of reality. We can, for example—as shown by Kendler's path-analytic diagram of the origins of depression—study the interrelationship of a diverse range of causal attributes, from genes to life events and psychological attributes such as low self-esteem.

I should add a word of caution with respect to the role of correlation in research. The interventionist model requires that noncausal correlative connections between the putative cause and effect be eliminated, and the model sets rigorous conditions for detection of a causal relation. It should not be misunderstood as a green light for *aconceptual research,* reporting mindless significant correlations or correlations from studies that are purely technology driven.

Several authors have emphasized a need for increasing stability of psychiatric explanatory models (for example, the notions of explanatory invariance or continuum of stability). It is not difficult to agree with this desideratum, but it is more difficult to specify the concrete steps needed in this direction.

The conceptual aspects of science have an important, even crucial role to play. Only by asking the right questions can we expect substantive empirical gains, if only by falsifying the involved hypotheses. What counts as "conceptual" and as a "right question" is, of course, heterogeneous and context dependent. Certainly, philosophical considerations belong here and are crucial, for example, in preparing a ground for taxonomic discussions—richly illustrated in the present volume. By emphasizing the aspects of cognition and behavior that exhibit low conditionality, interdisciplinary collaboration with psychology, developmental psychology, cognitive science, and basic neuroscience may stimulate the formation of new models and hypotheses.

An important set of conceptual constraints in psychiatric research stems from clinical knowledge, more specifically from familiarity with the patient's experience, expression, and lived world. As it was argued in the phenomenology section, such familiarity is itself embedded in a certain conceptual matrix (that is, the clinician's grasp of modes and forms of normal experience). Paradoxically and regrettably, today's psychiatry appears to have lost this foundational familiarity. In a recent article, Nancy Andreasen, an emblematic figure of the operational paradigm, laments a profound neglect and ignorance of descriptive psychopathology in contemporary psychiatry. She concludes that "research in psychopathology is a dying (or dead) enterprise," an unintended by-product of the operational turn in psychiatry (Andreasen 2007). It is, however, difficult to see how psychiatry, in the absence of phenomenological constrains on its phenotypic categories, can meaningfully address the questions of etiology.

Levels of Explanation

Several contributions of this volume talk about explanatory levels, and nearly all mention a paradigmatic model of vision developed by David Marr. Marr, a psychologist with sophisticated mathematical insights, was a revolutionary researcher, fascinated by the then-emerging possibilities of modeling the brain functions by computer simulations. Partly because of his influence, the notion of "levels" has today become widespread in psychology and cognitive science, and often with different meanings.

In the current cognitive literature, we may find references to at least three levels. The most abstract level is the *phenomenal* level (namely, the level of conscious experience). Next, there is a functional *cognitive* level, describing what a given brain function actually performs (for example, a detection of a figure in a visual display). There is then a *computational level* (that is, a certain "software"-like set of computing rules and algorithms, actually running the "how" of the system's performance—not unlike in a personal computer). Finally, there is the level of the system's "hardware," or *physical implementation,* which happens to be biological (neuronal) but, could, in principle, be otherwise (for example, instantiated by a computer or trained pigeons).

One, famous attempt to implement cognitive models in psychiatry is worth mentioning here. A model of thought insertion, a Schneiderian first-rank symptom of schizophrenia, was developed by Christopher Frith and colleagues (1992). Thinking a thought, said the theory, involves a cognitive computational mechanism through which an "efferent copy" of *intended* thought (a copy of the thought *sent forward* to a comparator) is on-line compared with the *actual,* articulated conscious thought. In the case of a breakdown of the efferent copy—or comparator—systems, the patient experiences unintended thoughts, which he delusionally explains as being inserted to his mind from the outside. This hypothesis, subsequently modified by the authors, stimulated a lot of empirical research and provoked a lively philosophical debate, summarized in an instructive manner by Shaun Gallagher (2004).

An attractive feature of layered cognitive architecture is the assumption of a certain autonomy of levels and hence a possibility of investigating the same phenomenon from different perspectives. Yet this picture of level-independence is being regularly questioned. For example, in an excellent introductory book about consciousness, John Searle (1992) writes that *it is misleading to ascribe computations to the brain.* The *possibility* of *describing* the brain (by us) in computational terms should not lead us to believe that what the brain really does is computing. That would correspond to claiming that the water of a river flowing down to the sea is computing its own trajectory. The water obeys physical laws (for example, gravitation) and, correspondingly, the brain obeys physiological principles.

Another issue is the "hardware" implementation. Some authors argue that the human behavior or mind and the human body or brain are not linked contingently in a way that would permit us to *mimic the behavior at whim* by instantiating it in any sufficiently complex system. Thus, for example, the very nature of human perception is not independent of the fact that human bodies are mobile and have the size that they have.

Reduction, Physicalism, and Complexity

It is a part of scientific activity to translate, when appropriate, the higher levels to their lower counterparts in the search of reductive explanations. In general, it seems that a heuristic approach is currently most appropriate in psychiatric research: "We must take our levels as we find them—as heuristic aggregations where generalizations are findable and causal processing traceable. This heuristic approach to levels, complements the heuristic search for causal simplifications" (Schaffner, this volume). Kendler concluded elsewhere (2005) that we have to accept a "patchy" version of reductionism, that is, seek reductions not as means to achieve a grand etiological scheme, but more pragmatically, where it makes sense to do so (that is, makes a difference) and where it is possible. The breathtaking tale of studying "the reductionist's delight," the feeding behavior of *Caenorhabditis elegans,* emphasizes the limits of monofactorial, one-to-one, reductive explanations. Yet less-reductive alternatives are available: interactions, aggregations of causal influences, and dynamic complex system approach.

The feasibility of reduction of the experiential, phenomenological level to its assumed substrate is the central point of the mind-brain debate. An issue closely related to the mind-body question, and not fully explored in the present volume, concerns the nature, reality status, or specification (individuation) of major psychiatric symptoms. Some authors see such symptoms as readily reducible to presumably underlying neurocognitive dysfunctions or deficits (namely, as meaningless signals from a dysfunctional substrate). In other accounts, illustrated by Frith's model of thought insertion mentioned above, the cognitive deficit is *shaping the experiential content* of the symptom. Josef Parnas and Louis Sass suggest yet another route, where the symptoms are seen as *meaningfully* and mutually implicative phenomena, inherent in the stream of consciousness, with causal properties. The authors propose to reorient the focus taxonomy and etiological research from isolated florid symptoms (mental contents) to their generative sources in the altered *structures* of consciousness, postulated to constitute the conditions of the formations of symptoms and, hence, of causal significance and closer to the substrate level in biological terms.

A belief in the possibility of a final reduction of meaning, behavior, and experience (and everything else) into the level of subatomic entities and forces of fundamental physics is called *physicalism*. It is possible to distinguish two main emphases in physicalism: the epistemologic or explanatory, constitutive of the final reductionist ambition of science, and a more metaphysical aspect, about what and how it exists. There is often a tension between these two, because a skeptical view of the prospects of physicalist reduction (for example, in this volume, Campbell's Martians figuring out why a group of people on Earth meets in a specific room on every Monday at noon) does not imply any automatic rejection of the metaphysical claims of physicalism, which is, perhaps, today's mainstream metaphysics. This other aspect may, however, be questioned on its own premises. A reader interested in the debate of physicalism in relation to the mind-brain issue is referred to an older, but excellent, easily accessible book by David Chalmers (1996).

The "level" talk becomes complicated through the notion of *environment*. In the case of brain-mind, we may expand the issue by pointing to not only the role of the *natural* world but also the *cultural* and *social* milieu, "surrounding" the mind. These surroundings are not, strictly speaking, *exterior to the mind*. To talk about "surroundings" implies a spatial relation, in which there is a clear border at which the mind stops and the world begins. Yet it is possible to argue against such a clean division. This line of argument, called "externalism," claims that it is impossible to confine the mind to the skull (for example, that the *actual existence* of a content, for example, a concept or a mental function cannot be said to "be in the head"). It is important to realize that the claim that "*meaning ain't in the head*" (Putnam 1998) is not only metaphorical but also concrete, with full existential weight. Not only are mind, meaning, and action always ecologically deployed but the ecological filaments of the mind are also constitutive of its individuality and concrete existence. (See Clark [1998] for a highly accessible introduction to externalism, and Nöe [2006].) That is what the phenomenological concept of being-in-the-world signifies. Similar ideas surface in the notions of complexity, networks, and ecological niche.

The notions of complexity, compositional relations, and emergent dynamic patterns are today in vogue. We observe emergent dynamic patterns everywhere in the surrounding world (for example, when water starts to

boil, when whirls are formed in a fast-flowing river, or when a child succeeds in taking her first walking steps).

The models accounting for these phenomena, originally developed in
chemistry and mathematics, are here illustrated with biological studies.
Intuitively, these models appear as promising nonreductive avenues for
studying brain behavior in context. Yet it is unclear how such models—
with their own requirements and a need of advanced mathematic knowledge—may become applied to psychiatric data. We need to think carefully what kinds of phenomena are suited as explananda (that is, the phenomena to be accounted for by the modeling) and which variables may be
adequate to be considered as explanatory or control parameters. Thus, the
very possibility of this new causal paradigm will be a challenge to psychiatry. We will need to rethink carefully which variables may have an a priori importance and limited conditionality.

Perhaps the onset of an illness, considered as an emergent new order of
experience, might be appropriate candidate for trying out complex nonlinear models. The transition to psychosis may, in certain cases, be considered (at least metaphorically [Bovet and Parnas 1993]) as an emergence of
a new stable coherence. Some candidate variables of potential explanatory
value may include known genetic factors, developmental achievements or
delays, developmental disarray (variability) or coherence, emotional dispositions, neurocognitive dysfunctions, and preonset phenomenology of
the disorder in question.

Final Words

Our goal in this book has been to expose you to first-rate philosophical
thought addressing a range of issues central to the science and practice of
psychiatry. Philosophy is not like natural sciences in striving for a definitive resolution of an issue—of proposing *the answer*. Rather, the goal has
been to stimulate readers to think more clearly and more deeply about the
problems before you. As was stated in our introduction, whether we like
it or not, all of us have had working philosophical frameworks—perhaps
unexamined—for nearly all the questions that have been explored in this
book. If you have taken a step back to ponder those frameworks, to question and reexamine your positions, then this book will have succeeded in
its aims.

REFERENCES

Andreasen, N. C. 2007. DSM and the Death of Phenomenology in America: An Example of Unintended Consequences. *Schizophrenia Bulletin* 33:108–112.

Bennett, M. R., and P. M. S. Hacker. 2003. *Philosophical Foundations of Neuroscience.* Oxford: Blackwell.

Bovet, P., and J. Parnas. 1993. Schizophrenic Delusions: A Phenomenological Approach. *Schizophrenia Bulletin* 19:579–597.

Chalmers, D. J. 1996. *The Conscious Mind: In Search of a Fundamental Theory.* Oxford: Oxford University Press.

Clark, A. 1998. *Being There: Putting Brain, Body, and World Together.* Cambridge, MA: MIT Press.

Frith, C. 1992. *The Cognitive Neuropsychology of Schizophrenia.* Hove, Sussex: Lawrence Erlbaum Associates.

———. 2004. Comments on Shaun Gallagher. *Psychopathology* 37:20–22.

Gallagher, S. 2004. Neurocognitive Models of Schizophrenia: A Phenomenological Critique. *Psychopathology* 37:8–19.

Kendler, K. S. 2005. Toward a Philosophical Structure for Psychiatry. *American Journal of Psychiatry* 162(7):243–252.

Noë, A. 2005. *Action in Perception.* Cambridge, MA: MIT Press.

Putnam, H. 1988. *Representation and Reality.* Cambridge, MA: MIT Press.

Sadler, J. Z., O. P. Wiggins, and M. A. Schwartz, eds. 1994. *Philosophical Perspectives on Psychiatric Diagnostic Classification.* Baltimore: John Hopkins University Press.

Searle, J. 1992. *The Rediscovery of the Mind.* Cambridge, MA: MIT Press.

Spitzer, M., F. A. Uehlein, and G. Oepen. 1988. *Psychopathology and Philosophy.* Berlin: Springer-Verlag.

Spitzer, M., and B. A. Maher, eds. 1990. *Philosophy and Psychopathology.* Berlin: Springer-Verlag.

INDEX